Psychiatry for the Developing World

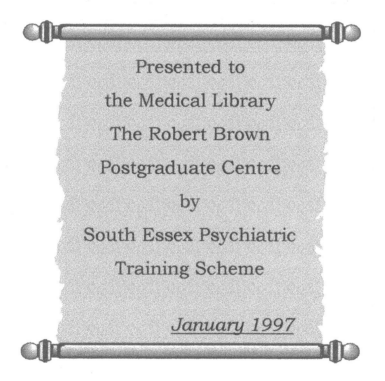

Edited by

DIGBY TANTAM, ALICE DUNCAN
AND LOUIS APPLEBY

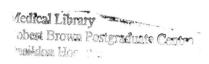
Psychiatry for the Developing World

GASKELL

Gaskell is an imprint of the Royal College of Psychiatrists, 17 Belgrave Square, London SW1X 8PG

British Library Cataloguing in Publication Data

Psychiatry for the Developing World

I. D. Tantam II. A. Duncan
III. L. Appleby

ISBN 0-902241-86-9

Distributed in North America
by American Psychiatric Press, Inc.
ISBN 0-88048-643-0

Phototypeset by Dobbie Typesetting Limited, Tavistock, Devon
Printed by Henry Ling Limited, The Dorset Press, Dorchester

Contents

Section IV. Training and research

Contributors

Moruf L. Adelekan, Dip Psych, FMCPsych, Senior Lecturer, Department of Behavioural Sciences, University of Ilorin, Ilorin, Nigeria

Louis Appleby, MRCPsych, Senior Lecturer, The Department of Psychiatry, School of Psychiatry and Behavioural Sciences, Withington Hospital, West Didsbury, Manchester M20 8LR

Mario Argandoña, Chief, Treatment and Care Programme on Substance Abuse, World Health Organization, 1211 Geneva, 27-Switzerland

Stephen W. Brown, MRCPsych, the David Lewis Centre for Epilepsy, Mill Lane, Warford, Nr. Alderley Edge, Cheshire SK9 7UD

Kennedy Cruickshank, MD, MRCP, Department of Public Health and Epidemiology, University of Manchester

Alice Duncan, MB BS, MRCPsych, Consultant Psychiatrist, Stockton Hall Psychiatric Hospital, The Village, Stockton-on-the-Forest, York YO3 9UN

Michael Farrell, MRCPsych, Senior Lecturer and Consultant Psychiatrist, National Addiction Centre (The Maudsley/Institute of Psychiatry), Addiction Sciences Building, 4 Windsor Walk, London SE5 8AF

Tom Fryers, FFCM, Director of Public Health, South Cumbria Health Authority, Priors Lea, Abbey Road, Barrow-in-Furness, Cumbria LA13 9JU

Robert Giel, MD, Emeritus Professor, Department of Social Psychiatry, Academische Fienkenhuis Groningen, Oostersingel 59, 9700 RB Groningen, Holland

Giovanni de Girolamo, Servizio Salute Mentale USL-27, Viale Pepoli 5, 40123 Bologna, Italy

David Goldberg, FRCPsych, Professor of Psychiatry, Institute of Psychiatry, De Crespigny Park, Denmark Hill, London SE5 8AF

Oye Gureje, FMCPsych, Senior Lecturer, Department of Psychiatry, University of Ibadan, and Honorary Consultant Psychiatrist, University College Hospital, Ibadan, Nigeria

A. Jablensky, DMSc, FRCPsych, Professor and Chair, Department of Psychiatry, Royal Perth Hospital, University of Western Australia, Nedlands, Western Australia 6009

Sudhir K. Khandelwal, MD, MNAMS, Additional Professor, Department of Psychiatry, All India Institute of Medical Sciences, Ansari Nagar, New Delhi 110 029, India

Graeme McGrath, MRCPsych, Consultant Psychiatrist, The Rawnsley Building, Central Manchester Hospitals and Community Care Trust, Oxford Road, Manchester MI3 9BX

Malik Mubbashar, FRCPsych, DPM, Director, WHO Collaborating Centre, Department of Psychiatry, Rawalpindi, Pakistan

R. Srinivasa Murthy, Professor of Psychiatry and Head of Department, Department of Psychiatry, National Institute of Mental & Neuro Sciences, Bangalore, 560 029, India

John Orley, MBM, CHB, Senior Medical Officer, Division of Mental Health, World Health Organization, Geneva, Switzerland

Tariq Saraf, MB BS, MRCPsych, Research Registrar, The Rawnsley Building, Central Manchester Hospitals and Community Care Trust, Oxford Road, Manchester MI3 9BX

John Strang, FRCPsych, Professor and Director of the Addiction Research Unit, National Addiction Centre (The Maudsley/Institute of Psychiatry), Denmark Hill, London SE5 8AF

Digby Tantam, FRCPsych, Chairman, Section of Psychological Medicine, School of Postgraduate Medical Education, The University of Warwick, Coventry CV4 7AL

A Venkoba Rao, FRCPsych, Emeritus Professor of Psychiatry, 'TILAK' 506 K.K. Nagar, Madurai 625 020, India

Preface

The history of psychiatry for the developing world has been a reprise of the history of contact between the developing world and Westernised countries. After an initial reaction of strangeness, during which the differences between the two worlds was emphasised (the reported absence of depression in Africans was an example of this), came a realisation that psychiatric disorders, and human predicaments, were more notable by their ubiquity than by their culture boundedness. This phase coincided with a marked increase in the numbers of psychiatrists from developing countries travelling abroad for training, and with the first generation of textbooks for psychiatrists in developing countries.

We are now in a third phase. Many developing countries have established excellent services and training programmes, although they rely much less heavily on trained medical and other professional staff than do the services in developed countries. Descriptions of some of these services are given by Malik Mubbashar in the first chapter. Even when countries are still unable to train more than a few psychiatrists, sending doctors abroad for training is no longer quite as attractive as it was. There is a new recognition that psychiatric services have to be developed locally, to suit local circumstances, and psychiatric textbooks must reflect this. At the same time, many developed countries have re-discovered their own cultural and ethnic pluralism. MacLuhan's global village has arrived, and the traveller abroad who spots an amazing artefact or participates in a wholly new cultural experience is likely to return home and find the artefact on sale in the high street and the experience happening at the local community centre.

Psychiatrists in every country have to be increasingly aware of the effects of culture on disorder, and on the acceptability and uptake of treatment. The important difference between the psychiatrist in the developed and in the developing world is economic: what funds are available, and what infrastructure exists to support psychiatric practice. Roads and not rituals are likely to determine psychiatric care. The psychiatrist may have received the highest level of training, may attend international conferences (although may not have access to many journals), may even have a video machine (courtesy of overseas aid) and the videos to show (courtesy of a recent trip to a WHO conference); but it may prove impossible to transport them to the staff or members of the public who need to see them, or to show them because of the intermittent electricity supply.

Psychiatry for the developing world is therefore a mix of basic service provision with a high level of theory and training, and requires the psychiatrist to struggle constantly against practical obstacles. We believe that a textbook for the developing world should reflect both these aspects: a sophisticated world view, and a practical attitude. The textbooks that are widely used in the developed world seem to us to be insufficiently practical, and the smaller number of textbooks that have been written for developing countries are often out of date in the theoretical approaches that they advocate. We have therefore edited this new textbook specifically directed to psychiatrists in developing countries which, we hope, will have achieved this combination of good theory and realistic practice.

The book is designed to be comprehensive since we realise that its readers may not always have access to a full range of other books and journals. Multiple authorship has contributed to comprehensiveness by enabling us to choose experts in particular fields, and by enabling representation from different countries. All the contributors have knowledge of psychiatry in the developing world as well and, wherever possible, we have chosen contributors who have also practised in a developing country. The contributors come from Asia, Africa, South and Central America, the Caribbean, and Europe and we anticipate that the book will be relevant to all these parts of the world. Indeed, we expect that the book will find a place in every country where psychiatric education and traditions have been influenced by British psychiatry. The core of the book is provided by chapters developed from lectures and seminars on the Manchester course for the Diploma in Psychiatry which attracts visiting trainees in psychiatry who originate from all over the world. We expect it to be used primarily by trainee psychiatrists but also as an educational resource for their trainers.

It has been long in gestation as few clinicians in developing countries, however senior they are, have the time and resources for authorship that their colleagues elsewhere take for granted. We are grateful to Gaskell Press, and indeed to many of our contributors, for their patience. There has been one unexpected bonus of the delay, since it has enabled us to use the tenth edition of the *International Classification of Diseases* as the diagnostic standard throughout the book. Our contributors deserve our thanks, too, for their tolerance of our many editorial enquiries. We hope that these have been as helpful in practice as we intended them to be. We have deliberately tried to avoid changing the style of any contributions, and so the chapters represent the richness of English as it is spoken, and written, throughout the world.

Section I.   General principles

1 Epidemiology of mental disorder in developing countries

MALIK H. MUBBASHAR

Three-quarters of the world's population live in developing countries, most of which have gained independence from colonial Western rule during the last four to five decades. As part of the continued colonial heritage in these countries, their health services in general, and mental health services in particular, were originally modelled on those in the West. These, for the most part, comprised large custodial hospitals working in isolation, neither aware of or sensitive to the needs of the community. Then, as in the West, the psychopharmacological revolution of the 1950s and the social psychiatry movement in the 1960s had a far-reaching and lasting impact, resulting in the establishment of psychiatric units in general hospitals for the first time and helping to establish psychiatry as a discipline with a firm scientific foundation.

These modern developments, however, were confined to the major urban centres, serving 10–15% of the total population. The majority of the population, i.e. those living in rural areas, did not benefit from such changes. Furthermore, mental health professionals made few efforts to enhance the community's awareness of the role of behavioural and psychosocial factors in health and disease generally, so that until recently, behavioural sciences were not included in the curricula of medical schools. In addition, preventive activities were not accorded priority. Thus the development of services in developing countries left the majority of the population either unserved, under-served or inappropriately served.

Rates of disorders in developing countries

Although mental health services have been developed in many countries, research activities have not often been incorporated in their planning. This has led to a lack of reliable epidemiological data regarding the extent and distribution of mental disorders in the developing world. In addition, research has been hampered by the myth that psychiatric disorders are an urban and Western phenomenon, and the scarcity of manpower trained in research methods, epidemiology and bio-statistics. In addition, there has been a lack of proper, validated, indigenous instruments free of the cultural bias inherent in some Western research instruments. Investigators have studied populations of varying age and sex composition, and have used different methodologies including diagnostic criteria. The result has been widely differing prevalence and incidence figures. When research data are available, they can be used for a number of purposes, as shown below.

Planning and evaluation of health services

In order to make decisions on the allocation of resources, health service planners need to decide first whether resources are to be spent on physical disorders (e.g. diarrhoea) or psychiatric disorders; and second, which of the latter are to be given priority.

An important consideration is the efficiency of intervention strategies and the relationship between their costs and benefits. There are various techniques of economic appraisal available which can assist in this process of decision-making and enable more and better mental health care provision given the limited resources available. However, the power of such analyses should not be exaggerated and they should be used to aid rather than dictate decisions. It is likely, for instance, that in an evaluation of mental health care it will be difficult to measure all costs and benefits.

The various types of economic appraisal available include cost-only studies (e.g. Cassell *et al*, 1972), cost-effective analyses, cost-utility analyses (e.g. Drummond, *et al*, 1987) and modified cost-effective analyses (e.g. Glass & Goldberg, 1977; see also Chapter 2). The latter is the most commonly adopted as it measures costs and outcomes at several levels.

Aetiology

Epidemiological data are helpful in delineating not only the aetiological factors that initiate a disorder, but also those that maintain it or cause relapse, thus providing opportunities to devise intervention strategies for primary, secondary and tertiary prevention.

Nosology

Studies of a particular disorder can generate valuable information about the distribution and frequency of particular signs and symptoms, as well as the frequency of their concurrence. This will help in studying the appearance of the disorder in a particular culture and relating this to aetiology, management and outcome.

Outcome and prognosis

Multi-centre epidemiological studies carried out in developing countries have shown that the incidence (the rate of new cases in a defined area and time span) and the prevalence (the rate of all cases of a disorder in a defined area and time span) of mental disorders are similar to what is seen in developed countries. It has been shown that the point prevalence of severe incapacitating mental disorders is around 1 % while the life-time risk of such disorders is approximately 10% (Basheer, 1961, 1973; Bash & Bash-Liechti, 1973; Dube, 1970). There are therefore at least 40 million individuals in developing countries suffering from severe mental disorders (mainly schizophrenia), related psychotic disorders, and dementia.

The importance of schizophrenia is enhanced in developing countries because 50% of their population is under 15-years-old and the annual population growth is 2–3%. Since the age of the highest risk of developing schizophrenia is 25–30 years, and the proportion of the population in this age group in developing countries is rising, simple projections show that the number of individuals suffering from schizophrenia will have increased by 80% by the year 2000 to a total of 23 million.

According to estimates by the World Health Organization (WHO), one-third of total disability is caused by mental disorders, a significant number of which are preventable. An outstanding example of this is epilepsy, the prevalence of which varies from 5–30% in developing countries, compared to 0.9%–1.2% in developed countries. This translates into about 25 million people affected in the developing world. Another example is mental retardation: the prevalence of severe mental retardation among those below 18 years of age is estimated to be about 3 per 1000 while the prevalence of mild and moderate retardation is estimated to be more than 50 per 1000 (WHO, 1986).

Mental disorders such as neurosis, personality disorder and adjustment disorders are much more difficult to detect. Precise figures for their incidence and prevalence are not available, but are estimated to be of the order of 5–10% in the general population of developing countries. Substance abuse is also widely prevalent in many developing countries but it is extremely difficult to obtain reliable figures for it, partly because of the lack of policies governing the sale of psychotropic drugs. However, recent WHO estimates suggest that alcohol dependence and drug abuse are rising.

Surveys conducted in the general population show the prevalence of psychiatric disorder to be about 15% while studies in Western general hospital settings have shown that 20–30% of all individuals reporting to health care facilities suffer from psychiatric disorder. In the developing world, the presentation of emotional and psychological problems often takes the form of somatisation which can result in mis-diagnosis, mis-management, waste of already meagre resources, and lack of satisfaction for both care-seekers and care-givers.

Another common mode of presentation is the acute psychotic episode, the annual incidence of which is 0.5 per 1000 population. This was once commonly misdiagnosed as schizophrenia, leading some earlier studies to report a much higher incidence of schizophrenia in developing countries. The patient usually presents to emergency departments, placing pressure on services to remove him or her from the community – this is not only inappropriate and costly in the short term, but also detrimental to the development of primary care-based facilities in the long run.

Many preventable aetiological factors for mental disorder are found in developing countries. Infections and infestations may contribute to the development of mental illness in the developing world, particularly in the presence of dwindling food supplies, poor drinking water and declining standards of living. Rapid industrialisation and urbanisation bring in their wake large scale migration, unemployment, overcrowding and the break-up of traditional family support systems.

Mental health care delivery systems

Mental health services in developing countries have suffered from two limitations: administrative difficulties and cultural differences. Both are discussed in detail below.

Administrative difficulties

The establishment of mental health services in developing countries is made difficult by many factors. To start with, a low national priority is accorded to health, particularly mental health. In many developing countries, budgetary allocations for health vary from 0.84 to 3% of gross national product, and only a fraction of this allocation is earmarked for mental health services. Mental health planning and legislation are also often ignored or relegated to low priority by health planning bodies. Finally, difficulties also arise from the lack of trained manpower and the lack of infrastructure required for its effective use when it is available.

Cultural relevance

Cultural difficulties stem largely from the application of the Western model of health care delivery, whose assumptions, concepts and methods have evolved in a cultural setting profoundly different from what is found in developing countries. This is particularly evident in the separation of body, mind and spirit by Western models, the separation of thought and feelings, and the consideration of health and disease as separate entities rather than dimensions of a single continuum. As a result, mental health professionals trained in the West can find it difficult to communicate with patients. The problems patients present are often classified according to intrapsychic processes which are incomprehensible in developing countries. Modern psychiatry tends to emphasise certain emotions like fear and sadness to the relative exclusion of others such as jealousy and hatred. This leads people living in developing countries to view psychiatry as alien.

In addition, treatment of most mental disorders has been almost exclusively with medication and has not been designed to address the full spectrum of causes that may produce, maintain and enhance a patient's problem (Kleinman & Sung, 1976).

Innovations in mental health services

Reorganisation of health services, including psychiatric services, has been a focus of attention over the last few decades, as existing facilities are inadequate and inappropriate to meet the needs of their communities. The starting point for indigenous, innovative approaches to mental health care is provided by WHO's recommendations:

(1) a national mental health policy, formulated by professionals from the field of mental health, public health administration, economics, education and social sciences. The policy should be reviewed regularly, and should clearly delineate objectives and priorities, fixing timetables to achieve these. These objectives should be realistic and cognisant of material and human resources available in the country
(2) a national mental health programme, which should be adequately financed to allow: (a) the setting of mental health cells in national and regional health administration to implement national mental health policy, educate the public, and collect, analyse and publish data about mental health; (b) the recruitment, training and employment of personnel; (c) the adequate provision of drug treatments; and (d) a network of facilities including transport
(3) mental health services should be integrated with general health services, and with non-medical community agencies. Their organisation should be decentralised
(4) basic mental health care should be provided by non-specialists; specialist mental health workers should devote a greater part of their time to training and supervising these workers.
(5) mental health legislation should be reviewed or new legislation passed.

The Alma-Ata declaration (WHO, 1978), envisaging health for all by the year 2000, with primary health care and intersectoral collaboration as its guiding principle, represented a historic point of reference, whereby health services recognised the need to provide universal care in an acceptable and affordable manner. For developing countries, this means the building up of an organisational infrastructure and a manpower base, and the identification of priorities for health care. Steps taken to achieve these goals in mental health were slow to start, but in the 1980s, with the guidance and collaboration of the WHO, many developing countries implemented national mental health policies and programmes. These aim to prevent and treat mental disorders and disabilities, using mental health technology and behavioural science to the benefit of the population as a whole, with special emphasis on the needs of rural populations. Community participation in the development of mental health services and self-help should be encouraged, and emphasis laid on the harmful effects of broken homes, juvenile delinquency, drug abuse, and rapid social changes such as industrialisation and urbanisation. The proper mental development of children through parental guidance, school education and social interaction outside the home is another important objective.

A clinical referral system to specialist care should also be established as part of a mental health programme. Essential drugs for common mental disorders such as depression, psychosis, epilepsy, mental retardation and addictions should be provided at rural health centres in adequate quantity; their regular supply should be ensured. At all levels of mental health care, from teaching hospitals to basic health units, an information system should be developed to record all patients seen, their demographic data, mode of presentation, diagnosis, source of referral and treatment.

Innovative strategies of mental health care in Pakistan

The National Mental Health Programme in Pakistan illustrates the strategies that can be used to meet the mental health objectives outlined above. The programme was formulated at a multi-sectoral workshop in 1986 and was officially included in the seventh five-year development plan for 1988–93. One of its major components was to evolve alternative mental health delivery systems utilising existing facilities. A community-based rural mental health programme was first set up in the Rawalpindi division and is now being replicated nationally, in a multi-phase approach.

The priority in the first phase was to evaluate the needs and demands for mental health services in the community; to gauge the knowledge, attitudes and practices prevalent in the community; and to educate the community by mass programmes using, for example, mosques and social congregations. Training of primary health care personnel, school teachers and the community was then undertaken. By 1994, more than 840 primary care physicians and more than 3500 multi-purpose health workers, lady health visitors, and birth attendants from all over the country had been trained. Furthermore, more than 80 middle-level health administrators and managers had by then been sensitised to the need to initiate mental health programmes in their areas of jurisdiction, and taught ways of achieving this. In addition, activities intended to expand manpower began in all medical schools whose aim was to offer training in social sciences equivalent to that in biological sciences.

The next phase of the programme involved activities in inter-sectoral collaboration and for this purpose a school mental health programme was set up in 1987. Initially, the education administrators were shown how mental health principles could be used to improve the quality of education. Secondly, training packages were developed for school teachers. The response of teachers and children was overwhelming, the formation of an All-Pakistan teachers' movement for mental health being one result. School children prepared wall charts and posters with mental health slogans, and acted as an important source of referral of the mentally ill to health care facilities. Furthermore, teachers now say that they feel closer to the children and know more about them as people. It has been claimed that absenteeism has gone down by 50% and children have started paying more attention to personal hygiene (Mubbashar *et al*, 1989).

The third phase was the development of indicators for evaluating the impact of the school mental health programme on knowledge, attitudes and super/stitions in the community. Studies designed to achieve this are in the process of being analysed. Another innovative activity has been collaboration between traditional healers or faith healers and mental health professionals. Faith healers have been provided colour-coded case identification cards, the same as those being used by multipurpose health care workers. Faith healers claim that although their results with hysteria are better, they are pleased to have the help of health care facilities in the management of epilepsy, drug dependence and some other disorders, and are serving as an important source of referral to health professionals. Furthermore, more than 70 social welfare officers all over the country have incorporated mental health principles into the performance of their duties.

Conclusion

Epidemiological principles form an important basis for a national mental health programme. The Pakistan programme has been discussed here in some detail as an illustration of this but it should be noted that national mental health programmes have been devised in other countries of Asia (e.g. India, Thailand and Sri Lanka) and in Africa (e.g. Uganda, Botswana, and the Seychelles).

References

BASHEER, T. (1961) Survey of mental illness in Wadi Halfa. *World Mental Health*, **13**, 181.
────── (1973) Childhood psychiatric disorders in Sudan. In *Proceedings of Pan African Psychiatric Conference, Khartoum, 20–25 Nov.*
BASH, K. W. & BASH-LEICHTI, J. (1973) Psychological Testing and Psychiatric Morbidity in Iran. *International Mental Health Resources News*, **15**, 1.
CASSELL, W. A., SMITH, C. N., GRUNDERG, F., *et al* (1972) Comparing costs of hospital care. *Hospital and Community Psychiatry*, **23**, 197–200.
DRUMMOND, M. F., STODDART, G. L. & TORRANCE, G. W. (1987) *Methods for the Evaluation of Health Care Programmes.* Oxford: Oxford University Press.
DUBE, K. C. A. (1970) Study of prevalence and biosocial variables in mental illness in rural and an urban community in Uttar Pradesh, India. *Acta Psychiatrica Scandinavica*, **46**, 327.
GIEL, R. & HARDING, T. (1976) Psychiatric priorities in developing countries. *British Journal of Psychiatry*, **128**, 513–522.
GLASS, N. J. & GOLDBERG, D. (1977) Cost benefit analysis and the calculation of psychiatric services. *Psychological Medicine*, **7**, 701–707.
KLEINMAN, A. & SUNG, B. (1976) *Why do Indigenous Practitioners Successfully Heal?* Paper presented at the conference on the healing process. East Lansing (MI): Michigan State University.
MUBBASHAR, M. H. (1989) *Eastern Mediterranean Region Health Services Journal*, **6**, 14–19.
WHO (1978). *Primary Health Care Report of the International Conference on Primary Care.* Alma-Ata USSR, 6–12 September 1978. *Health For All Series*, **1**.

2 The economics of mental health care in the developing world

GRAEME McGRATH and TARIQ SARAF

The World Health Organization (WHO, 1981, 1984) estimates that about 40 million people in the world have significant disabilities secondary to chronic mental health problems. If disabilities secondary to associated neurological illnesses and psychosocial stressors are included, this figure climbs to a staggering 200 million. The majority of those so disabled are to be found in the developing countries, and this at least in part must reflect the widely disparate distribution of resources between developed and developing countries. The losses of human capital and productivity so engendered are enormous, but may not be proportionally as great in the developing countries with respect to the level of disability as the potential for wealth and production generation in developing countries may be relatively less per able bodied person.

There is increasing political and administrative will towards the provision of mental health care services, which are coming to be seen as essential in developing countries (Segall, 1983). It is well established that mental health problems and associated psychosocial disabilities are a source of significant drain on national resources, but on the other hand providing essential preventive and curative services in response to this immense morbidity is bound to be an expensive proposition, possibly beyond the limited resources of many developing countries.

The problems are multifold. One of the major drawbacks for proper planning and evaluation of service development is the complete lack of reliable information and statistics concerning indicators of need and the quantity of available resources being utilised. Secondly, there is no generally acceptable set of intervention techniques or model of service delivery that is consistent with the meagre manpower available to run the service. A number of pilot programmes have been initiated with little or no economic evaluation at all (Mubbashar, 1989). In addition, evaluation of new health care programmes is costly, and so diverts resources from the (perceived) most urgent requirements for health care.

Health planners in the developing world continue to entertain the idea that provision of mental health services is not an urgent matter. Even when they realise its importance, there is a belief, not based on any formal evaluation, that provision of such a service is a costly exercise without concomitant rewards. Even where a policy commitment exists, no discrete guidelines for budgetary allocations are available to the health planners. The consequence is inevitably the continuing neglect of mental health services in developing countries.

In any society intense competition for resources with other economic and social sectors ensures that health does not traditionally enjoy a high priority. Health budgets generally increase very little year on year, and this is especially true in developing countries. Furthermore, within the health services, despite limited resources, there is observable failure to utilise such resources optimally. The consequent wastage, often as much as 50% of committed resources, includes ineffective or inefficient use of existing personnel, low motivation and morale, low productivity and inequitable distribution of health care (Ghosh, 1982; WHO, 1989). Health services are generally planned unrealistically or allocated disproportionately, especially in regard to the increasing disparity between the private and public sectors. Furthermore, planning is often focused around an urban-based, hospital-based and cure-orientated service, mimicking the developed countries. Most planning decisions are guided by 'unaided intuition' or political expediency without appropriate evaluation of the real or felt needs of the populace. It is a common practice to replicate models developed in the Western world and in the context of developed social and educational infrastructures, without suitable modifications and without giving appropriate consideration to the particular attitudes and service utilisation patterns of the local population (see Chapter 1). Finally, health and the development of health services cannot be considered in a political vacuum. This is particularly glaring in the case of provision of mental health services, where strong political and administrative will and commitment is essential for any increased budgetary allocation.

The value of economic analysis

There is a constant tension between the needs for health care and the demands of other sectors of social spending, for example education, sanitation and water supplies. In addition difficult choices have to be made between alternative forms of health care, for example between the provision of mental health services and other health services.

The application of economic principles and analysis can be a useful tool in this situation, the underlying asumption being that introducing an effective mental health service into at least the primary care system of a society could actually reduce overall health costs, thus benefiting the society providing such services. This 'cost offset' effect (McGrath & Lowson, 1987) is due to a substantial proportion of patients with mental health problems not being identified at the primary care level in developing countries. They may, as a consequence, undergo unnecessary and expensive medical investigations and 'placebo' treatments on account of failure of the health workers to detect these emotional problems (McGrath & Lowson, 1987). Application of appropriate techniques of health economics would help define the most cost-effective options from a multitude of available models of intervention. Mental health, unlike other areas, does not generally require costly technology; rather it depends more on sensitive deployment of personnel who have been properly trained in psychosocial skills. Those areas which do incur expenditure include cost of training activities, teaching materials, appointment of personnel at national and regional levels, in addition to the cost of provision of essential psychoactive medications and establishing proper referral and supervisory services (WHO, 1990).

General principles of health economics

The cost of using resources for one purpose can be defined as the loss of benefits that could be accrued from using the same resources in other ways. This is what economists call the opportunity cost, a concept which lies at the core of economic thinking.

No society will ever be able to meet all conceivable needs, and this means that hard decisions will inevitably have to be made between alternative uses of available resources (this is true whether resources are artificially restricted by government intervention or provided to the limits which taxation or other revenues will allow). Allocation of resources to any treatment programme means that the community inevitably foregoes the opportunity to use those same resources for other activities. Thus the economic definition of cost is the sacrifice of benefits foregone. Costs must not be seen as implying a merely financial cost; for example societies may value concepts such as quality of life, equitable distribution of care or maximising dignity and programmes that do not address these may be seen as costly. There is a useful distinction to be made between 'hard' (monetary) and 'soft' (non-monetary) costs and benefits (Glass & Goldberg, 1977). Nor are costs incurred only by those providing health care; costs (both 'hard' and 'soft') are incurred by patients, families and other public sector agencies.

Given the accepted scarcity of resources, the pursuit of economic efficiency implies that societies and their governments should choose the patterns of social spending (including health care) which yield the maximum total benefit to society for the same expenditure.

Some economic terms

A *benefit* is anything to which an individual or society would be willing to commit resources (i.e. pay some sum in cash, goods or services) to obtain, whereas a *cost* is anything to which an individual or society would be willing to commit resources to avoid (see Tables 2.1 and 2.2).

Benefits from symptom improvement may be monetary (e.g. money earned by return to work, improvement in productivity for society), but will also include non-monetary factors such as improved use of leisure time, extension of life, increased quality of life and reduction in the burden of care to others.

Demand is an indication of desire to obtain a commodity, and in health care is closely related to the presentation of health problems to the caring services. In health care services the commodity in demand is 'better health'. Health is viewed by health economists as a 'fundamental commodity', i.e. one for which

TABLE 2.1
Types of costs and benefits

Type	Costs	Benefits	Measures
Capital			Area
Land			Volume
Buildings	Use for health care	Release for other use	Number
Transport			Number
Expenditure			
Labour			Profession
Supplies			Type, number
Support	Current expenditure	Revenue released	
Support			Type, number
Services			
Throughput	Extra work for staff	Reduced cases	
		Work	Bed-days
Staff training	Less opportunity	More opportunity	Numbers trained
			Training hours
Personal			Scales of burden
			and quality of life
Satisfaction	Reduced	Increased	
Convenience	Reduced	Increased	
Time	Reduced	Increased	Time lost
Expense	Reduced	Increased	Monetary where
			relevant (e.g. fares)
Health			
Disability	Increased	Reduced	Symptom measures
Pain	Increased	Reduced	Health status scales
Boredom	Increased	Reduced	QALYs
Restriction	Increased	Reduced	
Productivity	Loss	Gain	Output
			Earnings

demand is generated for its own sake. The demand for health care is considered to be secondary to the demand for better health.

Utility represents the satisfaction gained from the caring services, so the greater the utility the greater will be the demand.

Need, in economic terms, is not the same as the individual's subjectively perceived need for health care, but instead is based on the assumption that the individual consumer of health care lacks relevant information on which to make judgements about the effects of treatment options open to him. The doctor decides on the quantity and type of health care required by the patient. Thus, the patient's needs involve expert assessment and decision.

TABLE 2.2
Stages of option appraisal

Define the problem
Set the appraisal objective
Outline possible options
Identify costs and benefits
Measure costs and benefits
Assess equity
Eliminate impracticable options
Make final choice

Needs are therefore not absolute, but relate to the end being sought, involve the values of a third party (which must be made explicit in any assessment study) and can be ranked and costed.

Marginal cost is the cost of producing an extra unit of output. Fixed costs are those incurred irrespective of the quantity of output (e.g. land, buildings), variable costs vary with the level of output (e.g. special investigations performed) and average costs are fixed plus variable costs divided by the total units of output (e.g. number of patients treated). The marginal cost relates to the average cost whereby if one additional unit of output costs less than the average then the overall average costs are reduced; if the unit costs more than the average, then costs are increased. For example, if patients are added into spare capacity then the marginal costs are low, and may be much less than the average if overheads have already been included. On the other hand if new buildings or equipment are required then the marginal cost may be much greater than the existing average cost.

Marginal analysis implies that choices in health care are not usually couched in terms of whether or not one should devote any resources at all to the care of (say) neurotic patients in general practice, but whether we should give more or less resources, and to what form of treatment. In this case it is the incremental (or marginal) costs and benefits of expansion or contraction of a treatment programme that are relevant, not the costs and benefits of the whole existing programme. If the evaluation concerns setting up an entire service then marginal costs coincide with total costs.

Economic factors in evaluation

The fact that a course of action may be 'cheaper' (in monetary terms) is not a sufficient reason for preferring it. 'Economising' in the sense of choosing the cheapest alternative is merely cost-cutting and ignores possible benefits from seemingly more expensive alternatives. Apart from the fact that cheaper services may be more expensive in the long run (for example by failing to provide appropriate training to meet future needs, or to provide a durable working environment) a more expensive course of action may be preferred, as it may be:

1. more effective
2. less dangerous or causing fewer side-effects
3. more equitably distributed
4. more acceptable to patients
5. easier to administer

These are all economic reasons for preferring one course of action over another. Indirectly the value of the ('soft') benefits achieved is the excess ('hard') cost of the preferred course of action over its cheaper alternative. This demonstrates that economic evaluation is, and should always be, complementary to clinical evaluations (Drummond, 1980).

It should be noted that compared to developed countries, in relatively poor developing countries monetary costs and benefits will have a greater value in comparison to non-monetary costs and benefits. The consequence is that poorer countries may concern themselves less with issues such as equitable provision of services and increasing quality of life for all members of society and more with concentrating resources on those with the greatest economic potential.

Measuring costs and benefits

It is important that the lists of costs and benefits should be as comprehensive as possible. Items should be mentioned even if they cannot be measured or valued. This is particularly significant for mental health problems, as a large number of benefits and costs pertaining to patients, families and society are not always overt or regularly considered clinically when deciding on diagnosis or treatment. They would include the amount of distress experienced by the patient or others, inconvenience to family, and disruption of normal functioning. Many of these factors reflect the patient's 'quality of life' and it has become increasingly popular to consider this as an important outcome measure (Rosser, 1983; McEwen, 1984; Holland, 1985; Teeling Smith, 1985); Morris (1991), for example, recommends quality of life as an important factor in deciding which antidepressant to choose. A useful criterion for defining costs is to consider the opportunities lost in using resources for one particular purpose. It is also important not to count the same cost twice. Table 2.1 illustrates some of the important possible types of costs and benefits and their measures.

Types of economic appraisal

A number of techniques are available for economic appraisal, depending upon the particular questions being asked (Drummond *et al*, 1987). A technique suitable for one type of evaluation is not necessarily suitable for another. The various techniques do, however, only differ in terms of measure of outcome; they employ the same costing principles and methodology.

Cost-only studies

These studies collect information on all the costs of alternative programmes of treatment. They are not of much help to health planners and professionals, as efficiency does not imply obtaining the cheapest option but the most effective option for the resources available, and this requires some measure of outcome as well as cost.

Cost-effectiveness analysis (CEA)

This is the most frequently used technique of economic appraisal in the health care setting. It is essentially concerned with the 'how' of policy but does not provide any information on whether to pursue any particular policy or how much of a policy. It does, however, help to define how a fixed budget can be used to meet a particular health services' target. CEA involves measures both of the outcome and the costs. It does not require a value to be placed on outcome except that it should be measurable in physical units along a single dimension. An example might be increase in life expectancy measured as life-years gained. The cost per unit of outcome can be calculated and compared across programmes. One limitation of CEA is that it can only be used to compare services for individuals with similar needs and thus comparable outcome measures. For an example of CEA comparing home with hospital treatment for similar patients see Fenton *et al* (1982).

Modified cost-effectiveness analysis (MCEA)

In MCEA, outcome is measured on a number of dimensions (Glass & Goldberg, 1977). This requires separate comparison of costs and of each dimension of outcome, for example health status, satisfaction with treatment and convenience of the service. A service model which scores highly on each dimension of outcome may be the most efficient despite being the most expensive. For equivalent outcomes it is clearly preferable to choose the cheaper option if available. However, if one method is the most effective and also the most expensive, it is not possible to determine from MCEA whether it is the most efficient and therefore preferable alternative.

Cost-utility analysis (CUA)

In CUA, evaluation of various options involves placing a value on each outcome. The value of outcome is expressed in terms of utility, which is measured by an individual's preference for a particular state of health or change in health state. This is the basis of 'quality of life' measures, which in effect provide a weighting factor which can be multiplied by life expectancy to produce a measure known as 'quality adjusted life years' (QALYs; Drummond, 1987; Teeling Smith, 1985). Some economists hope that QALYs will be a universal measure for comparing all health outcome whatever the condition or treatment. Once a utility measure is defined, the alternative options of service delivery could be compared in terms of their cost per QALY produced: the alternative with the lowest cost per QALY is the most efficient, as it results in achieving the greatest output from a given amount of resources.

Cost-benefit analysis (CBA)

Cost-benefit analysis addresses the question of whether it is worthwhile to pursue a particular policy. This is of particular importance at times of resource allocation, when some choice has to be exercised in deciding which policies to pursue and, equally important, which not to pursue. This technique helps in deciding between various competing objectives, unlike the CEA which addresses the question of evaluating alternative ways of reaching some already defined objective. In the context of developing countries this question assumes the role of a key paradigm at times of resource allocation when the planners have to compare provision of mental health services with the alternative of doing nothing at all. CBA requires that all the costs and benefits of a particular project to the community should be identified in monetary units. The net benefit to the society can then be calculated by simply subtracting the total costs from the total benefits. Programmes with a net benefit would be expected to raise the welfare of the community if undertaken. Cost-benefit is the most powerful form of economic analysis but its application in health care, especially mental health is particularly fraught with practical difficulties, notably how to estimate indirect and non-monetary costs to the individual and society.

It can be very difficult to reduce monetary and non-monetary factors to a common denominator for inclusion in cost-benefit comparisons. Goldberg & Jones (1980) suggest separating hard from soft costs and benefits in a form of 'modified cost benefit analysis'. An example of such an analysis in practice can be found in the comparison of a traditional in-patient psychiatric ward with a community 'hostel ward' (Goldberg *et al*, 1985; Hyde *et al*, 1985; Bridges *et al*, 1988).

Drummond (1980) defines four questions to which economic appraisal can address itself:

1. What is the cost of a treatment?
2. What is the benefit gained from a treatment?
3. What is the most efficient way to treat a given condition?
4. Is the treatment worthwhile?

The third question assumes that treatment will be given (i.e. the treatment objective is not itself in question) and hence the CEA can be used to compare alternative forms of treatment. The fourth question, "Is the treatment worthwhile?", is often taken for granted, but logically should precede question three. It is a question which addresses very different issues, and suggests that the only answer lies in the CBA. It is unusual to find this question posed for treatment programmes that are not already in existence (although it should be), but it is useful, for example, in asking how much more (or less) of an already existing treatment or screening programme can be justified.

Option appraisal

Option appraisal is an important economic exercise which should be employed at all stages of health service planning and development. It essentially implies stating and costing as many alternatives for a given objective or resource usage as possible. It is especially relevant to planners in developing countries where a wider range of options may be available as there may be no pre-existing established services, and where planners and mental health professionals have to make crucial decisions regarding the allocation of resources to achieve the most rational and efficient methods of service provision. Option appraisal is undertaken by a systematic examination of all the advantages and disadvantages of every possible way of solving a problem (or at least every way that planners can imagine that could be implemented). Efficiency in this context implies maximising the benefits of an intervention over its costs.

Option appraisal could be reduced to several simpler stages as illustrated in Table 2.2. The first stage is to define the problem in terms of a health or health service deficiency. Thereafter, objectives of the appraisal should be set. This could take many forms depending on what is the limiting factor. In the case of developing countries, the usual form the objective would take is to increase benefit for a fixed cost, for example, to work out the most efficient method of spending half a million rupees for reducing psychosocial disability in school children with visual deficits. Clearly such objectives are regulated by the degree of political and administrative commitment to any particular cause and to the differential values societies place on different priorities of their health. After setting the objective, all possible solutions to it should be outlined. This should be as broad a list as possible including options such as 'doing nothing' and 'continuing as at present'.

When undertaking an option appraisal in developing countries it is appropriate to give consideration to traditional health systems. These may be of particular importance in rural areas, examples being faith healers and Islamic Tibb (Young, 1983; Kapor, 1979). In some areas over 60% of the rural population use traditional practices in addition or in preference to those of Western medicine. One essential consideration in option appraisal is the equitable distribution of resources. In the context of developing countries this entails redistribution of health care resources from urban (predominantly hospital-based) care to rural primary care facilities, which are responsible for the health care needs of more than 70% of the population.

Comparing developing with developed countries

In developed countries with well-established health care provisions for the majority of the population and clinical problems, changes in service delivery usually involve adjustments to services which already exist. The choice is therefore how much of what type of treatment to provide and not whether to have mental health care services at all. Thus the costs that need to be considered are the marginal costs of such changes, usually in the context of relatively large budgets, and the opportunity costs are usually considered in terms of which area of service development can be postponed or done without for each new area of development. More recently, in an era of increasingly tight budget control and escalating costs, the same decisions have had to be made about marginal cuts in service. Even so, the decisions are usually made on the grounds of 'efficiency' (i.e. getting the maximum amount of perceived care for the money available) or 'cost-effectiveness' (getting the cheaper of two options that provide the same level of perceived care). It is rare to find decisions based on cost-benefit calculations where the benefits of service provision can be demonstrated to outweigh the costs. In developing countries, where the luxury of high spending on health services is unavailable, and in many cases services may not exist at all, the choices may be more radical ones. The choice of restricting the available mental health service to, for example, drug treatment of the most common and disabling conditions (schizophrenia, depression, epilepsy) may be a very real option to be considered if very few resources are available. It may be more beneficial to overall mental health in a population to provide other forms of basic health care, social services or education than to offer a traditional mental health service. At the very least, treatments that are introduced have to be demonstrably cheap, effective and likely to more than pay for themselves in terms of increased productivity or other social benefits that cannot be provided more efficiently by other means. There is a very real need to demonstrate a positive cost-benefit ratio, and without such a demonstration it would be very difficult to justify the expenditure of scarce resources.

Health services research

With their key health services at an early evolutionary stage this is one of the most crucial areas of research and evaluation for developing countries (see Chapter 1). An important task for health planners and professionals is to evaluate a selection of culturally appropriate and economically feasible models of health delivery. Very often Western models are replicated with resultant wastage and alienation. Simple operational research with careful appraisal of available and newer options could easily lead to much desired management of meagre resources for greater benefit of a greater number of the population. Associated areas identified in a WHO report (1989) include health personnel management problems like utilisation, low productivity, labour market forces leading to manpower imbalance and broadly irrelevant and expensive training of health personnel.

Indicators of need

Good quality statistics are essential for proper design of service provision. Most developing countries estimate their service needs on Western epidemiological data. At the other extreme some have undertaken ambitious and expensive data collection programmes. Application of the principles of economic analysis is a useful tool in identifying the most suitable and cost-effective method of estimating needs by comparing methods such as case registers, key informant interviews, or community surveys.

Indicators of cost

This is required as an essential first step in any rational planning. All developing countries need to calculate cost indices for various services, for example the cost of individual consultations, the relative cost of services provided by professionals with different levels of training, the total cost of a day spent as a hospital in-patient and so forth. That the list of costs can be extended almost indefinitely is no justification for avoiding the costing exercise, as this is an essential first step in economic appraisal.

Case study. Allocating resources to psychotropic drugs in developing countries

Cost-benefit calculations can be applied to the provision of psychotropic drugs. The assumption made in this exercise is that a significant level of psychiatric morbidity has been identified, and that epidemiological studies have provided estimates, however crude, of the prevalence and severity of the most common disabling diagnoses which are likely to respond well to established medication, namely major depressive disorder, schizophrenia and manic depressive illness.

A large proportion of the health budget, especially in the private sector, is spent on the provision of expensive medicines. There is an urgent need to establish priorities in this area. The WHO has already prepared a list of essential psychoactive drugs in consultation with developing countries. There is a need for a cost-effectiveness analysis in these countries before actual policy implementation. The case of phenobarbitone, an anticonvulsant, is of special interest. The majority of epileptics in developing countries are under the care of mental health professionals, and despite some clinical reservations the economic benefits of using a relatively cheap drug such as phenobarbitone as compared to other more expensive anticonvulsants need to be carefully studied.

The problem of allocating resources to psychotropic drugs involves first an assumption that resources are going to be allocated at all to such drugs. This requires an option appraisal exercise that may compare services with alternatives such as non-provision (and thus allocating resources to non-medical services, non-psychiatric services or other forms of mental health care). Once this assumption is made, then it follows that only those drugs giving the greatest cost–benefit ratio should be bought and used. This applies to each group of psychotropic drugs (e.g. antidepressants, major tranquillisers) separately, but it is also necessary to build into the decision-making process a procedure for ensuring that different groups of drugs are bought in the right amounts and in the right combination to ensure the optimal cost–benefit ratio overall. This means that the first step must be to find a means of determining both the costs and benefits of individual drugs in such a way as to allow direct comparison between groups of drugs. Thus, the antidepressant exhibiting the greatest benefit per unit cost may, for the sake of argument, be imipramine, whereas the best neuroleptic might be chlorpromazine. It must then be possible to determine not only how much imipramine to buy but also what proportion of the available resource to spend on each drug to maximise the cost–benefit ratio overall.

Costs

These can be estimated in a fairly straightforward way for each drug. It is necessary to estimate the size of the population that can be expected to be treated using each drug. This would be the same as the prevalence of each disorder if the aim is to provide equal care across the population. If it were decided that some groups took priority, for example treatment were to be restricted to potential wage earners, then the size of these smaller populations would have to be estimated.

These figures could then be used to generate costs in two areas; first, direct costs, that is the cost of providing the number of courses of treatment required by the identified suffering population; second, indirect costs, primarily the costs of treating side-effects or complications of treatment. In practice the latter may be predominantly medical treatment of overdose and drug dependency. Each of these could be estimated from the average cost of providing the medical service (this should in fact be the marginal cost of treating each additional patient unless totally new services are set up) multiplied by the estimated number of patients requiring treatment.

These costs are all expressed in monetary terms and can be summed up to provide an estimate of total cost for each drug separately.

Benefits

The most important benefits to quantify in terms of determining the optimal cost–benefit ratio to a developing country planning on purchasing psychotropic medication are those accruing directly to the economy of the country. The most immediate benefits of treatment and symptom relief (and possible saving of life) are of comparatively less importance except in so far as they are related to return to work or reduction in other costs (medical or social). Theoretically, if the working population is increased by an effective treatment then there is a cost in providing employment for those newly available for work, and this should be included in the estimate of costs.

The benefits of return to work can be estimated in one of two ways. The first is to estimate the size of the working population. This is no easy task in developing countries where the productive working population is not easy to define. In rural farming economies women may do much or all of the productive work but in areas of industrial development most work is done by migrant men. This working population is then divided into the gross national product (GNP) or gross domestic product of the country. This puts a value on the return to work of each working person treated. Ideally, some method should be found to put an equivalent value on benefits which indirectly contribute to productivity, for example women caring for children allowing others to work or other caregivers returning to work when the dependent person's illness is treated. It should also be noticed that in areas where the economy is close to subsistence levels (i.e. production only caters for local needs) increasing employment may have little or no effect on GNP.

The second, and perhaps easier method is to concentrate on populations of professionals who are selected as having most economic potential and estimating the benefit of return to work for each individual in each group, using known figures for productivity. Even in this case it may be necessary to 'weight' the benefits using other non-monetary factors. For example civil servants or doctors may contribute indirectly (e.g. by doctors treating patients who then return to work) or have a value considered comparable to monetary contributions (e.g. civil servants contributing to the running of the country or its services).

Non-monetary benefits of treatment are primarily relief of symptoms (including potential saving of life from suicide). Some value may be placed on factors such as the social satisfaction gained from a society taking greater care of its sick members or the political benefits of having an improved health service or mental health care facilities. In developing countries such benefits are of relatively low priority, and only relevant to the first stage of selecting appropriate drugs for purchase, finding the best drug in each category. Quality of life should be a consideration in the prescribing of anti-depressants (Morris, 1991), but this must be defined locally, by the treated population. Again the needs of individuals may have to be weighted against the overall gains for the population. In many developing countries the increase in quality of life (for a given allocation of resources) of the population as a whole which might be achieved by preferentially treating those with the greatest economic potential, thus improving the economic position of the country, may outweigh that produced by treating everyone regardless of their productive capacity.

As a basis for making choices between drugs each could be assigned a value on a scale of clinical benefit. A suitable scale might be (although published data on even the most widely used drugs may not provide this information):

0. Drug has not been shown to be better than a placebo
1. Drug provides minimal relief to most patients or substantial relief to a minority
2. Drug provides considerable symptomatic relief to the majority of patients
3. Drug is life-saving or has a major effect on adaptation of at least half of patients
4. Drug is life-saving or has a major effect on adaptation of the large majority of patients.

A further elaboration would be to draw up a scale of the amount by which symptoms can be expected to be relieved in the treated population (i.e. not assuming all patients respond equally). The scale above is then corrected by the percentage of patients expected to gain that level of improvement (i.e. the scale is effectively made into a two-stage evaluation). This, however, is still restricted to a simple measure of global improvement. A more comprehensive method of evaluating benefits would be to ascribe a similarly derived weighted value to each symptom or group of symptoms where improvement is expected. This would be similar to the method of assessing risk factors (see below).

There are other indirect costs and benefits which may need to be considered. For example, treating mental illness in adults may have the effect of increasing fertility, improving child care (and perhaps reducing infant mortality or morbidity), perhaps making more of the population available for education. These could potentially be included in the analysis by making assumptions about costs and benefits and performing sensitivity analyses, but it should be remembered that there may be wide ranging effects on the population or the country that have not been predicted.

The risk factor

Risk can be viewed as a negative benefit (i.e. the estimated benefits accruing from the use of a drug should be reduced by a 'risk factor'). The method of estimating risks needs to be comparable both within and between the groups of psychotropic drugs being compared.

The risks from taking drugs include the severity of side-effects (including mortality risk), toxicity and the risk of dependency. These could be assessed for each individual agent by drawing up a list of all known risks, allocating a severity value to each, and then multiplying this by the probability of occurrence of each risk to produce a series of 'risk factors' for each drug. Published information on each drug will give some help in estimating both the severity and probability of each risk factor, but it is likely that to some extent these will have to be given arbitrary values based on local knowledge and judgement. The mean value of these risk factors then gives an overall risk factor for each agent. Thus for two comparable antidepressants the table might look something like Table 2.3. It should be noted that despite the lower risk of death from overdose in antidepressant 'B' the risk factors taken overall still favour antidepressant 'A'. This demonstrates that all possible factors need to be included in the appraisal – it is very common for psychotropic drugs to be sold on the basis of one 'major' benefit without taking the whole spectrum of risks into consideration (Jelley & Owen, 1991).

Both benefit and risk factors will be affected by rates of compliance (acceptability of the treatment to patients), and if possible known or estimated compliance rates should be included in the calculation. In general it would be acceptable, albeit crude, to reduce overall estimated benefit and risk in proportion to compliance. Risk factors should also be adjusted to take into account the overall effectiveness of the drug in treating the target condition (for example if a drug produces symptomatic relief in only 60% of patients but side-effects in all).

Corrected benefits

The risk factor so obtained can be used as a weighting which is then applied to the measured benefits. The symptomatic benefits for each drug are thus calculated by multiplying the value for benefit, however obtained, by the risk factor for that drug. This provides a value for benefit that can be used in the cost–benefit ratio, which in turn provides a direct way of choosing between different drugs in the same category (for example selecting the best antidepressant).

Whichever way of assessing benefits is adopted, the values obtained for each drug, corrected by the risk factors, would then be multiplied by the number of patients in the identified population to be treated, to give the overall benefit factor for this drug.

TABLE 2.3
Determining 'risk factors' for two different antidepressant drugs

		Antidepressant A		Antidepressant B	
Risk	Severity (1–10)	Probability of occurrence	Risk factor	Probability of occurrence	Risk factor
Dry mouth	1	0.9	0.9	0.9	0.9
Constipation	1	0.4	0.4	0.6	0.6
Postural hypotension	2	0.3	0.6	0.4	0.8
Cardiac arrhythmias	6	0.04	0.24	0.06	0.36
Epileptic fits	6	0.01	0.06	0.008	0.05
Death from overdose	10	0.004	0.04	0.002	0.02
Mean risk factor	0.37		0.45		

Risk factors are for illustration, only a small sample of the range of risk factors is included.
The figures for risk factor are arbitrary, for illustration only.

Allocating resources

Once a list of preferred drugs in each category has been drawn up, it is then necessary to decide how much of each to purchase with the available resources. The procedure outlined above provides a method for choosing between similar drugs. It is more difficult to compare treatments for different conditions. In practice all psychotropics can be considered of roughly equivalent effectiveness in treating specific conditions, but difficulties arise between different groups of psychotropic medication. An example might be trying to calculate comparable benefit and risk factors for an antidepressant which is wholly effective in, say, 60% of cases of depression with a neuroleptic which is partly effective in 80% of cases of acute psychosis.

'Available resources' should not be judged simply as an arbitrary amount of money to spend on drugs. Instead, it is more appropriate to perform a marginal analysis of the changes in benefits and costs for each increase in the amount spent. Thus, the question to be answered should be 'How much of each drug should be purchased for each increase in spending' rather than 'How much should be spent overall'. This way of approaching the problem not only allows a rational way of determining how to spend any increase in funding, but also provides a way of determining when to stop spending increasing amounts on drugs (i.e. the point at which there are diminishing marginal returns).

The first stage would be to select one illness category, for example major depressive disorder. Then the costs and benefits (expressed per 1000 patients to be treated) are fed in, and the process repeated for each drug considered appropriate for treatment. At this stage only a few drugs need to be considered, i.e. those of known efficacy and relatively low cost. Newer antidepressants may be excluded without formal evaluation. On the other hand, if the algorithm was programmed into a computer then relevant computation would be rapid and inexpensive, so all drugs could be included.

The result at this stage would be a series of values representing a cost–benefit ratio per 1000 patients with a particular illness for each drug. This would allow the optimal drug choice to be made in that category. Once the measurement of costs and benefits has been standardised then similar figures for drugs in other illness categories can be directly compared, so that for purposes of example imipramine could prove to be the 'best' antidepressant and chlorpromazine the 'best' oral neuroleptic agent.

The next stage, of deciding which proportion of each drug to include in a limited budget (and more importantly deciding on changes in relative proportions with increasing marginal spending), can be done by running the same algorithm, but this time including only the 'best' drug in each illness category for which treatment is to be offered, and making the base *at risk* population group 100 000. Thus, the same population group is used for each different drug and illness. The aim of such a procedure is to *maximise* the cost–benefit ratio across the whole budget, and also for each increase in budget.

Conclusions

As a general principle it is irrational to plan, or change, the provision of health care services without considering costs, benefits and the overall efficiency of the service being provided. This is especially relevant to developing countries where relatively small changes in service provision can have large effects on outcome, and may utilise a large proportion of the country's GNP.

The consideration of economic factors as central in health care planning is a relatively recent phenomenon even in the developed world, and many problems remain to be solved if economic appraisal is to become a commonly used tool in provision of health services. Nevertheless, much can be done already, and this chapter has attempted to illustrate some ways in which economic thinking can help towards the provision of rational, useful and efficient health services in the developing world.

References

BRIDGES, K., GOLDBERG, D., HYDE, C., *et al* (1988) The application of modified cost-benefit analysis in the evaluation of a hostel ward for chronic psychotic patients. In *Cost and Effects of Managing Chronic Psychotic Patients* (eds D. Schwefel, H. Zoliner & P. Potthof). Berlin & Heidelberg: Springer-Verlag.

CULYER, A. J. (1991) The promise of a reformed NHS: an economist's angle. *British Medical Journal*, **302**, 1253–1256

DRUMMOND, M. F. (1980) *Principles of Economic Appraisal in Health Care*. Oxford: Oxford University Press.

——, STODDART, G. L. & TORRANCE, G. W. (1987) *Methods for the Economic Evaluation of Health Care Programmes*. Oxford: Oxford University Press.

FENTON, F. R., TESSIER, L., CONTANDRIOPOULOS, A. P., *et al* (1982) A comparative trial of home and hospital psychiatric treatment: financial costs. *Canadian Journal of Psychiatry*, **27**, 177–187.

GHOSH, B. (1982) *Health Services Management – an Indian Casebook*. Bangalore: Indian Institute of Management.

GLASS, N. J. & GOLDBERG, D. (1977) Cost-benefit analysis and the evaluation of psychiatric services. *Psychological Medicine*, **7**, 701–707.

GOLDBERG, D. & JONES, R. (1980) The costs and benefits of psychiatric care. In *The Social Consequences of Psychiatric Illness* (eds L. Robin, P. Clayton & J. Wing). New York: Brunner/Mazel.

——, BRIDGES, K., COOPER, W., *et al* (1985) Douglas House: a new type of hostel ward for chronic psychotic patients. *British Journal of Psychiatry*, **147**, 383–388.

HOLLAND, G. (1985) *Techniques of Health Status Measurement Using a Health Index*. London: Office of Health Economics.

HYDE, C., BRIDGES, K., GOLDBERG, D., *et al* (1985) The evaluation of a hostel ward: a controlled study using modified cost-benefit analysis. *British Journal of Psychiatry*, **151**, 805–812.

JELLEY, M. & OWEN, J. H. (1991) The words used to sell psychotropic drugs. *Psychiatric Bulletin*, **15**, 755–756.

KAPOR, R. (1979) The role of traditional healers in mental health care in rural India. *Social Sciences and Medicine*, **13**, 13–27.

McEWEN, J. (1984) The Nottingham Health Profile: a measure of perceived health. In *Measuring the Social Benefits of Medicine* (ed G. Teeling Smith). London: Office of Health Economics.

McGRATH, G. J. & LOWSON, K. (1987) Assessing the benefits of psychotherapy: an economic approach. *British Journal of Psychiatry*, **150**, 65–71.

MOONEY, G. H. & DRUMMOND, M. F. (1982) Essentials of health economics (series of six articles). *British Medical Journal*, **285**, 949.

MORRIS, J. (1991) The need to consider quality of life as an outcome of antidepressant therapy. *Psychiatric Bulletin*, **15**, 755–756.

MUBBASHAR, M. H. (1989) *When Wisdom Guides*. 2nd Upjohn Lecture of Spring Quarterly Meeting of Royal College of Psychiatrists. Leeds: England.

ROSSER, R. M. (1983) A history of the development of health indicators. In *Measuring the Social Benefits of Medicine* (ed G. Teeling Smith). London: Office of Health Economics.

SEGALL, M. (1983) Planning and politics of resource allocation for Primary Health Care: promotion of a meaningful national policy. *Social Sciences and Medicine*, **17**, 1947–1960.

TEELING SMITH, G. (1985) *Measurement of Health*. London: Office of Health Economics.

WORLD HEALTH ORGANIZATION (1975) Organisation of mental health services in developing countries. Sixteenth Report of the WHO Expert Committee. *WHO Technical Report Series*, **564**.

——— (1981) *Social Dimensions of Mental Health*. Report of WHO Working Group. Geneva: WHO.

——— (1984) Mental health care in developing countries: a critical appraisal of research findings. *WHO Technical Report Series*, **698**.

——— (1989) Management of human resources for health. Report of a WHO Expert Committee. *WHO Technical Report Series*, **783**.

——— (1990) *The Introduction of a Mental Health Component into Primary Health Care*. WHO Monograph. Geneva: WHO.

WIG, N. N., SULEIMAN, M. A., ROUTLEDGE, R., *et al* (1980) Community reactions to mental disorders: a key informant study in developing countries. *Acta Psychiatrica Scandinavica*, **61**, 111–126.

YOUNG, A. (1983) The relevance of traditional medical cultures to modern primary health care. *Social Sciences and Medicine*, **16**, 1205–1211.

3 Diagnosis and classification

A. JABLENSKY

Imagine a typical working day of a psychiatrist in the out-patient department of a University Hospital in a developing country. There may be over a hundred men, women and children waiting in front of the office to see the doctor; some of them must have travelled over considerable distances, having spent the night camping near the hospital. Most of them come in family groups, large or small, and quite a few are obviously physically sick. Apart from about a dozen familiar faces coming for a follow-up visit, the doctor has never before seen these people. As no one ought to be turned back, there will be less than five minutes per 'case', though some would be given more, and some less time. It is the family group that states both the problem and its presumed cause (only rarely is the visit a dyadic doctor–patient situation) and expects to be told what the cure should be. Often, the expectations include an injection, or at least a prescription for pills to be taken home from the hospital pharmacy.

How can the doctor make the best possible use of these few minutes, in order to recognise and diagnose the problem, decide on the appropriate course of action, explain conclusions, advise on treatment, and reassure both patient and family? Following scrupulously the rules of good history taking, interviewing, diagnosis, differential diagnosis and formulation, developing a management plan and choosing a treatment, as taught in postgraduate training, is simply not possible. With practice, every doctor learns to short-circuit the standard examination and assessment procedures and develops for this his/her own rules of thumb. Nowhere is the pressure to use modified and abbreviated psychiatric assessment techniques greater than in the developing countries and it is unfortunate that up to date little has been done to evaluate systematically alternative strategies in settings typical of such countries. Nevertheless, there is some knowledge and a good deal of unpublished practical experience which throw light on the problem of diagnosing and classifying mental disorders in the developing countries.

Even if a conscious decision is made to dispense with formal psychiatric diagnosis, one still does implicitly classify the problems one way or another, unless doctor–patient encounters are allowed to result in completely random outcomes. Classification is a fundamental cognitive activity and the relevant question is not whether diagnosis and classification can be circumvented but

27

whether the concepts and tools serving these functions are appropriate and effective in the conditions under which psychiatry is practised in the developing countries.

Purposes and properties of diagnosis and classification

Functions

Making a diagnosis has been defined as follows: "The psychiatrist interviews the patient, and chooses from a system of psychiatric terms a few words or phrases which he uses as a label for the patient, so as to convey to himself and others as much as possible about the aetiology, the immediate manifestations, and the prognosis of the patient's condition" (Shepherd *et al*, 1968). In the past 20 years psychiatric diagnosis has also acquired the capacity to convey something about the rational choice of treatment.

Diagnosis and classification are interrelated: choosing a diagnostic label usually presupposes some ordered system of possible labels, and a classification is the arrangement of such labels in accordance with certain specified principles and rules. According to Feinstein (1972), medical classifications perform three principal functions:

(a) denomination, i.e. assigning common names to groups of phenomena;
(b) qualification, i.e. enriching the informativeness of a name or category by adding relevant descriptive features such as typical symptoms, age at onset, severity;
(c) prediction, i.e. a probabilistic statement about the expected course and outcome of the named entity, as well as a statement about its likely response to treatment.

From the point of view of cognitive psychology, diagnosis and classification are tools helping to achieve economy of memory (or 'reduction of the cognitive load'); ease of manipulation of objects, by simplifying the relationships among them; and generation of hypotheses (Rosch, 1976). There are many different ways in which classifications can be constructed. The philosopher Carl Hempel (1959) postulated that the categories of a classification should be 'mutually exclusive and jointly exhaustive' of the universe of observations; there is also the widespread view that, ideally, the classification of mental disorders should be based on aetiology.

These conditions have never been met fully by psychiatric classifications, or, for that matter, by any medical classification. Medical, including psychiatric, classifications are eclectic in the sense that they are organised along several different, co-existing principles (e.g. causes, presenting symptoms or traits, age at onset, course) without a clear predominance of one or another of these principles, and they tend to mutate as knowledge progresses or social conditions change. In spite of their apparent logical inconsistency, medical classifications survive and evolve because of their essentially pragmatic nature: almost daily

Terminology

Classification: denotes 'the activity of ordering or arrangement of objects into groups or sets on the basis of their relationships' (Sokal, 1974), i.e. it refers to the process of creation of categories.

Classificatory system: the product of the classification process.

Identification: the act of assigning a particular object to one of the classification categories (in the instance of medical classification this is the act of making a diagnosis or *diagnostic identification*).

Semiotics: sometimes used to denote the description and classification of symptoms and signs in psychopathology.

Taxonomy: signifies the study of various strategies of classification.

Nosology: denotes the system of concepts and theories that support the classification of symptoms, signs, syndromes and diseases.

Nosography: the activity of describing and assigning names to diseases and morbid conditions.

Nomenclature: classification of names of diseases and morbid conditions within a particular branch of medicine.

they are put to the test of usefulness in therapeutic or preventive decision-making and in clinical prediction. This process ensures a natural selection of useful concepts by weeding out impracticable or obsolete ideas.

The diagnostic process

Making a diagnosis is a procedure which involves a chain of behavioural interactions and cognitive activities on the part of both the examiner and the subject. Four elements are usually distinguished (Shepherd *et al*, 1968): (a) the interviewing technique of the psychiatrist; (b) the perception of the patient's speech and behaviour; (c) the inferences and decisions made by the psychiatrist on the basis of what he has perceived; and (d) the attachment of a particular diagnostic label to the patient. Even a brief reflection on what is implied will reveal a host of different factors that may influence each one of the interacting elements: the nature of the encounter situation between the doctor and the patient, the interviewing style, the patient's behaviour, the interviewer's past experience, knowledge and personality, the explicit or implicit theory behind the interpretation of observations, and the classificatory framework available – to mention only a few.

Essentially, the process is one of hypothesis generation and hypothesis testing, with iterations and feedback 'loops' determined by the interviewer's cognitive appraisal of the information flow (Elstein *et al*, 1978). It is also important to note that the process is sequential, and that the output of each stage serves as the input to the next. Both errors of commission (e.g. a misinterpretation of a believer's statement about God guiding her thoughts as a delusion of control) and errors of omission (e.g. failing to register the psychomotor signs of depressive mood in a patient denying depressive feelings), therefore, have cumulative effects in the course of the diagnostic interview and may result in a misclassification. As diagnosticians generally tend to 'narrow down' on a diagnostic hypothesis fairly early in the interview (Eddy & Clanton, 1982), the initial part of the process, in which the basic facts about the case have to be elicited and aggregated, is of critical importance, especially under time pressure.

Interviewing guides and schedules

A great variety of instruments have been developed to aid the diagnostic process by ensuring a systematic coverage of all relevant (and sometimes irrelevant) areas of history and psychopathology. Standardised interviews (in the sense of containing item definitions and rating scales) may be fully structured or semi-structured: the former list all questions in the format in which they should be asked, while the latter provide a mix of mandatory questions and optional probes, thus allowing some flexibility and judgement on the part of the interviewer.

An example of a highly structured diagnostic interview is the Composite International Diagnostic Interview (CIDI; Robins *et al*, 1988) which contains over 400 algorithmically arranged questions linked to the diagnostic criteria of DSM–III–R (American Psychiatric Association, 1987) and ICD–10 (World Health Organization, 1992). The interviewer is not allowed to deviate from the script of the interview or to use judgement whether a symptom is present or not. The CIDI has been shown to produce reliable diagnostic assessments in diverse settings (Wittchen *et al*, 1991) and is currently being tested in a WHO cross-cultural study.

The Present State Examination (PSE; Wing *et al*, 1974) is one of the most widely used semi-structured interviews which covers 140 psychopathological symptoms. Its flexibility is ensured by the availability, in the course of the interview, of a number of cut-off points at which the inquiry may be discontinued if, on the evidence of defined probe questions, the interviewer is satisfied that no symptoms in a given area of psychopathology are likely to be elicited. A recent, tenth edition of the PSE is now available (Wing *et al*, 1990).

It should be pointed out that none of the diagnostic interview schedules available today have been designed for use in the developing countries, and that very few would meet the logistic requirements, such as brevity and flexibility (the cultural constraints are discussed below). The brief version of the PSE is probably closest to such requirements because of its flexible format (an 'ultra-short' 10-item screening version as well as a syndrome checklist are also available) and the existence of approved translations in over 20 languages. (Information on the different language versions may be obtained from the WHO Division of Mental Health, Geneva, Switzerland.)

Reliability and validity of diagnosis

Disagreement on the diagnostic classification of cases when different clinicians are presented with the same patient information is a well documented and investigated phenomenon. Experimental methods have been applied to partition disagreement according to sources (Shepherd *et al*, 1968) and it has been shown that each of the four elements of the diagnostic process can contribute, to a greater or lesser extent, to poor agreement on diagnosis.

The psychometric concept of reliability refers to that proportion of the total variance of a measurement which is true variance, i.e. reflects the differences among objects rather than differences among observers or measuring instruments and procedures. When applied to the diagnostic process in psychiatry, an index of reliability informs us about the extent to which the identification of any individual symptom, syndrome, or disease concept is replicable across independent raters and settings or stable over time (inter-rater and test–retest reliability).

A range of statistics are at present available to quantify reliability in psychiatric research and practice, the most widely used being Cohen's kappa (Spitzer *et al*, 1967) and the intra-class correlation coefficient (Bartko, 1991). However, simple measures such as the pairwise agreement ratio (PAR) are fully appropriate for monitoring diagnostic agreement in everyday clinical practice or training, when, for example, K raters assess the presence (p) or absence (a) of a particular symptom or a particular disorder in a patient. If m raters choose alternative p, and n raters choose alternative a, there will be $m(m-1)/2$ pairs agreeing on p, and $n(n-1)/2$ pairs agreeing on a. The pairwise agreement ratio A will be:

$$A=[m(m-1)+n(n-1)]/K(K-1)$$

Validity of a diagnostic concept, or of a system of classification, is a more complex concept, and there is no simple statistic that would quantify it. The four types or aspects of validity of psychometric tests – construct, content, concurrent, and predictive – can also be applied to psychiatric diagnosis and classification but, as pointed out by Kendell (1989), practical utility for the management of patients is often the overriding concern when the validity of a diagnostic or classificatory concept is at issue. However, a diagnostic category which (i) is based on a coherent and explicit concept (construct validity), (ii) refers to verifiable observations for establishing its presence (content validity), (iii) can be corroborated by independent procedures such as biological or psychological tests (concurrent validity), and (iv) predicts future course of illness or treatment response (predictive validity), is more likely to be practically useful than a category failing to meet these criteria. Few, if any, of the current diagnostic concepts in psychiatry meet all four criteria, and a number of them are of uncertain validity when applied outside the culture in which they were generated.

The establishment of the validity of a clinical syndrome is, therefore, a multi-stage process which should include at least six strategies (Kendell, 1989): (i) identification and description; (ii) demonstration of boundaries between related syndromes; (iii) establishing a distinctive course or outcome; (iv) establishing a distinctive treatment response; (v) establishing that the syndrome 'breeds true' in families; (vi) demonstration of an association with a histological, psychological, biochemical or molecular abnormality. To these should be added: (vii) establishing the transportability of the syndrome across cultures and populations. While, for example, dementia associated with Alzheimer's disease has been adequately investigated with regard to (i), (iii), (v), and (vi), there is less than certainty regarding (ii), practically nothing on (iv), and unresolved questions regarding (vii). The balance would be far more problematic with diagnoses such as neurasthenia, multiple personality disorder, or telephone scatologia (DSM–III–R).

Requirements for a 'state of the art' classification system

In addition to allowing the reliable identification of its constituent categories or rubrics, a good diagnostic and classificatory system today is expected to meet a variety of needs of its potential users, clinicians, researchers and administrators:

(1)   The system should be capable of discriminating well not only between syndromes but also between patients, disorders, impairments, and disabilities in individual patients. This implies that several independent axes will be needed, as well as special provisions to record co-morbidity.

(2)   The rules of inclusion/exclusion of any given diagnostic category, and the symptom hierarchies implied (e.g. should depression or anxiety take precedence in the diagnosis if both are present?) should be formulated so as to minimise the risk of serious treatment or management errors. For example, misclassifying a depressive illness as a transient, mixed anxiety and depressive reaction which may be treated with reassurance and anxiolytics is a more costly error than misclassifying an anxiety state as depression and treating it with an antidepressant.

(3)   The system should be adaptable to the different cognitive styles of its users. In particular, it should allow the clinician to use the class of knowledge usually described as clinical experience or judgement, and enable valid decisions to be made under the conditions of uncertainty, incomplete data, and time pressure which occur far more commonly than is assumed by the designers of diagnostic systems.

(4)   The system should be adaptable to different settings and should perform well in in- and out-patient services, primary care, emergencies, and the courtroom. In addition, it should be 'user-friendly', i.e. sufficiently simple and clear in its overall organisation, to allow entry at different levels for different users, including non-professional health workers.

(5)   The system should be meaningful in different cultures. Characteristic symptoms and behaviours occurring in different cultural contexts should be directly identifiable, without the need of interpreting them in terms of 'Western' psychopathology, and there should be provisions for diagnosing and coding the so-called culture-bound syndromes without forcing them into the conventional rubrics of the classification.

A final requirement which is rarely considered concerns the social needs and self-esteem of those who are diagnosed, i.e. the mental health care 'consumers' and their families. Psychiatric diagnoses should be amenable to presentation and explanation in lay terms, including concepts which are meaningful and non-stigmatising within the particular culture. The avoidance or reduction of stigma associated with psychiatric diagnosis is an overriding concern that needs to be taken into account when developing, adapting, or translating diagnostic classifications.

Culture, diagnosis and classification

The notion of culture and psychiatry

The concept of culture is difficult to define. At the opening of a major international conference on transcultural psychiatry some 30 years ago, Aubrey Lewis (1965) pointed out that social scientists had been using over 160 different definitions of the term 'culture' in the English language only. Although it is unlikely that unanimity will ever be achieved among anthropologists, sociologists, psychologists, social geographers and historians in defining such a complex and multifaceted idea, culture may be conceptualised for the purposes of mental health research and care as 'the ideas, values, habits, and other patterns of behaviour which a human group consciously or unconsciously transmits from one generation to another and hence usually treats as traditional or worthy of reproduction' (Murphy, 1982).

One of the first psychiatrists to realise the fundamental importance of the study of culture for the scientific understanding of mental disorders was Kraepelin (1904) who advocated a systematic approach ('comparative psychiatry') to the description of psychiatric illnesses in different peoples and nations. Drawing on contributions from two separate sources – one in clinical and epidemiological psychiatry and another in the social sciences – the related but not fully identical disciplines of cross-cultural psychiatry, transcultural psychiatry, and ethno-psychiatry emerged in the period between the two World Wars.

The emic–etic distinction

The study of culture and mental illness has been characterised by the co-existence of two opposing viewpoints on the nature of the relationship between culture and mental disorders. The emic approach (the term is derived from 'phonemic', as analogy) tends to regard each culture as a singularity and insists that psychiatric disorders can only be understood from the perspective of the particular culture in which they occur. In contrast, the etic approach (the term is derived from 'phonetic') assumes that the building blocks of psychopathology and the basic patterns of causation are more or less similar across the cultures and that the role of culture is to facilitate or inhibit the expression of various forms and configurations of psychopathological disorders.

When carried to its extreme consequences, the emic position would deny the mere possibility of a 'common language' in psychiatry, as each culture would have its own and specific psychiatric semiotics and classification. The etic approach, on the other hand, easily merges into standard medical thinking, in which culture plays no role except as a background or noise in the diagnostic system. Fortunately, few psychiatrists or social scientists today would subscribe to the pure versions of either of the two approaches which may be more properly described as forms of ideology rather than scientific theory.

The 'new cultural psychiatry'

The idea of culture as mainly exerting a 'pathoplastic' influence, or giving no more than a particular 'colouring' to psychiatric syndromes, has been challenged by the 'new cultural psychiatry' (Kleinman, 1988; Littlewood, 1990). According to the proponents of this point of view, diagnosis cannot be independent of the context in which it is made – not so much because of problems of reliability but because the majority of the mental disorders are not 'things' that can be detached from the network of cultural beliefs and social interactions in which they occur. Diagnoses, therefore, cannot be compared across cultures; they require an ethnographic interpretation.

Kleinman (1988) has described as 'the category fallacy' 'the reification of one culture's diagnostic categories and their projection onto patients in another culture, where those categories lack coherence and their validity has not been established'. Although this, and other critical positions of the 'new cultural psychiatry' regarding the contextual aspects of psychiatric diagnosis are valid warnings against the uncritical adoption of Western diagnostic systems by psychiatrists in the developing world, or against ethnic or racial bias in psychiatric diagnosis (Adebimpe, 1981), no convincing evidence has so far been presented that 'a distorted view of pathology and an inappropriate use of diagnostic categories' (Kleinman, 1988) is the large-scale result of the international use of new diagnostic and classification systems. Neither has, however, the universal validity of all current diagnostic concepts in psychiatry been demonstrated.

Universals versus relativity

One of the key questions in the theory of psychopathology is 'which manifestations of mental morbidity are universal characteristics of the psychobiological make-up of the species and which manifestations are the product of particular circumstances of culture, social conditions and history? Do we have the means of distinguishing between them?' A definitive answer to this question has not been provided, although it is of critical importance to the validity of the diagnostic concepts and classifications which are in daily use in different parts of the globe.

A hypothesis, deriving from the influential phenomenological theory of Jaspers (1963), is that the primary *forms* of abnormal experience which are not psychologically understandable or reducible to other experiences, such as primary delusions, hallucinations, subjective thought disorders, or affective disorders are universal and culture-free, while their *content* and subjective meaning (persecution, bewitchment, guilt) are provided by the culture and the learning history of the personality. The argument can be extended to the analysis of syndromes and disease entities in which certain elements would be psychobiological universals and others would be precipitations of culture.

This hypothesis is testable: if the same syndrome can be reliably identified in different or contrasting populations and cultures and is found to meet the requirements of several of the validating strategies referred to above, it is likely to be a 'universal' syndrome. As a corollary, the finding of a single culture in which a predicted syndrome does not occur would raise serious doubts about the generalisability of the concept. Schizophrenia has been extensively investigated from this point of view (Jablensky *et al*, 1992) and the research data so far available suggest strongly that its incidence and basic symptomatology are very similar across cultures. It would be extremely misleading, however, to conclude that schizophrenia is 'culture-free' because its relatively more favourable course and outcome in the developing countries as compared to the West, documented in the WHO studies, is more likely to be an effect of the social environment than of a different biological basis.

The majority of the other psychiatric disorders have not been as systematically investigated across cultures but the cumulative evidence from clinical and epidemiological research indicates that manic and depressive illnesses (Sartorius *et al*, 1983), acute psychotic disorders, anxiety disorders, and the organic brain disorders occur and can be diagnosed in all cultures (Murphy, 1982). The evidence is very limited, however, with regard to personality disorders, impulse and habit disorders, gender identity and sexual preference disorders, developmental disorders, and the entire group of behavioural and emotional disorders with onset in childhood and adolescence. 'Universals' are unlikely in these areas.

Culture-bound syndromes

A large number of disorders typically occurring in certain cultures but not in others, and recognised as such by the members of those cultures, have been described and tentatively systematised (Yap, 1974). These disorders usually present complex, often dramatic, sequences of behaviour which, as a rule, involve other members of the community and evoke collective coping responses. An example is '*latah*' (South-East Asia), a state characterised by attacks of extreme suggestibility, imitative behaviour, and vocal tics, which may occur in epidemic waves. Another is '*susto*' (Mexico and Central America) which is characterised by anxiety, depression, and multiple somatic symptoms and complaints. The list of these conditions is indeed open-ended and, while their ethnographic description may be a worthwhile goal on its own, their status in relation to psychiatric classifications is far from clear. Some, but not all, of the syndromes described up to date can be subsumed under the concepts of depression, dissociative disorders, or generalised and phobic anxiety (Murphy, 1982), but 'Western' diagnostic systems have generally ignored them. It is a legitimate point to ask why the concept of a 'culture-bound syndrome' should be applied exclusively to non-Western phenomena, when many of the 'disorder' categories in DSM–III–R, DSM–IV (APA, 1994), and ICD–10 clearly meet the same general descriptive criteria. Examples include anorexia nervosa, parent–child relational problems, academic problems, phase of life problems, late luteal phase dysphoric disorders, and probably many others.

The concept of culture-bound syndromes, therefore, presents a dilemma which neither of the two influential current classifications has resolved. One solution would be to distribute these states as 'inclusion terms' under the appropriate general rubrics of mood disorders, anxiety states, or dissociative states. However, such a classification could only be provisional, since little is known about the pathophysiological basis, course and outcome of many of these states. Another possibility would be to include them, with annotations, in an appendix to the diagnostic classification. The first alternative may be preferable because it avoids relegating the syndromes to a residual category.

Diagnosing and classifying mental illness in developing countries

Mental health care in the developing countries is provided under conditions which would be regarded as extreme constraints in the more affluent parts of the world. The population:health workers ratio is orders of magnitude greater than in most of the industrialised countries. The population:psychiatrists ratio may be as high as 1–2 million per specialist in some developing countries, while it is 10 000 (or less) to one in many European countries and North America. Psychiatrists are usually located in the big cities, and distance and financial means often determine who receives care and who does not. Existing psychiatric facilities are often legacies of the past, and the big mental hospital may still be the main resource for both acute and long-term care. Mental health care is rarely regarded as a priority by the authorities and budgets are meagre. Diagnostic technology is hardly available, treatment resources are severely restricted, peer consultation may be non-existent, and a young psychiatrist may experience an acute sense of professional isolation and helplessness.

On the other hand, there are important resources: families are highly supportive of their sick members, there is less stigma attached to mental illness, and much of the burden of mental morbidity is shouldered by a great variety of informal agencies such as native healers, herbalists and priests, or by highly structured traditional medicine systems such as Ayurveda or Unani. Most individuals and families in traditional communities have shared beliefs about the nature of mental illness and expectations of its treatment which may favour recovery and re-socialisation. The epidemiology and ethnography of mental illness in the developing countries is, by and large, unchartered land offering exciting opportunities to the research-minded psychiatrist or social scientist.

Against this background, the goal of validly diagnosing and classifying mental disorders in developing countries places a greater number of additional demands on the clinician than is usually the case in the developed countries. These include:

(a) culturally appropriate interviewing techniques and at least some knowledge of the local languages and dialects, which may be numerous;
(b) understanding of the patients' values and beliefs system and of their position and role in the family and the community;
(c) knowledge of the variation in the presenting features of mental disorders in the culture;
(d) a heightened 'index of suspicion' for somatic and cerebral organic pathology which may accompany mental and behaviour disorders in a large proportion of the cases.

The general purposes and objectives of diagnosis and classification in the developing countries, i.e. description of the important clinical features, identification of causes (where possible), prediction of future course and treatment response, and communication about the patient, are not different from those that apply everywhere but there are at least two points of special emphasis. First, the diagnosis may be the most important piece of information on a patient seen in the facility briefly but likely to appear again at some unspecified time in the future. An informative, possibly multiaxial, and carefully recorded diagnosis, therefore, will enable at least a modicum of clinical management and monitoring under the existing constraints and limitations.

Secondly, in each developing country there usually is an acute need for basic epidemiological data on mental morbidity which should help to improve service provision and also may be used for research. Special epidemiological surveys are costly to design and conduct, and the routine diagnostic information should be usable for epidemiological purposes.

Current diagnostic systems

The development of a common language

In reviewing the field more than 30 years ago, Stengel (1959) noted that "the lack of a common classification of mental disorders has defeated attempts at comparing psychiatric observations and the results of treatments undertaken in various countries or even in various centres in the same country". Subsequently, the World Health Organization initiated an international programme for standardisation of psychiatric diagnosis, classification and statistics which ultimately resulted in the ICD–8 glossary of mental disorders (WHO, 1967), and was followed by ICD–9 (WHO, 1978) which incorporated the glossary into the 'official' body of the classification. Concurrent developments in the US led to the formulation of 'operational' criteria for diagnosis (Feighner *et al*, 1972; Spitzer *et al*, 1978) and to the third revision of the *Diagnostic and Statistical Manual*, DSM–III (APA, 1980). The wide acceptance of the operational diagnostic criteria and DSM–III was a stimulus for WHO to develop a new version of ICD which should combine the advantages of the operational diagnostic criteria with a broader international appeal and a greater clinical relevance. Jointly with the Alcohol, Drug Abuse and Mental Health Administration (ADAMHA) of the US, WHO completed a review of the major advances in all areas of psychiatric diagnosis and classification, and produced a draft version of ICD–10 following extensive consultations with over 160 experts from some 40 countries (Jablensky *et al*, 1983). ICD–10 was officially endorsed for international use by the World Health Assembly in 1990; field trials and reliability studies carried out by a worldwide network of research centres helped to complete a final version of ICD–10 (WHO, 1992).

DSM–III–R (R=revised) is still the official classification in the US, and the recently published DSM–IV (APA, 1994) was developed with the explicit aim of reducing further the discrepancies that exist between ICD–10 and DSM–III–R.

Overall structure of ICD–10

Mental and behavioural disorders in ICD–10 are organised in ten 'blocks', each comprising conditions defined primarily by:

(i) demonstrable aetiology (F0: organic and symptomatic mental disorders; F1: psychoactive substance use disorders);

(ii) symptom patterns (F2: schizophrenia, schizotypal and delusional disorders; F3: mood disorders; F4: neurotic, stress-related and somatoform disorders);

(iii) associated physiological function or other physical features (F5: behavioural syndromes associated with physiological disturbances and physical factors);

(iv) behaviour and trait patterns (F6: disorders of adult personality and behaviour);

(v) type and course of psychological impairment (F7: mental retardation; F8: disorders of psychological development); or

(vi) age at onset (F9: behaviour and emotional disorders with onset usually occurring in childhood and adolescence).

In addition to the F symbol allotted to the mental disorders in ICD, related disorders are indexed by two digits, the first denoting the 'block' and the second the group. For example, vascular dementias are indexed by the alphanumeric code F01. The majority of groups of disorders are subdivided further: thus multi-infarct dementia is F01.1 and subcortical vascular dementia is F01.2.

Chapter V of ICD–10 has 100 3-symbol alphanumeric positions which, if subdivided, permit the coding of 1000 diagnoses. Only part of this capacity (715 different diagnoses) has been used in the actual classification, the rest being reserved for future needs.

Each ICD–10 diagnosis is supplied with a clinical description (a glossary-type annotation of the essential features of the category) and diagnostic guidelines, specifying the criteria required for making a diagnosis, as well as any inclusion/exclusion rules and terms. The guidelines are designed for the clinician; they are less detailed than the diagnostic criteria for research and indicate the number and type of symptoms that should usually be present before a firm diagnosis is made.

Alternative presentations of ICD–10

The ICD–10 system was conceived as a 'family' of classifications. The 'core' classification contains the clinical descriptions and diagnostic guidelines described above. A special version, ICD–10 Diagnostic Criteria for Research, has been developed which includes detailed and precise rules for including and excluding patients into and from each of the major diagnostic categories. In addition, there is an abridged version (short glossary) containing annotations of the rubrics only, which is incorporated in the volumes containing the entire international classification.

Although the ICD–10 'core' is a syndromological axis, the system is designed for multiaspect (multiaxial) use. The annex to Chapter V contains a list of physical conditions often associated with mental and behavioural disorders which may be used as an aetiology/physical co-morbidity axis, as well as a list of factors influencing health status and contact with health services which provides much of the required contents for a psychosocial axis. However, an explicit multiaxial schema is under development, which will contain five axes: psychiatric syndromes; developmental conditions; concomitant physical morbidity; abnormal psychosocial situations; and disabilities.

A condensed version of ICD–10 for use in the developing countries and in primary care has been proposed by Cooper (1988). The schematic representation of this proposal is shown in Table 3.2.

New features and concepts in ICD–10

The overall structure of ICD–10 is simpler and clearer than that of ICD–9, although the number of diagnostic categories has been increased considerably. The ten 'blocks' of disorders are arranged in a sequence which loosely corresponds to a diagnostic hierarchy of aetiology and severity. Thus, the organic and symptomatic disorders of known aetiology and the substance misuse disorders appear at the top of the hierarchy and must be diagnosed first (if present) or excluded. They are followed by the schizophrenic and other psychotic disorders, the mood disorders, the neurotic and stress-related disorders, etc. This order of broadly defined severity also implies that if syndromes from two or more different levels of this hierarchy are present, the one belonging to the higher level of severity should be given precedence as the main diagnosis (however, the remaining syndromes should be recorded too).

The traditional distinction between psychoses and neuroses as major classes of morbidity has been abandoned in ICD–10, and the two terms appear only as descriptive adjectives. Other terms which have been avoided in ICD–10 include 'psychogenic' and 'psychosomatic', while terms such as 'organic' have been given a more precise definition.

The list of conditions and diagnoses includes a number of new diagnostic concepts for which sufficient validating evidence has been established in the last two decades (examples are subcortical vascular dementia; dementia in HIV disease; schizotypal disorder; recurrent brief depressive disorder; or enduring personality change after catastrophic experience). The entire section on disorders of psychological development reflects the new thinking and research data in this area. However, the new features of particular relevance to psychiatric diagnosis in developing countries are: (i) the acute and transient psychotic disorders; (ii) the reactions to severe stress and adjustment disorders; and (iii) the somatoform disorders. Their implications for diagnostic practice in the developing countries are discussed in the next section.

DSM–III and DSM–III–R

The third revision of the *Diagnostic and Statistical Manual* of the American Psychiatric Association (APA, 1980) was a turning point in the history of psychiatric classification in that: (i) it accomplished a transition from a

TABLE 3.2

Proposed condensation of ICD–10 categories for primary care (Cooper, 1988)

A	B	C	D
1 Dementias	1 Organic and symptomatic disorders	1 Organic and symptomatic disorder	1 Severe (psychotic) mental disorders
2 Transient and symptomatic organic disorders			
3 Disorders due to alcohol	2 Alcohol and drug disorders	2 Alcohol and drug disorders	
4 Disorders due to drugs			
5 Schizophrenic disorders	3 Schizophrenia and related disorders	3 Severe (psychotic) mental disorders	
6 Paranoid, acute and other disorders			
7 Affective disorders	4 Affective disorders		
8 Neurotic (anxiety) disorders	5 Neurotic and stress disorders	4 Neurotic, stress and personality disorders	2 Neurotic, stress and personality disorders
9 Somatoform disorders			
10 Psychophysiological disorders			
11 Stress reactions and adjustment disorders			
12 Adult personality disorders	6 Adult personality and behaviour disorders		
13 Other abnormality of adult behaviour, emotion or impulse			
14 Disorders with onset specific to or usually associated with childhood or adolescence and development	7 Disorders of childhood, adolescence and development	5 Disorders of childhood, adolescence, and development	3 Disorders of childhood, adolescence and development
15 Developmental disorders			
16 Mental retardation	8 Mental retardation	6 Mental retardation	

statistical classification to a clinical diagnostic manual; (ii) it introduced explicit diagnostic criteria and multiaxial evaluation; and (iii) it aligned psychiatric classification with contemporary advances in psychiatric research.

Mental disorders in DSM–III are grouped into 17 major diagnostic classes (a total of over 350 different diagnostic categories) and each class contains subgroups arranged in loose hierarchies. Although many of the DSM–III diagnostic criteria are debatable, their use has increased the reliability of diagnostic assessment in both routine mental health care and research. Some of the criteria have been criticised for being unwieldy or unnecessarily restrictive. For example, the DSM–III diagnosis of schizophrenia requires the presence of either overt psychotic symptoms or of prodromal signs plus a decline in functioning for a period of at least six months, a demand which tends to bias the diagnosis towards chronic, poor prognosis cases.

The other innovation, a multiaxial coding system, consists in the provision of five axes for assessing and recording aspects of the case that may be important for prognosis, treatment and management:

Axis I: clinical psychiatric syndrome;
Axis II: personality and specific developmental disorders;
Axis III: physical disorders; Axis IV: psychosocial stressors;
Axis V: highest level of adaptive functioning during the past year.

Multiaxial assessment has been shown to be feasible in routine clinical practice (Mezzich *et al*, 1982), yet it has been noted (APA, 1991) that its actual use is short of the initial expectations.

A number of modifications, none of them substantial, have been introduced following several years of field experience with DSM–III, resulting in the revised version, DSM–III–R. Many of the changes consist in a relaxation of the diagnostic hierarchy inclusion/exclusion rules – for example, panic disorder is now diagnosable even if it occurs in the context of a depressive episode (which would 'override' the diagnosis of panic disorder in the original DSM–III). Among other things, DSM–III–R is a slight improvement in the compatibility with ICD–10, although some discrepancies remain. It should be noted that both DSM–III and DSM–III–R make use of the ICD–9 numerical codes for disorders, and that a cross-reference manual exists on the correspondences in coding. However, while DSM–III or DSM–III–R diagnoses can be 'translated' into ICD–9, the reverse process is not possible because of the greater specificity and narrower scope of DSM diagnoses.

DSM–III has been criticised for its cultural limitations. According to Kleinman (1988) "DSM–III is so organized that every conceivable psychiatric condition is listed as a disease to legitimate remuneration to practitioners from private medical insurance and government programs". However, regardless of the obvious examples of diagnostic labels that would only have meaning in the US context, DSM–III has been extremely successful worldwide, including some of the developing countries. Thus, it has been positively received by psychiatrists in Latin America (Alarcon, 1983), and has performed satisfactorily in a field trial in Botswana (Ben Tovim, 1985). It seems that DSM–III and DSM–III–R owe their success not so much to the validity of their diagnostic criteria but to the fact that by providing them, they met a widely felt need of psychiatrists worldwide.

DSM–IV

Following the release of ICD–10, the DSM system has been put into yet another cycle of reorganisation. A preliminary version was published (APA, 1991) which suggested that the overall format of 17 major diagnostic classes, as well as the multiaxial scheme, were unlikely to be changed. However, DSM–IV draws from a wider base of expertise and empirical databases than DSM–III, and a large number of specific modifications of the diagnostic criteria have been articulated, many of them in the direction of greater DSM–IV/ICD–10 compatibility.

DSM or ICD?

Although this would be seen as an awkward question by both the DSM–III/IV and ICD–10 designers, it may be a real dilemma for psychiatrists in developing countries. In fact, no comparative trials have been conducted up to date to assess the advantages and disadvantages of the two systems, and the similarities between them make it unlikely that either system would prove definitively superior, were such trials to take place. As ICD codes are mandatory for national statistics, DSM users should be familiar with the ICD system as well. Either or both systems may be used in clinical practice and teaching, but it should be kept in mind that ICD–10 was developed with the participation of developing world psychiatrists and has undergone field trials in a large number of developing countries. It has, therefore, a wider cross-cultural basis.

Special problems of diagnosis in developing countries

Organic and symptomatic mental disorders

The proportion of these cases in an unselected series of out-patient attendances or admissions in a developing country is likely to be substantially higher than in other parts of the world (at least 20% in Botswana; Ben Tovim, 1985). The underlying pathology would vary according to geographical area but the presenting syndromes include delirium (e.g. with malaria, viral encephalitis, epilepsy), dementia (e.g. with trypanosomiasis, HIV disease), and a variety of psychotic, mood, anxiety, or dissociative disorders (ICD–10 rubric F06) which arise in association with acute or subacute physical illness. Epilepsy, usually untreated, is a common problem in most developing countries. A psychiatrist in a developing country is by definition a neuropsychiatrist.

Schizophrenia

The incidence of schizophrenia in the developing countries is similar to that observed in the developed countries, and the diagnosis can be made on the basis of the same symptoms and signs as elsewhere, including Schneiderian first-rank symptoms. Catatonic syndromes are more frequent in the developing countries, and acute onset is relatively more common. According to ICD–10, a schizophrenic syndrome of a duration of less than one month should be classified as an acute schizophrenia-like psychotic disorder. However, even when the duration of the episode exceeds one month, the probability of recovery and complete remission is significantly higher than for a similar clinical picture in the West.

Acute and transient psychotic disorders

These are states of rapid onset ('out of the blue'), few, if any, prodromal signs, dramatic and variable presentation, and short duration. Often, but by no means always, they arise in response to psychosocial or physiological stress, there is no characteristic family history, and the premorbid personality is inconspicuous. Repeated episodes are possible but the tendency to recur is significantly lower than in schizophrenia or affective disorder.

Acute psychotic disorders which are different from schizophrenia or manic–depressive illness have been described as bouffée délirante (Magnan & Legrain, 1895) in French psychiatry, and as cycloid psychoses (Kleist, 1928) in German psychiatry. They are similar to, or identical with the psychogenic psychoses (Wimmer, 1916; Stromgren, 1968) described by Danish psychiatrists. For reasons which are not properly understood, these illnesses represent a very small fraction of psychiatric morbidity in the industrialised countries today but they are relatively common in the developing countries. Their correct and timely recognition is important because of their benign prognosis which is very different from the prognosis in schizophrenia or mood disorders. ICD–10 contains a major rubric (F23) with 5 subdivisions and diagnostic guidelines which should help to differentiate the typical polymorphic acute states from those including some of the symptoms but not the pattern of course of schizophrenia. Since very little is known about their aetiology, pathophysiology, and genetics, this group of disorders should be a rewarding field for clinical and epidemiological research.

Mood disorders

Manic states seem to be more frequent in the developing countries than in the West and may be precipitated by stress (Rack, 1982). Depression more often gives rise to diagnostic difficulties because of the variation in the presentation of the depressive affect and experience in different cultures. Its psychic component may not be conceptualised and described as such and various somatic complaints come to the foreground. Since depression is a universal form of experience, many languages possess a rich vocabulary of metaphors which convey the depressive affect, and the heart is often the 'seat' of depression in many cultures (the heart may be 'burning', 'sinking', or 'squeezed'). Contrary to previous opinion, feelings of guilt and low self-esteem are not infrequent in non-European cultures (Jablensky *et al*, 1981).

Neurotic, stress-related, and adjustment disorders

This group of disorders is of particular relevance to psychiatry in primary care because of their frequency and characteristic presentation. Anxiety states are by far the most common, and with the exception of agoraphobia which is claimed to be rare, they present the entire range of syndromes described in current classifications. Anxiety and depression often co-exist and it may not be possible to distinguish them reliably. As a rule, both present commonly with physical symptoms and complaints, and ICD–10 offers a range of diagnostic categories and guidelines for such somatoform disorders (F45). A dilemma which may arise is whether to classify a condition as an anxiety state, e.g. generalised anxiety disorder (F41.1), or as a somatoform autonomic dysfunction (F45.3), considering the overlapping features. The ICD–10 guidelines emphasise the descriptive aspects of diagnosis and F45.3 should be preferred if the patient's focus is on the physical symptoms rather than on intrapsychic anxiety. An important consideration here is that the appearance of anxiety and depression as predominantly somatic complaints is part of a cultural code and represents illness behaviour sanctioned by the environment (Kleinman, 1988). An attempt on the part of the psychiatrist to 'reframe' the patient's complaints in terms of subjective feelings is likely to be culture-alien to both the patient and his family and may fail to elicit the response appropriate to the effective treatment and management of the problem. Both cultural sensitivity and common sense are required in the choice of the appropriate 'paradigm' in such cases, and there seem to be no hard and fast rules.

The dissociative disorders are another important diagnostic group for which ICD–10 offers detailed provisions to replace the former practice of lumping them together under the term hysteria.

The ICD–10 section F4 also contains diagnostic rubrics and guidelines for reactions to severe stress and adjustment disorders, a group of conditions of great epidemiological and social importance in view of the mass experiences of migration, resettlement, war and natural catastrophe stress.

Personality disorders

Particular caution is needed to avoid the 'category fallacy' with regard to the diagnosis of personality disorder in cultures and social contexts characterised by different norms and sets of values than those in which present classifications originated. Cultures may have strikingly different concepts of the self and of the interrelationship between the self and the others (Markus & Kitayama, 1991), and there is little evidence to support the cross-cultural validity of the specific personality disorders as described in DSM–III–R Axis II or ICD–10. On the other hand, very little research has been carried out into the personality disorders occurring in non-European cultures.

The risk of a diagnostic bias, or of 'medicalising' essentially social problems, is particularly great with regard to diagnoses such as antisocial personality disorder and borderline personality disorder (DSM–III–R), and dissocial personality disorder and emotionally unstable personality disorder (ICD–10). As pointed out by Alarcon (1983), "vast segments of the Latin American population, a young population indeed, may acquire or use some of the features described in the diagnostic criteria as the only way to social survival . . . in some countries, failure to accept social norms has been elevated to the category of collective enterprise".

Flow charts as aids to management

In most developing countries provision of mental health care to the majority of those in need is only possible in the context of primary health care and through the involvement of non-professional health workers or personnel of limited training. The function of the psychiatrist in such contexts will be largely one of a trainer, supervisor and consultant. Field research carried out by WHO (Harding, 1980) has demonstrated the feasibility of this approach and helped to develop tools which should enable such primary health care workers to make appropriate management decisions without making a formal psychiatric diagnosis. A series of flow charts has been constructed on the basis of cross- cultural survey data (Essex & Gosling, 1983) in which the great variety of presenting complaints typical of primary care settings in developing countries is compressed into eight categories: (1) violence to others; (2) violence to self; (3) delusional (including hallucinations); (4) withdrawn behaviour; (5) abnormal speech; (6) abnormal behaviour; (7) anxiousness; and (8) depression.

An algorithm has been written for the sequence of decisions following the initial categorisation of each presenting problem, leading to actions such as drug treatment, advice to patients and families, home visits, or referral.

Evaluation studies in India, Egypt, Uganda, Lesotho, and Tanzania have demonstrated that the flow chart approach is feasible and acceptable and that inter-observer agreement on problem categorisation by primary care workers is higher than 70%. The actual use of the flow chart method, however, has been less widespread than expected. As pointed out by Essex & Gosling (1983), its success will depend on "whether or not the medical establishment will accept and promote a system for mental health training in developing countries which is radically different to everything that has preceded it".

Conclusion

Diagnostic skills are as essential to the practice of psychiatry in the developing countries as they are in the developed countries. In the former, however, a number of cultural, social, geographical, and service organisation factors pose requirements and constraints which challenge, and in some instances invalidate, the transfer and application of both concepts and techniques from Western psychiatry. Although the balance of the evidence from cross-cultural research suggests that the major forms and patterns of mental morbidity are similar across the cultures, their content, characteristic presentation, course and outcome, and response to treatment vary and are determined to a significant degree by the context in which they occur. Knowledge about culture and cultural variation in psychiatric morbidity must, therefore, be more fully integrated into the training of psychiatrists worldwide.

New classifications of mental disorders, and especially ICD–10, are a step forward in the development of assessment tools that are sensitive to this variation. However, much of the field of psychiatric diagnosis and classification in developing countries is unexplored and represents an important and attractive area for scientific endeavour.

References

ADEPIMBE, V. R. (1981) Overview: white norms and psychiatric diagnosis in black patients. *American Journal of Psychiatry,* **138**, 279–285.

ALARCON, R. D. (1983) A Latin American perspective on DSM–III. *American Journal of Psychiatry,* **140**, 102–104.

AMERICAN PSYCHIATRIC ASSOCIATION (1980) *Diagnostic and Statistical Manual of Mental Disorders* (3rd edn) (DSM–III). Washington: APA.

——— (1987) *Diagnostic and Statistical Manual of Mental Disorders* (3rd edn, revised) (DSM–III–R). Washington: APA.

——— (1991) *DSM–IV Options Book: Work in Progress.* Washington: APA.

——— (1994) *Diagnostic and Statistical Manual of Mental Disorders* (4th edn) (DSM–IV). Washington: APA.

BARTKO, J. J. (1991) Measurement and reliability: statistical thinking considerations. *Schizophrenia Bulletin,* **17**, 483–489.

BEN TOVIM, D. I. (1985) DSM–III in Botswana: a field trial in a developing country. *American Journal of Psychiatry,* **142**, 342–344.

COOPER, J. E. (1988) The structure and presentation of contemporary psychiatric classifications with special reference to ICD–9 and 10. *British Journal of Psychiatry,* **152**, Suppl. 1, 21–28.

EDDY, D. M. & CLANTON, C. H. (1982) The art of diagnosis. Solving the clinicopathological exercise. *New England Journal of Medicine,* **306**, 1263–1268.

ELSTEIN, A. S., SHULMAN, L. S. & SPRAFKA, S. A. (1978) *Medical Problem-Solving: an Analysis of Clinical Reasoning.* Cambridge, MA: Harvard Press.

ESSEX, B. & GOSLING, H. (1983) An algorithmic method for management of mental health problems in developing countries. *British Journal of Psychiatry,* **143**, 451–459.

FEIGHNER, J. P., ROBINS, E., GUZE, S. B., *et al* (1972) Diagnostic criteria for use in psychiatric research. *Archives of Psychiatry,* **26**, 57–63.

FEINSTEIN, A. R. (1972) Clinical biostatistics. XIII: On homogeneity, taxonomy and nosography. *Clinical Pharmacology and Therapeutics,* **13**, 114–129.

HARDING, T. W. (1980) Mental disorders in primary health care – a study of their frequency and diagnosis in four developing countries. *Psychological Medicine,* **10**, 231–241.

HEMPEL, C. G. (1959) Introduction to problems of taxonomy. In *Field Studies in the Mental Disorders* (ed. J. Zubin). New York: Grune & Stratton.

JABLENSKY, A., SARTORIUS, N., GULBINAT, W., *et al* (1981) Characteristics of depressive patients contacting psychiatric services in different cultures. *Acta Psychiatrica Scandinavica,* **63**, 367–383.

———, ———, ERNBERG, G., *et al* (1992) *Schizophrenia: Manifestations, Incidence and Course in Different Cultures.* Psychological Medicine Monograph Supplement 20. Cambridge: Cambridge University Press.

JASPERS, K. (1963) *General Psychopathology.* Manchester: Manchester University Press.

KENDELL, R. E. (1989) Clinical validity. *Psychological Medicine,* **19**, 45–55.

KLEINMAN, A. (1988) *Rethinking Psychiatry.* New York: The Free Press.

KLEIST, K. (1928) Ueber zykloide, paranoide und epileptoide Psychosen und ueber die Frage der Degenerationspsychosen. *Schweizer Archiv für Neurologie und Psychiatrie,* **23**, 1–35.

KRAEPELIN, E. (1904) Vergleichende Psychiatrie. *Zentralblatt für Nervenheilkunde und Psychiatrie,* **27**, 433–437.

LEWIS, A. (1965) Chairman's introductory remarks. In *Transcultural Psychiatry CIBA Foundation Symposium* (ed. by A. V. S. de Reuck & R. Porter). London: Churchill.

LITTLEWOOD, R. (1990) From categories to contexts: a decade of the 'new cross-cultural psychiatry'. *British Journal of Psychiatry,* **156**, 308–327.

MAGNAN, V. & LEGRAIN, V. (1895) *Les Dégénérés.* Paris: Rueff.

MARKUS, H. R. & KITAYAMA, S. (1991) Culture and the self: implications for cognition, emotion, and motivation. *Psychological Review,* **98**, 224–253.

MEZZICH, J. E., COFFMAN, G. A. & GOODPASTOR, S. M. (1982) A format for DSM–III diagnostic formulation: experience with 1111 consecutive patients. *American Journal of Psychiatry,* **139**, 591–595.

MURPHY, H. B. M. (1982) *Comparative Psychiatry.* Berlin: Springer.

RACK, P. (1982) *Race, Culture and Mental Disorder.* London: Tavistock.

ROBINS, L. N., WING, J. K., WITTCHEN, H. U., *et al* (1988) The Composite International Diagnostic Interview: an epidemiologic instrument suitable for use in conjunction with different diagnostic systems and in different cultures. *Archives of General Psychiatry,* **45**, 1069–1077.

ROSCH, E. (1976) Classification of real-world objects: origins and representations in cognition. In *La Mémoire Sémantique* (eds S. Ehrlich & E. Tilsving). Paris: Bulletin de Psychologie.

SARTORIUS, N., DAVIDIAN, H., ERNBERG, G., *et al* (1983) *Depressive Disorders in Different Cultures*. Geneva: WHO.

SHEPHERD, M., BROOKE, E. M., COOPER, J. E., *et al* (1968) An experimental approach to psychiatric diagnosis. *Acta Psychiatrica Scandinavica*, Suppl 201.

SOKAL, R. R. (1974) Classification: purposes, principles, progress, prospects. *Science*, **185**, 115–123.

SPITZER, R., CONEN, J., FLEISS, J. L., *et al* (1967) Quantification of agreement in psychiatric diagnosis. A new approach. *Archives of General Psychiatry*, **17**, 83–87.

——, ENDICOTT, J. & ROBINS, E. (1978) Research diagnostic criteria: rationale and reliability. *Archives of General Psychiatry*, **35**, 773–782.

STENGEL, E. (1959) Classification of mental disorders. *Bulletin of the WHO*, **21**, 601–663.

STROMGREN, E. (1968) Contributions to psychiatric epidemiology and statistics. *Acta Jutlandica*, **40**, 1–86.

WITTCHEN, H. U., ROBINS, L. N., COTTLER, L. B., *et al* (1991) Cross-cultural feasibility, reliability and sources of variance of the Composite International Diagnostic Interview (CIDI). *British Journal of Psychiatry*, **159**, 645–653.

WIMMER, A. (1916) *Psykogene Sindssygdomsformer*. Copenhagen: Gads Vorlag.

WING, J. K., COOPER, J. E. & SARTORIUS, N. (1974) *The Measurement and Classification of Psychiatric Symptoms*. London: Cambridge University Press.

——, BABOR, T., BRUCHA, T., *et al* (1990) SCAN: Schedules for Clinical Assessment in Neuropsychiatry. *Archives of General Psychiatry*, **47**, 589–593.

WORLD HEALTH ORGANIZATION (1967) *Manual of the International Statistical Classification of Diseases, Injuries, and Causes of Death, 1965 revision* (8th edn) (ICD–8). Geneva: WHO.

—— (1978) *Mental Disorders: Glossary and Guide to their Classification in Accordance with the Ninth Revision of the International Classification of Diseases* (ICD–9). Geneva: WHO.

—— (1992) *The Tenth Revision of the International Classification of Diseases and Related Health Problems* (ICD–10). Geneva: WHO.

YAP, P. M. (1974) *Comparative Psychiatry: a Theoretical Framework*. Toronto: University of Toronto Press.

Section II. Treatment

4 General principles of assessment and investigation

R. SRINIVASA MURTHY

India, with a population of 890 million has only 20 000 mental hospital beds and about 5000 general psychiatric hospital beds. This is less than Holland, whose population is about 15 million. Until about two decades ago mental health care available to the population was either non-existent or only of the institution-based type.

The situation was similar in other developing countries. Since then, there have been dramatic advances in the understanding of the mental illnesses and their treatment. Specifically, the availability of the large number of drugs (neuroleptics, antidepressants, lithium) has made treatment a reality; the growing primary health care infrastructure in developing countries has raised both the awareness in the general public as well as the possibility of care in settings other than mental hospitals; the acknowledgement of the frequency and the morbidity of acute psychosis, schizophrenia, depression, and other mental disorders in developing countries has increased their importance in public health; and the World Health Organization (WHO) has given a big push to the development of appropriate models of care relevant to developing countries. As a reflection of this, a growing number of mental health programmes are being implemented (e.g. India, Pakistan, Iran, Egypt, Tanzania, Nepal, Yemen), with the main emphasis on decentralisation and integration of mental health care with primary health care.

Levels of care

The decentralisation "of mental health services implies that mental health care should be made available at the community, district, and regional levels through psychiatric in- and out-patient units linked to the general medical facilities. . . Integration of mental health care into the general health service means that the mental health component should be incorporated into the work of the primary health worker, the community health centre, district and regional health centres and hospitals." (WHO, 1975).

In this chapter, we shall consider assessment and investigation of patients with psychiatric disorders at each level of the decentralised service. Most of our description will be based on the Indian experience but it will be readily applicable to other developing countries. The Indian health care system is summarised in Table 4.1.

The village level

The health functionaries working at this level are non-physicians, providing mental health care as part of other general health care duties which could range from nutrition education, through conducting home deliveries, to dispensing a limited range of drugs for common ailments. Four types of assessment should be possible at this level:

(1) *Early identification of illnesses and referral.* This is the most important level. A number of simple tools are available to carry out this task, e.g. the questionnaire

TABLE 4.1
India's health care system

Level	Catchment area	Medical staff	Other staff	Mental health targets
Village/ sub-centre	500–3000	Nil	2 MPWs (2 health supervisors cover 4 village dispensaries)	Use MPW manual to: 1) manage psychiatric emergencies 2) maintain treatment initiated at higher level 3) diagnose and treat grand mal fits 4) liaise with teachers over children with conduct disorder 5) counsel patients with substance abuse 6) refer more serious cases
Primary health centre 2–10 general beds	30 000	2 general physicians	20–25 MPWs and nurses, including 1 health educator	Supervise MPWs Neurologically assess, diagnose and manage all psychiatric disorders using algorithms Treat acute confusional states Counsel for psychosocial problems Conduct epidemiological surveys Refer if necessary
District hospital 30–50 psychiatric beds	1–2 million	1 psychiatrist Other physicians	1 Community psychiatric nurse Possibly social worker Other non-psychiatric staff	Consultation to lower levels Treat severe, disturbance or life-threatening conditions ECT or high dose medication Refer
Teaching and other large hospitals	Regional centre	Psychiatric department	Range of support staff	Specialist care Occupational therapy Psychotherapy

MPW: multi-purpose health worker.

developed by Kapur & Isaac (1978), which comprises 15 simple questions and allows the health worker to identify severe mental disorders in patients and refer them for further help.

(2) *Severity.* The health worker should know whether emergency action has to be undertaken. The important symptoms to look for are: fever (measured with a thermometer); a history of fits; a high alcohol intake; and suicidal or homicidal intent. If any of these are present, the health worker should arrange for the patient to be seen immediately at the primary health centre or beyond.

(3) *Follow up.* Visits should be scheduled for patients maintained on treatment for psychosis, depression, epilepsy or neurotic problems. Multi-purpose workers should be trained to ask specific questions about the presence of giddiness, blurring of vision, dryness of mouth, excessive salivation or drowsiness, and to make a simple examination for extrapyramidal signs (rigid limbs, expressionless face, tremors of hands).

(4) *Psychosocial factors.* Health professionals at this level should be capable of assessing psychosocial factors by enquiring about stress, personality, family life, and social circumstances.

All of these assessments can be taught using available manuals and training programmes ranging from 1–2 days to one week.

The primary health centre/dispensary level

Patients seen at this level include patients who refer themselves, presenting in most cases with symptoms of depression or anxiety (Harding *et al*, 1980), and those referred from the village centres. Primary health centres should include facilities for physical examination, a thermometer, a sphygmomanometer, and a means of testing vision. Laboratory services required include simple investigations of blood, urine, sputum and stools so that anaemia, diabetes, infection including tuberculosis, and parasite infestation can be detected. Chest X-ray should also be available. Patients may need to be admitted for some of these tests to be performed or when a more detailed clinical assessment, with repeat assessment of level of consciousness and temperature is necessary. In persons with multiple somatic complaints the most relevant investigations are haemoglobin, stool for helminthiasis, visual acuity, blood pressure measurement and urine examination for diabetes. Drug-induced psychoses should also be assessed at this level. The common drugs to be checked for are chloroquine, anti-tuberculosis drugs, steroids, antihypertensives, and oral contraceptives.

More specialised investigations, e.g. electroencephalogram (EEG) or computerised axial tomography (CAT) scans are not usually available. However, this limitation can be overcome by taking a careful clinical history, and making use of a family member as an informant. In addition, a thorough physical examination and repeated assessment over a period of a few days may lead to a fuller understanding of the problems.

The district level

Usually, there is a psychiatrist at this level along with other specialists like physicians, paediatricians, gynaecologists and surgeons. The mental health team normally contains a psychiatric nurse, and in addition there may be a clinical psychologist or a psychiatric social worker. District hospitals normally have between 50 and 200 beds. In most, psychiatric patients are admitted to general wards along with patients with organic disorders. A wide variety of assessments and investigations are usually possible. However, sophisticated facilities such as EEG, CATscan, and blood culture may not be available.

Some patients may refer themselves to the district centre. Others will be referred from the physicians in the primary health centre and will include: persons with organic psychosis (e.g. typhoid encephalopathy), undiagnosed 'fits', psychosis related to head injury or alcohol intake, metabolic disorders with psychiatric problems (e.g. uraemia), and chronically mentally ill persons. The psychiatrist will have to use the following specific approaches to assessment: thorough clinical history and mental examination, the opinion of other medical, surgical specialists, physical investigations, psychosocial evaluation of the personality of the patient, the family situation, occupational history, and observation in the ward facility.

The specialist centre

The levels of care discussed above are all that are required by most patients, but a few may have to be referred onto the specialist centre. At this level there should be a full-fledged department of psychiatry with a multidisciplinary mental health team and sophisticated facilities for investigation. Assessment of the most complicated problems including personality disorders, marital problems, undifferentiated forms of psychoses, or organic mental disorders are all possible.

An important aspect of work at this level is consultation/liaison with other specialities. This aspect of mental health care requires a wide experience of medical problems presenting as mental disorders, the skill of communicating with the other specialists, counselling skills to deal with adjustment reactions or other emotional responses to myocardial infarction, surgery, childbirth, or the discovery of life-threatening or terminal illnesses. The psychiatrist at this level will have to involve and maximise the roles of other members of the mental health team. The availability of specialised investigations makes complete understanding of organic problems possible.

Evaluation of levels of care approach

Sakalawara Project: an evaluation of the primary level of health care

This project was initiated by the National Institute of Mental Health and Neuro Sciences, Bangalore (NIMHANS) in 1976 to develop feasible models of mental health care. It was carried out in 120 villages (75 000 people in total) in Karnataka State, around the Rural Mental Health Centre of NIMHANS at Sakalawara. A survey of the magnitude of mental health problems, existing pattern of utilising care, the burden of illness and the impact of a domiciliary care programme was undertaken in the rural population using a simple questionnaire for identifying priority conditions like psychosis and epilepsy.

Between 3 and 5% of the adult population of the village were interviewed and the results were cross-validated against other accepted methods of psychiatric care findings (Kapur & Isaac, 1978). This method was shown to be effective in identifying persons with psychosis, epilepsy and mental retardation.

The feasibility study showed that more than 90% of the psychotics and nearly 80% of the epileptics identified in the villages had been ill for more than two years at the time of detection, with varying degrees of disability in personal, social and vocational functioning. While nearly 100% of the identified patients had sought previous consultation with more than one traditional healer, only a few had sought help from the mental health care agency (NIHMANS) despite it being not very far away. Many people who had made contact with the mental health care agency had been lost to follow-up, and had suffered unremitting symptoms and secondary disability.

People with psychiatric disorders identified in the survey were offered treatment. It was found that a majority of those with psychosis and epilepsy could be adequately cared for in their home setting, that most were prescribed 5–6 drugs, and that only 4% required hospitalisation. The feasibility study also showed that improvement in identified patients served to motivate other ill people in the same village and nearby villages to get regular help.

This feasibility project led to the development of training programmes and manuals of instructions for primary centre health workers and doctors. The training strategy was field-tested at two primary health centres in Karnataka State following which regular training programmes in basic mental health care were developed and manuals of instructions for medical officers and multipurpose health workers were finalised.

The WHO collaborative study on strategies for extending mental health care (1975–81)

This study involved seven developing countries, namely Brazil, Colombia, Egypt, India, the Philippines, Senegal and Sudan. The Raipur Rani block in Haryana State, North India, was the Indian project area. The focus of this project was the evaluation of new community mental health services which involved the integration of mental health with general health services. Community mental health care within primary care services did not exist in any of the study areas before 1975. The research team at each centre designed, in collaboration with local health authorities, a set of interventions in response to local expressed needs for mental health care. These interventions were focused on priorities selected according to clearly defined criteria. The nature of the interventions varied according to the characteristics of each area. Systematic efforts were made to evaluate the impact of the interventions by comparing baseline observations with repeat observations made after 18 to 24 months of intervention.

Information on provision of care through a case register, regular data on drug use, referral of cases, evaluation of training programmes and descriptive accounts of community reactions were collected in each centre. The study area in India covered a total population of 60 000, with one primary health centre, one dispensary, and a few subcentres with four doctors and over a dozen health workers (Wig *et al*, 1981).

The reports of the project demonstrated that it was possible to define priority conditions; identify appropriate management for these conditions at primary care settings; and to enumerate tasks necessary for doctors, health workers and the community. In addition, training strategies for health personnel were developed and these training programmes led to appreciable changes in the attitude and knowledge of health staff. These changes included an increased recognition of the link between somatic symptoms and psychological problems, an increased awareness of the extent of mental health problems, and knowledge about correct indicators and dosages of certain essential psychotropic drugs. After training there was a considerable increase in the diagnostic sensitivity of the health workers with very little decrease in specificity. The primary health care personnel could also use a limited range of psychotropic drugs appropriately. Nearly four per thousand of the population started receiving care through the existing health facilities. The repeat 'key informant' attitude- studies showed a positive shift in community attitudes.

Though the data available from the project is limited, it did show that it was possible to deliver mental health care through general health services in several developing countries. Similar experiences have been reported from Tanzania, Guinea-Bissau, Pakistan, Nepal, Iran and many other developing countries (Schulsinger & Jablensky, 1991; Mubbashar *et al*, 1986; WHO, 1990*a*,*b*).

In India, larger population models covering one to two million people have been developed from the lower level pilot studies described here. The feasibility and the value of providing mental health care at different levels has been established, and the skill mix of staff required is becoming understood. With experience it can be expected that even more effective supervision, task definition, and training will enable more patients to be treated at lower levels of the health care system, ushering in a new era for mental health especially for the developing countries.

References

HARDING, T. W., DE ARANGO, M. V., BATTAZAR, J., *et al* (1980) Mental disorders in primary health care: a study of their frequency and diagnosis in four developing countries. *Psychological Medicine*, **10**, 231–241.

KAPUR, R. L. & ISAAC, M. (1978) An inexpensive method of detecting psychosis and epilepsy in the community. *Lancet*, ii, 1089.

MUBBASHAR, J. J. H., MALIK, S. J., ZAR, J. R., *et al* (1986) Community-based rural mental health care programme – report of an experiment in Pakistan. *EMR Health Services Journal*, 14–20.

SCHULSINGER, F. & JABLENSKY, A. (eds) (1971) The national mental health program in the United Republic of Tanzania. *Acta Psychiatrica Scandinavica Supplementum*, 364.

WORLD HEALTH ORGANIZATION (1975) Organisation of mental health services in developing countries. *Technical Report Series*, 564.

—— (1990*a*) *The Introduction of a Mental Health Component into Primary Health Care*. Geneva, Switzerland: WHO.

—— (1990*b*) A new era in mental health. Ch. 17. In *EMRO – Partner in Health in the Eastern Mediterranean 1949–1989*. pp 296–303. Alexandria, Egypt: WHO.

WIG, N. N., SRINIVASA MURTHY, R. & HARDING, T. S. (1981) A model for rural psychiatric services – Raipur Rani experience. *Indian Journal of Psychiatry*, **23**, 275–290.

5 Psychotherapy and traditional healing

DIGBY TANTAM

The epidemiology of emotional disorders in the developing world has been considered elsewhere in this book (Chapter 1). Emotional disorders – depression, psychosomatic disorders, anxiety and anxiety-related disorders – are no less common than in the developing world (see Table 5.1), and no less likely to lead to medical consultation, although the presentation may be of a physical rather than a psychological symptom. Psychotherapy is the treatment of choice in the developed world, either alone or in conjunction with psychotropic drugs. What about the developing world? Although traditional methods of treatment, which are to be found in every society, are often described as a form of psychotherapy, medical practitioners have made much less use of psychological methods of treatment in developing countries. It is sometimes assumed, erroneously in our view, that they are too time-consuming to be applicable to countries with an over-burdened health service, even though it is often just these countries who have shortages of imported goods, including psychotropic drugs, but have no shortage of human power.

In order to consider whether or not psychotherapy should be included in psychiatric services in developing countries, it is necessary to be clear about what it is, whether it works, how much it costs, and how to train people to use it. These questions cannot be answered completely satisfactorily for the developed world, let alone the developing world, but in the subsequent sections we shall consider what evidence is currently available. Most of it is relevant to the first question, i.e. what psychotherapy is.

What is psychotherapy?

A typical definition of psychotherapy would be that psychological treatment in which the relationship between the therapist and the patient is one of the main factors in improvement. The therapeutic relationship is also important in physical treatment, where it accounts for the placebo effect, and in social treatment, in which relief is provided through an increase in social provision or a reduction in social demand but also through 'support'. Much of what is attributed to 'mind' in Western psychology may also be attributed to the action of the 'soul' or 'spirit', to possession by other 'spirits', or to influence from others

57

TABLE 5.1
Emotional disorders in non-Western countries

Country	Prevalence		
	General population	Primary care	Psychiatric clinic
Botswana[1]	12.4% depression 11% panic disorder 12.9% anxiety		
Ethiopia[2]		<6.8% rural } unexplained <16.2% capital } somatic	
Kenya[3]		20% anxiety and depression 20.7% unclassified	
China[4]			17.2% major depression 17% other emotional disorders

1. Hollifield *et al* (1990).
2. Dormaar *et al* (1977).
3. Ndetei & Muhangi (1972).
4. Altschuler *et al* (1988).

by sorcery or magic. There is no consensus about how these different words are to be used, and we shall use the term 'psychological' in this section to include 'spiritual' and 'magical'. Not all traditional healing is 'spiritual' and therefore only some traditional healing is included in our definition of psychotherapy. Traditional herbal and dietary treatments are excluded, although the widespread internal or external use of decoctions of Koranic scriptures by those attending Islamic healers we consider to be psychological. We also consider abreaction with amylobarbitone or ether to be a psychological treatment since the medication is used to make a person more suggestible to the effects of a psychological treatment, not for any direct effect. Exorcism, which we consider a psychological treatment, may involve dancing or the use of incense smoke, and these may have a similarly disinhibiting metabolic effect.

The term 'treatment' is included in the definition to emphasise that psychotherapy is applicable to illnesses, and not just to life-problems or relationship strains. Psychotherapy has been successfully used in the treatment of florid psychotic symptoms (Kingdon & Turkington, 1991) as well as in the reduction of the burden on relatives of psychotic patients; in the reduction of fits in epileptic patients (see Chapter 11); in the treatment of sexual dysfunction; for anxiety-related disorders such as hysteria or obsessive–compulsive disorder; and for habit disorders such as anorexia, or substance abuse. However, its main indication is the treatment of anxiety, depression, or both, and in the treatment of psychosomatic disorders such as irritable bowel syndrome.

Schools of psychotherapy

Psychotherapy may be carried out in private conversations between two people (individual psychotherapy), in families, in 'stranger groups' which may be as small as five people or as large as 150, or in communities. In this section we will concentrate on individual psychotherapy since that is the type of therapy that fits most easily with a doctor's normal pattern of consultations. There are numerous techniques and schools of individual psychotherapy, and even more traditional healing techniques which might be termed psychotherapy.

Relationship orientated treatment: psychoanalysis and psychodynamic therapy

Freud posited a basic existential conflict between relationships with others and the satisfaction of personal desires, assumed to be self-seeking and appetitive. At some crucial phase of development, which Freud himself considered to occur at the Oedipal period at about 5 to 7 years of age, the conflict is internalised: one part of a person identifies with others, but other parts wish to control or destroy these others. Intrapyschic barriers are erected to exclude the appetites from consciousness, but if they fail, which they may for a variety of reasons, emotional disorder may result: anxiety or depressed mood reflect the internal damage and the content of the disorder is a symbolic transformation of the conflict itself.

Psychoanalysts consider that an important first step in treatment is diagnosis. Since patients are unconscious of their appetites, they cannot be asked about conflicts and so the conflict is inferred from an analysis of the links between the patient's utterances ('associations'). The next step is to explain to patients what desires and impulses they are in conflict with, and how these desires might be spilling out into symptoms. If the patient gains 'insight', the symptoms may be relieved but as conflicts are usually mirrored in ambivalence in current relationships, insights usually have to be worked through by changes in relationships. Relationship difficulties are particularly likely to arise with the psychotherapist, on whom are 'transferred' many conflicting feelings from past relationships. The third element of therapy is therefore the development of the therapeutic relationship. Since this takes some time to develop, psychoanalysis is normally a long-term treatment.

Psychoanalysts have described a number of 'defence mechanisms' by which people balance these internal conflicts, and have linked these mechanisms to symptoms. In Bond & Vaillant's (1986) empirical study, there was a loose, but statistically significant, relationship between psychoanalysts' descriptions of defence mechanisms and subsequent vulnerability to psychiatric disorder. It is not known whether the predictive validity is greater than other personality theories, including folk theories.

Psychoanalytic influence is apparent in almost every twentieth century theory of psychotherapy, including such well-known approaches as transactional analysis, and group psychotherapy. It has also attracted considerable philosophical and literary interest which, in recent years, has tended to be critical rather than supportive (see Grunbaum, 1986).

The typical intervention is interpretation: translating the hidden meaning of a symptom, dream, or utterance so as to link past and present, or one relationship with another.

Cognitive–behavioural therapy

Since Watson (1919), it has been known that anxiety could be transferred from normally fear evoking stimuli to normally innocuous stimuli, and that once transferred anxiety would continue to be evoked. Watson considered that this might account for adult psychiatric difficulties, but it was not until 1958 that methods of psychotherapy based on a reversal of the process and an inhibition of the fear response were described (Wolpe, 1958). Learnt fear can be reduced more simply (but less predictably) than Wolpe believed, by exposure to the feared stimulus under conditions in which anxiety can diminish rather than be enhanced. Enhancement results from avoidance and some of the defence mechanisms described by psychoanalysts, and is one of an increasing number of convergences between psychoanalysis and behavioural treatment.

Simple operational or classical conditioning paradigms are no longer considered adequate explanations of the genesis of emotional disorders. Emotional responses 'modelled' by significant others may also be learnt by imitation (Bandura, 1969) and cognitive appraisal is now given a much greater role in learning processes. Ellis (1962) and Beck (1976) have each developed a psychotherapeutic approach in which the therapist assumes that faulty learning of cognitive responses and strategies have taken place, and sets out to correct them. They treat thought as just another behaviour, albeit one that is very influential. People may think the way they do out of habit, and not because thinking that way is the most effective or the most true to the situation. 'Negative automatic thoughts', as Beck terms them, of this irrational kind are especially important in the genesis of depression, but may also lead to anticipatory anxiety which contributes to the faulty learnt behaviour associated with anxiety-related disorders.

Cognitive–behavioural therapy rests on the assumption that faulty learning of emotional responses or automatic thoughts persists without effective challenge by a person, but responds rapidly to challenge by the therapist. This would seem to suggest that the relationship with the therapist is itself of importance to the treatment, but the theory does not contain an account of this. This is obviously a weakness. The great strength of the theory is that it generates clear explanations which are consistent with common-sense psychology.

Typical interventions are to identify negative automatic thoughts or anxiety-sustaining habitual behaviours, determine counter-evidence or alternative behaviours, and practise the latter during exposure to triggers which would normally evoke the former.

Problem-solving therapy

Problem-solving techniques are a systematisation of common-sense approaches to difficulties with the addition, in the case of interpersonal therapy, of research findings about the importance of social relationships in providing support through adversity. Time is spent delineating the problem, which often results in a change in how the patient sees it. A common consequence is that patients see that they are in a predicament: whichever action they take to solve the problem, this has an undesirable consequence. The predicament may be of any kind, but very often involves a relationship with another person, and usually involves conflict with that person. In interpersonal therapy, the emphasis is always on relationships. Sometimes exposing the conflict is enough to enable resolution, but otherwise possible solutions need to be explored. Patients may be unable to find any satisfactory solution either because they have restricted the range of solutions that they are prepared to consider, or because they have assumed, often erroneously, that action on their part will lead to catastrophe. Patients may therefore either be unable to see any possible solution, or feel that to do anything would be worse than doing nothing. Masterful inactivity may be an effective coping strategy sometimes, but it has clearly failed when a patient begins to suffer an emotional disorder because of a failure to resolve a predicament.

The focus on interpersonal conflict in the problem-solving approach is obviously common ground with the psychoanalytic approach, and the restrictive assumptions that the patient makes about possible solutions is common ground with cognitive–behavioural therapy. Therapists who use a problem-solving approach may thus make use of psychoanalytic understanding and interventions at times, as well as cognitive therapy techniques. However, the approach to the patient is different from either of these. The patient is assumed not to be bound by unconscious forces, early traumas, habitual fears, or automatic thoughts, but able to choose courses of action.

Typical interventions are to have the patient set targets, identify strengths and resources, brainstorm possible solutions, list pros and cons, and rehearse possible outcomes, perhaps in role play with the therapist.

Traditional healing

The time spent on eliciting the patient's symptoms and their history seems to vary from healer to healer. Divination may be used, for example by automatic writing, or the patient's horoscope may be ascertained, but accounts of traditional healing (e.g. Kleinman, 1980) often stress the very limited time spent in diagnosis. In close-knit communities patients and their difficulties may already be known to the healer, but it seems likely that in many cases the healer knows little of his or her patient other than what can be observed at the consultation. The explanation of the patient's problems may also be quite brief and indeed the patient may have only short periods of attention from the healer. However, patients may remain in the healer's shrine or clinic for a considerable time, talking to other patients and to any attendants that the healer might have.

Traditional healing, like psychotherapy, covers many different schools and no single treatment is typical of all of them. In Islamic cultures, the first line of treatment is often to give the patient a scripture written in Arabic or Arabic-looking script written with a water-soluble ink. The patient washes the script into a container and either drinks it, anoints the affected part with it, or both. Often the treatment is reinforced by herbs, or religious exercises. More severe problems may be treated by exorcism.

The lack of emphasis on diagnosis or history, the rather perfunctory and stereotyped nature of the spirit explanation, and the complete lack of attention to the actions of the patient leading up to possession are all contrary to other psychotherapeutic methods. It seems likely that explanation plays a rather smaller role in traditional healing than it does in other forms of therapy.

Common features of psychotherapy

Research evidence suggests that the similarities of Western treatments are greater than their differences. Frank (1989) proposes that four elements are present in all psychotherapies (Table 5.2) and also underlie the placebo effect. The healing setting may be a clinic or a holy place; the rationale may be medical, psychological (e.g. that symptoms emanate from a region of the mind called the unconscious), spiritual (e.g. that they are due to the effects of djinns), or in any other terms which are credible to the patient; and the healing ritual ideally requires careful observance, generates some anxiety, and involves unaccustomed behaviour, for example lying on a couch while talking to an unseen person, or speaking in tongues. Frank's four factors can be applied to the developing world just as readily as to the developed world, with one proviso. 'Confiding' seems to be a less important activity in at least some developing world cultures than it does in the West. Indeed, clients may assume that really potent healers do not have to ask about personal details, but know them without being told (a similar assumption is made about fortune-tellers in developed countries).

The healing setting

A medical clinic or dispensary provides many of the features of a suitable environment for psychotherapy, but special attention may be required to ensure adequate time for the consultation, privacy where that is required, and a lack of interruption. Often these features can only be provided in a special clinic set aside for the purpose. Privacy is often considered to be a crucial feature of psychotherapy, but the boundary is drawn differently in different cultures. In individualistic cultures, patients may wish to discuss issues with the psychotherapist which would not be revealed easily even to a spouse or a close family member. In other cultures it may be more important to keep secrets within the marriage, the family, or the clan. It is rare for patients to consult traditional healers on their own, and consultations are often carried out in the presence of others. However, most healers report that their higher status consultations are carried out in private, and this would seem to be a desirable goal for all psychotherapy.

The rationale, conceptual scheme or myth

There are many hundreds of psychotherapy theories, but psychoanalysis is the one that has been most influential in the developed world (see Table 5.3 for some

TABLE 5.2
Non-specific factors in psychotherapy (after Frank, 1989)

Placebo and psychotherapy counteract demoralisation by:
1. a healing setting
2. a rationale, conceptual scheme or myth
3. a ritual
4. an emotionally charged confiding relationship with a helpful person

TABLE 5.3
Some psychoanalytic defence mechanisms with definitions

Repression: a barrier against an unconscious impulse or memory
Regression: actions reminiscent of an earlier developmental stage
Reaction-formation: action counter to an unconscious wish
Isolation: breaking the links between thoughts and feelings
Undoing: acting in opposition to a previous action to forestall its consequences
Projection: attribute characteristics of self to others
Introjection: attribute characteristics of others to self
Turning against the self: impulse towards other acted out upon self
Reversal: impulse turned into opposite, e.g. love into hate
Sublimation: using a required task or duty as a release of internal conflict
Idealisation: denial of disappointment by others
Identification with the aggressor: appropriating aggression against the self

definitions). Behavioural and more recently cognitive–behavioural approaches have been more rigorously evaluated, however, and are, arguably, more effective in the treatment of emotional disorders (Miller *et al*, 1989). Cognitive–behavioural therapy has the further advantage that it is readily applicable to short-term treatment. Effective short-term treatments have also been developed from the existential traditions, e.g. interpersonal therapy (Klerman *et al*, 1984) and counselling or problem-solving techniques (Hawton, 1989).

Traditional healers learn their skills through apprenticeship rather than formal training, and may be as much recognised as healers because they have lived with another healer, or even because they are a healer's kin, as because of any particular technique which they espouse. Psychological treatment techniques used in traditional healing are thus difficult to systematise, and there has been much less interest in formulating theoretical schools, although professional associations do exist in some countries. Perhaps the concept that comes closest to a universal theory of traditional psychotherapy is that physical and psychological disorders are caused by possession by spirits or ghosts.

The ritual

Perhaps because of the lack of emphasis on explanation, traditional healing makes much greater use of ritual than other psychotherapy procedures. However, therapeutic rituals are an inescapable component of all psychotherapy. Every treatment has its own: cognitive therapists use diaries of their patients' moods, psychoanalysts use a couch, groups develop their particular customs. The importance of ritual is proportional to the mysteriousness of the therapy, and to the social distance between patient and therapist. Problem solving therapists try to demystify and therefore eschew ritual.

An important function of ritual is to arouse feeling. This may be achieved by placing the patient at a disadvantage, as in treating the patient on the couch in psychoanalysis or by blindfolding the patient during an exorcism; by the sympathetic arousal of feeling by chanting or dancing; by reinforcing feeling using re-enactment or rehearsal; or by using various disinhibiting techniques. These include incense, fasting, activity, or alteration of consciousness. Experienced psychotherapists can modulate the effects of the ritual to maintain emotion at an optimal level. If the patient seems too emotionless, it is possible, for example in a verbal therapy, to have the patient relive an experience by getting more and more details or by asking the patient to visualise the scene again, or by role playing the scene with the patient. Speaking in the present, referring to the relationship with the patient, using the names of the people that the patient is speaking about are also techniques which increase immediacy and therefore the intensity of feeling. Matter-of-factness, unemotional clarification, and reminders that the situation has passed may have the opposite effect of lowering arousal in a distressed patient.

Disinhibition may be produced chemically, by incense or intoxication, by fasting, by sleep deprivation, or by hypnosis. Hypnotic states can be induced in many people by focusing attention so much on a specific stimulus that it is withdrawn ('dissociated') from the situation and a person gives the appearance of being unaware of his surroundings. People in this state are unusually susceptible to influence ('suggestible') and may be commanded to undertake actions, although these will not be carried out if the subject objects to them. Hypnotised subjects may be commanded to recall otherwise inaccessible memories or to carry out therapeutic procedures such as self-talk after waking. There is considerable argument about the value of hypnosis. There is no good evidence that recall is any more reliable under hypnosis than at other times and, anyway, remembering is not of value in itself. What matters is accepting memories. Nor is there any reason to suppose that post-hypnotic commands will be obeyed any more successfully than other injunctions.

An emotionally charged relationship with a helpful person

Relationships are made up of social interactions, and social interactions of interchanges. The skills required to heighten emotion during the development of a helpful therapeutic relationship are commonly termed 'micro-skills' and those required to manage social interactions so that both emotions and tasks are addressed, 'interview skills'. These are considered in the next section.

Skills required of the psychotherapist in the developing world

Micro-skills

Micro-skills are summarised in Table 5.4. Many of these skills are culture specific. Attending skills in the West include looking at the patient for much of the interview but in other cultures this might be interpreted as challenging or socially inappropriate. Questioning in medical practice is normally best achieved by a progression from open-ended questions, in which patients are encouraged to define a complaint, a situation, or a concern in their own words, to the doctor using more and more narrowly focused questions, including closed questions which have either the answer 'yes' or 'no', to spiral down onto an agreed statement.

Patients may be reluctant to reveal their feelings in an interview, particularly when the presenting complaint is somatic. Doctors must be prepared to unearth feeling, and this can often be done by picking up a verbal cue indicating feeling

TABLE 5.4
Micro-skills

Attending
look at the patient
look relaxed
tolerate silence
follow verbal cues
invitation to talk
encouragement to talk with feeling

Questioning
open questions
closed questions
spiralling down

Responding to cues
verbal responding
non-verbal responding

Paraphrasing and summarising

Clarifying

Intervening

('My pain was agonising') or picking up a non-verbal cue, such as a deep sigh or a tremor in the voice. Bringing emotional factors into the forefront of the interview, and 'reframing' the problem as one that has a significant emotional component, can be accomplished by paraphrasing the patient's complaints in different terms. Paraphrases also allow patients to confirm or modify the doctor's understanding of their difficulty. A paraphrase, or summary, of the whole interview is often a useful closing technique. Additional micro-skills which are useful in treatment include clarification ('Is this what you mean?') and some of the range of interventions which have been touched on previously.

Interviewing skills

Interchanges, or micro-skills, need to be incorporated into an orderly social interaction which enables a task to be achieved as well as the therapeutic relationship to be furthered. Research, albeit mainly conducted in Western medical settings, suggests that there is an optional sequence of steps, which are shown in Table 5.5. These are applicable to any therapeutic interview or series of interviews, not only those with a psychotherapeutic purpose. Violation of these steps may be undertaken deliberately to arouse anxiety, or create uncertainty in the patient, but there is little evidence that this serves a useful purpose.

TABLE 5.5
Interviewing skills

Introducing oneself, if necessary, and indicating one's own
    understanding of the purpose of the interview
Data gathering
Establishing the patient's concern
Responding to the patient's concern
Anticipating future concerns or difficulties

It is important for doctors to introduce themselves to patients, but it may also be necessary to introduce the nature of the interview ('I'd like to talk about what's causing the giddiness in your head') and, if appropriate that it is to be conducted in private. If the interview is not to be conducted in a language familiar to the patient or to the doctor mention needs to be made of this. Many doctors in the developing world may find themselves in this situation routinely, but if the language gap is too great – if, for example, an interpreter is needed – we think it unlikely that satisfactory psychotherapy can be carried out.

Data gathering requires the micro-skills of attending, questioning, responding to cues, and paraphrasing. It would normally result in a succinct statement of the patient's symptoms, but this may not be enough to establish why the patient is consulting the doctor, and therefore what treatment the patient is requesting. This may need to be elicited at a further step. Lazare *et al* (1975) have suggested that all new patients should be asked 'What were you hoping that I would be able to do for you?' to elicit their request.

Relationship skills and personal qualities

The use of micro-skills and interviewing skills increases the likelihood that a therapeutic relationship will develop with the patient, but does not ensure that it will. Other factors also come into play. Some of these are skills, others personal qualities. 'The first lesson that we learn at medical school is to listen to the patient' (Smith, 1993) and this is, arguably, the single most important relationship skill in medical settings where the clinician is the repository of the patient's fears and secrets. Listening is not like overhearing: the attention with which doctors listen influences what they are told. Effective listening involves enabling patients to express half-baked theories, disturbing feelings, crazy ideas, therapeutic nihilism, antisocial comments, erotic thoughts, or criticism of doctors, their creed, or their beliefs. Any of these may be preferable to more socially compliant behaviour if this is adopted only to please the doctor. Listening to the patient's real thoughts and feelings requires the clinician to be able to empathise with the patient. On the basis of a literature review, Squier (1990) suggests that an empathic relationship between doctor and patient increases the potential of the consultation for relieving the patient's anxiety, increases patient satisfaction, and increases the patient's adherence to the treatment. Squier considers that empathy has two components: to think as if one was the other person, and to feel as if one was the other person (Table 5.6).

TABLE 5.6
Empathy (after Squier, 1990)

Components	Measures	Associated personal qualities
Taking other's perspective	Empathy Scale (Hogan, 1969)	Socially perceptive, likeable, good communicator, interpersonally effective, socially mature
Experiencing other's feelings	Questionnaire Measure of Emotional Empathy (Mehrabian & Epstein, 1972)	Emotional, easily aroused, socially interested, interested in helping others, volunteers to help others in distress

Empathic understanding may become more difficult when patients have been seen over a long period with little improvement; when patients are unable to give a clear account of their difficulties; when they have either negative or erotic feelings about the doctor or the process of treatment; when they re-evoke emotionally-charged memories by the doctor; or when the subject of the consultation is not clearly defined. Since all of these factors may apply to psychological treatment, particularly when it is long-term and relationship-focused, training in empathy is considered especially important for clinicians undertaking this work. A personal experience of being a patient in psychotherapy is often thought to be the best type of training.

Among the relationship skills that are associated with better outcome in psychotherapy, Beutler *et al* (1986) list a facilitative attitude which involves patients as collaborators: trustworthiness, expertise, and expectation of success. Facilitative attitudes include acceptance and tolerance of the patient's negative feelings. Collaboration requires that the patient is treated courteously, and that the obligations and ties that the patient has outwith the treatment are respected. Sue (1981) considers that trustworthiness is especially important in cross-cultural counselling, and that it includes "sincerity, openness, honesty, and perceived lack of motivation for personal gain". Trustworthiness requires that therapists adhere to accepted ethical guidelines. They should make regular appointments, stick to them and not be unexpectedly late or absent, and should meet the patient in an appropriate place. Therapists must also keep the details of the therapy confidential although taking care to keep appropriate records, must not normally contact others about the patient without the patient's agreement, and must maintain a professional attitude which means having no social or sexual contact with patients.

Possibly the most important factor after effective listening is an avoidance of coerciveness. The status of doctors can all too easily be abused. This might involve only imposing one's opinions or values on patients, but even this may be enough to impair the professional relationship. Much more serious exploitation does occur, and can be inadvertent. Patients must not be exploited financially. Therapists must be sufficiently aware of their own emotional responses to ensure that they do not exploit the patient emotionally either. Regular case discussions with peers or with a supervisor are desirable whenever a clinician is treating patients psychotherapeutically on a regular basis, in order to guard against this eventuality. Psychotherapists treating patients from unfamiliar cultures may need to have additional training to ensure that they are sensitive to that culture's traditions, and to any negative discrimination that members of that culture may experience.

Specific interventions

Schulsinger & Jablensky (1991) include three non-drug interventions in the five treatments that they consider appropriate for first (medical assistant) and second (psychiatric nurse, clinical medical officer) echelon mental health workers in Tanzania. These are environmental manipulation, which they consider especially appropriate for hysteria; interpersonal counselling, particularly for anxiety states; and problem solving "drawing heavily on the existing regulating mechanisms of the traditional community".

Psychiatrists or other specialists working in tertiary referral centres are likely to see patients with more entrenched problems or patients who are able to seek out more specialist treatment and who are more likely to expect verbally-oriented psychotherapy. There will be less opportunity to involve family members or influential community members in the treatment, or to pursue long-term treatment even if the clinician has the time to undertake it.

Kleinman (1980) suggests that effective treatments in psychiatry need to be assimilable into the explanatory model used by the patient. Psychotherapy has largely developed within Western explanatory models and, although there is an obvious potential for a merger with other traditions, this has not yet happened. Table 5.7 lists three Western explanatory models, each of which will apply to different patients or problems, but which will collectively be sufficient for most problems. The relationship model is closest to the explanatory model of spiritual possession: traditional healers often attribute possession to a failure of familial or spiritual duty, or to witchcraft by a disgruntled or envious neighbour or family member; relationship theorists ascribe emotional disorder to feelings like guilt, envy, or rivalry which arise in these interpersonal situations. In directive psychotherapy, clinicians use their authority to assuage anxiety or guilt. In the traditional setting, the healer also focuses on relieving the burden of the patient's bad spirit. Patients who do not respond to the directive approach are often at a turning point in their lives, and cannot choose which way to go. The psychotherapy sessions can become a protected, conflict- free domain in which the patient can rehearse action without suffering its consequences. Time spent in the healer's compound, and even the time spent travelling to it, may serve a similar function by giving time for reflection and rehearsal. It is possible that these similarities might make a relationship, or psychodynamic, approach more understandable to a patient with a traditional explanatory model than a purer cognitive or behavioural explanation.

Evaluation of psychotherapy: does it work?

There is very little evidence on this point from the developing world. In the developed world, meta-analyses of a mixed bag of psychotherapeutic approaches suggest that the average effect of psychotherapy is to reduce symptoms by about one standard deviation more than the spontaneous change of symptoms in the control group. This compares to an effect size of 1.3 for behavioural treatment of agoraphobia, an effect size of 1.1 for drug treatment of agoraphobia, and an effect size of 0.4 to 0.8 for the drug treatment of depression (all preceding figures in this paragraph are from Lambert *et al*, 1986). Elkin *et al*

TABLE 5.7
Three ways of tackling emotional disorder

1. Linking symptoms to a relationship problem, and resolving this by *direction* or *focal therapy*
2. Linking symptoms to habitual anxiety, and *unlearning* this using behavioural methods
3. Linking symptoms to negative thinking, and *confronting* this by cognitive or problem solving methods

(1989) found that the effect size of psychotherapy was lower than that of antidepressants in their sample of depressed patients, and that interpersonal psychotherapy was more effective than cognitive therapy in treatment.

Most of the principles considered in this chapter have not been specific to a particular psychotherapeutic approach and can better be considered to be elements in 'good clinical management'. The effect size of good clinical management is, perhaps surprisingly, of a similar order to that of brief psychotherapy and Andrews (1993) has commended the approach that has also been adopted in this chapter: systematic investigation, leading to specific training interventions.

There is no doubt that doctors differ in their ability to detect and manage psychiatric problems and a convincing amount of evidence (see below, Training) that training increases these skills. In the developed world where patients are seen as a first line by expensively trained medical practitioners, it makes sense to divert patients with emotional disorders to see a less expensive professional for treatment. Corney (1990) has reviewed the literature, and suggests that counsellors who may have no core professional skills are no more effective than the general practitioner for emotional disorders in general, but are more effective for postnatal depression. Professionals with behaviour therapy training are also more effective in the treatment of phobias and habit disorders, and those with cognitive therapy training accelerate the resolution of depression over standard general practitioner care. Catalan *et al* (1991) have also shown that the problem-solving approach is effective in general practice in the treatment of a mixed group of patients with anxiety-related disorders.

It is not clear how these results would apply to developing countries. Few evaluations of traditional healing have been carried out, but Whyte (1991) interviewed 170 Tanzanian families with a mentally disordered member about their treatment experience and found that traditional healing was the most expensive form of treatment and that it involved the greatest travelling. Only 19% of families said that it had benefited the disordered person 'more than a bit'. The comparable figure for hospitals and dispensaries was, however, only 24% and the outcome of traditional healing may have been better if more families of people with emotional disorders had been included.

It seems unlikely that an additional cadre of psychotherapists can be provided in the developing world, except in the most specialised centres. However, it does not appear that the complacent attitude that traditional healers do all that psychotherapists and counsellors do in the developed world is justified either.

The main thrust of a psychotherapy development should be to increase the detection, interviewing, and psychological management skills of the primary clinician.

Cost-effectiveness of psychotherapy

Detection of depression has been shown to accelerate recovery in general practice, and simple counselling can also reduce the use of psychotropic medication although with a slight, but manageable, increase in the duration of sessions with the doctor. Patients are more satisfied following consultations with more empathetic doctors, but it is not known whether this is likely to result in less need for consultations.

An indirect effect of psychotherapy training may be to reduce anxiety in response to patients. Doctors high on sympathetic anxiety have been shown to make more errors in decisions, to undertake invasive procedures for longer, and to order more investigations. Although the consequences of this have not been evaluated, it seems likely that there is a significant cost and that this would apply to a developing world setting.

Cost-evaluation of psychotherapy is in its infancy, but some offset studies have been performed which suggest that psychotherapy provision can reduce treatment costs, particularly the costs of physical treatment (McGrath & Lowson, 1987). This is likely to be an important consideration in the developing world where treatment resources are at a premium.

Training

The micro-skills and the interviewing skills described are common to many therapeutic methods and successful training programmes have been based on them. Training in their application to psychiatric interviews (Lieberman *et al*, 1989), psychotherapy interviews by the 'conversational method' (Goldberg *et al*, 1984), and first interviews by general practitioners (Gask *et al*, 1989) have all been shown to be effective. Gask *et al* concentrate on 'Feeling understood', 'Changing the agenda' and 'Making the link' and have demonstrated that they can be taught to general practitioner trainees and applied by them to interviews with patients with somatised psychiatric disorders.

Gask *et al*'s model is based on the 'microcounselling' method pioneered by Ivey (1971), in which the therapist's contribution is broken down into component 'macro-skills', each of which can be separately taught. Ivey has made 'attending behaviour' the initial element in the training of first interviewers (Table 5.4) and identified its micro-skills which can be 'taught in a few hours', and have been used in psychiatry training (Lieberman *et al*, 1989). Courses based on this have been given throughout the world and have been found to be of use specifically in a cross-cultural setting (Pedersen, 1985).

Kagan (1980) has pioneered methods of training in interpersonal sensitivity (one component of empathy) using videotapes of therapist–patient interactions to trigger a more accurate, retrospective account by therapists of their emotional responses to the patient, a process known as Interpersonal Process Recall. Kagan has also used brief videotaped sequences of 'interpersonal nightmares' enacted as if spoken by the patient to the viewer, as therapist.

Training in developing countries may be restricted by the availability of trainers. The World Health Organization is now making available instructional videotapes for use by, and slanted towards, clinical and medical officers in developing countries. The tapes feature experts from the developing world and one has been produced on psychotherapy (Chandrashekar & Tantam, 1993).

Playback of video recordings of actual patient interviews followed by peer discussion is probably the single most important factor in any interview training. However, this method is too unwieldy and intrusive to be of use in relationship training or supervision. Review of audio tapes or even process notes in conjunction with supervision, which may be with peers, is the preferred training method for training in longer-term treatment methods.

References

ANDREWS, G. (1993) Essential psychotherapies. *British Journal of Psychiatry*, **162**, 447–451.

ALTSCHULER, L. L., XIDA, W., HAIQING, Q., *et al* (1988) Who seeks mental health care in China? Diagnoses of Chinese outpatients according to DSM–III criteria and the Chinese classification system. *American Journal of Psychiatry*, **145**, 872–875.

BANDURA, A. (1969) *Principles of Behavior Modification*. New York: Holt, Rinehart & Winston.

BECK, A. T. (1976) *Cognitive Therapy and the Emotional Disorders*. New York: International Universities Press.

BEUTLER, L., CRAGO, M. & ARIZMENDI, T. (1986) Research on therapist variables in psychotherapy. In *Handbook of Psychotherapy and Behaviour Change*, 3rd edn (eds S. Garfield & A. Bergin). New York: John Wiley.

BOND, M. P. & VAILLANT, J. S. (1986) An empirical study of the relationship between diagnosis and defense style. *Archives of General Psychiatry*, **43**, 285–288.

CATALAN, J., GATH, D., ANASTASIADES, P., *et al* (1991) Evaluation of a brief psychological treatment for emotional disorders in primary care. *Psychological Medicine*, **21**, 1013–1018.

CHANDRASHEKAR, C. & TANTAM, D. (1993) *Psychological Treatment of Emotional Disorders. An Instructional Videotape for Medical Officers in Developing Countries*. Universities of Manchester and Warwick and World Health Organization.

CORNEY, R. (1990) Counselling in general practice – does it work? *Journal of the Royal Society of Medicine*, **83**, 253–257.

DORMAAR, M., GIEL, R. & VAN LUJIK, J. N. (1977) Psychiatric illness in two contrasting Ethiopian outpatient populations. *Social Psychiatry*, **9**, 155–161.

ELKIN, I., SHEA, T., WATKINS, J. T., *et al* (1989) National Institute of Mental Health Treatment of Depression Collaborative Research Program: general effectiveness of treatments. *Archives of General Psychiatry*, **46**, 971–982.

ELLIS, A. (1962) *Reason and Emotion in Psychotherapy*. New York: Stuart Press.

FRANK, J. D. (1989) The views of a psychotherapist. In *Non-specific Aspects of Treatment* (eds M. Shepherd & N. Sartorius). Bern: Huber.

GASK, L., GOLDBERG, D., PORTER, R., *et al* (1989) The treatment of somatization: evaluation of a teaching package with general practice trainees. *Journal of Psychosomatic Research*, **33**, 697–703.

GOLDBERG, D., HOBSON, R., MAGUIRE, G., *et al* (1984) The clarification and assessment of a method of psychotherapy. *British Journal of Psychiatry*, **144**, 567–580.

GRUNBAUM, A. (1986) Precis of 'The Foundations of Psychoanalysis: A Philosophical Critique'. *Behavioral and Brain Science*, **9**, 217–228.

HAWTON, K. (1989) Problem solving. In *Cognitive Therapy of Emotional Disorders* (eds P. Salkovkis, K. Hawton & D. Clark). Oxford: Oxford University Press.

HOGAN, R. (1969) Development of an empathy scale. *Journal of Consulting and Clinical Psychology*, **33**, 307–316.

HOLLIFIELD, M., KATON, W., SPAIN, D., *et al* (1990) Anxiety and depression in a village in Lesotho, Africa: a comparison with the United States. *British Journal of Psychiatry*, **156**, 343–350.

IVEY, A. (1971) *Microcounselling: Innovations in Interviewing Training*. Springfield, Illinois: Charles C. Thomas.

KAGAN, N. (1980) Influencing human interaction – eighteen years with IPR. In *Psychotherapy Supervision: Theory, Research, and Practice*. New York: John Wiley.

KINGDON, D. & TURKINGTON, D. (1991) The use of cognitive behavior therapy with normalizing rationale in schizophrenia – preliminary report. *Journal of Nervous and Mental Disease*, **179**, 207–211.

KLEINMAN, A. (1980) *Patients and Healers in the Context of Culture*. Berkeley: University of California Press.

KLERMAN, G., WEISSMAN, M., ROUNSAVILLE, B., *et al* (1984) *Interpersonal Psychotherapy of Depression*. New York: Basic Books.

LAMBERT, M., SHAPIRO, D. & BERGIN, A. (1986) The effectiveness of psychotherapy. In *Handbook of Psychotherapy and Behaviour Change* (eds S. Garfield & A. Bergin). New York: John Wiley.

LAZARE, A., EISENTHAL, S. & WASSERMAN, L. (1975) The customer approach to patienthood: attending to patient requests in a walk-in clinic. *Archives of General Psychiatry,* **32,** 553–558.

LIEBERMAN, S., COBB, J. & JACKSON, C. H. (1989) Studying the 'Grammar of Psychotherapy' course using a student and a control population. Some results, trends and disappointments. *British Journal of Psychiatry,* **155,** 842–845.

MCGRATH, G. & LOWSON, K. (1987) Assessing the benefits of psychotherapy: The economic approach. *British Journal of Psychiatry,* **150,** 65–71.

MEHRABIAN, A. & EPSTEIN, N. (1972) A measure of emotional empathy. *Journal of Personality,* **40,** 525–543.

MILLER, I. W., NORMAN, W. H. & KEITNER, G. I. (1989) Cognitive–behavioral treatment of depressed inpatients: six- and twelve-month follow-ups. *American Journal of Psychiatry,* **146,** 1274–1279.

NDETEI, D. & MUHANGI, J. (1972) The prevalence and clinical presentation of psychiatric illness in a rural setting in Kenya. *British Journal of Psychiatry,* **135,** 269–272.

PEDERSEN, P. (ed.) (1985) *Handbook of Cross-Cultural Counselling and Therapy.* New York: Praeger.

SCHULSINGER, F. & JABLENSKY, A. (1991) Essential methodology and technology of mental health care provision. *Acta Psychiatrica Scandinavica,* Suppl. 364, 16–41.

SMITH, R. (1993) Editorial: On not listening to patients. *British Medical Journal,* **306,** 410–411.

SQUIER, R. W. (1990) A model of empathic understanding and adherence to treatment regimens in practitioner–patient relationships. *Social Sciences and Medicine,* **30,** 325–339.

SUE, D. W. (1981) *Counselling the Culturally Different: Theory and Practice.* New York: John Wiley.

WATSON, J. B. (1919) *Psychology from the Standpoint of a Behaviourist.* Philadelphia: Lippincott.

WHYTE, S. (1991) Family experiences with mental health problems in Tanzania. *Acta Psychiatrica Scandinavica,* Suppl. 364, 77–111.

WOLPE, J. (1958) *Psychotherapy by Reciprocal Inhibition.* Palo Alto: Stanford University Press.

6 Physical treatment in psychiatry

ALICE DUNCAN

6.1 Electroconvulsive therapy

Electroconvulsive therapy (ECT) is the treatment by seizure induced by the passage of a small amount of electricity to the brain.

ECT remains a controversial treatment in public and medical circles; at an international level, the anti-ECT lobby has in some places succeeded in outlawing its use. However, if the number of patients receiving ECT has declined since the mid-1950s, this is mainly due to the major pharmacological breakthrough following the introduction of antidepressant drugs (see section 6.2 of this chapter).

ECT presents in two forms: the first is unmodified, or 'straight' ECT and is administered without the use of anaesthetics or muscle relaxants. It can cause major problems such as the patient's marked discomfort and distress, and fractures from the seizure's motor activity.

The second method, modified ECT, makes use of anaesthetics and muscle relaxants, thus reducing the risks of physical complications to those of the anaesthetic procedure. The most widely used muscle relaxant today is succinylcholine.

Modified ECT is the only currently acceptable method in developed countries, but unmodified ECT is still used in some developing countries. Reports from Nigeria, for example, suggest that ECT is still extensively used for all forms of functional psychosis (Ihezue, 1983; Odejide *et al*, 1987). However some developing countries, for example Jamaica in the West Indies, have significantly reduced the use of ECT. According to Hickling (1988) 60% of the admissions to the island's only psychiatric hospital were treated with ECT in 1969, compared to only 7% in 1979, and none by 1980.

Indications

ECT should be used in conditions where there are psychiatric, medical, social or humanitarian reasons for seeking rapid improvement of symptoms; where the risks of other treatments outweigh the risk of ECT and where there has been a good ECT response in previous episodes of the illness.

Depression

The most common clinical indication for ECT in developed and developing countries is severe depression. The Royal College of Psychiatrists (1995) has concluded that ECT procedure is an effective treatment in severe depressive illness. Kaplan & Sadock (1988), reported that over 80% of patients treated with ECT in the United States of America have a diagnosis of depression, with a response rate of 80–90%.

In depression, the strongest indications for ECT are an immediate to high risk of suicide, a significantly increased risk of physical harm to the patient's health because of refusal to eat and drink, or general self-neglect with increased risk of dehydration and infections. There are no specific tests at present to predict the outcome of treatment in depression, but certain symptoms are good indicators of a likely response to ECT. These include features of melancholia or biological symptoms (e.g. diurnal variation in mood; early morning wakening; loss of appetite, weight and libido; psychomotor retardation or extreme agitation; depressive delusions; hopelessness and accompanying depressive affect of doom). Also likely to respond to ECT are depressive illnesses presenting with obsessional, anxious or hypochondriacal complaints in someone not usually prone to this. ECT acts more quickly than antidepressants.

Mania

The use of ECT in the treatment of mania has been much less studied than in depressive disorders or schizophrenia. It may have some short-term therapeutic advantages and may be a reasonable alternative to lithium, but neuroleptic medication will also be required (Small *et al*, 1986). Clinical experience has also shown that ECT may be effective in acutely disturbed manic patients who have failed to respond to large doses of psychotropic drugs.

Schizophrenia

A number of studies have shown that ECT may have a place in the treatment of schizophrenia as an adjunct to neuroleptic medication. However, there is no conclusive evidence that ECT alone is an effective treatment for schizophrenia. Clinical experience has shown that ECT produces rapid and dramatic changes in acute catatonic schizophrenia, but that it is ineffective in mainly negative symptoms, defect state schiozphrenia. ECT is more likely to be used in the treatment of schizophrenia in developing rather than in developed countries.

Other psychiatric disorders

Clinical experience has shown that ECT is effective in other psychiatric disorders related to those already mentioned. These include schizophreniform and schizoaffective disorders, atypical psychosis and puerperal psychosis.

Puerperal psychosis deserves special mention as there is wide clinical experience attesting to the effectiveness of ECT treatment in this disorder; in comparison to drug treatment, it ensures a quicker return of the mother to her infant and is not a contra-indication to breast-feeding. These are significant advantages of ECT, especially in developing countries.

There are isolated reports of beneficial effects in the 'on/off' phenomenon of Parkinson's disease, and in resistant petit mal epilepsy when the frequency of attacks may be reduced. ECT may also be effective in the management of severe organic affective and psychotic conditions, in catatonia secondary to medical conditions, in hypopituitarism and in neuroleptic malignant syndrome.

Contraindications and other related issues

Raised intracranial pressure is always a contraindication to ECT. Conditions that are likely to be made worse by changes in blood pressure, cardiac rhythm or raised intracranial pressure which occur at the time of seizure even in a well modified fit, substantially increase the risks of complications. These include space-occupying cerebral lesions, cerebral aneurysm, recent intracerebral haemorrhage, retinal detachment, phaeochromocytoma, recent myocardial infarction (within three months) with unstable cardiac function, and aortic aneurysm. Other relative contraindications include any medical illness that would significantly increase the anaesthetic risk of the procedure such as severe respiratory infections. Extra care should be taken in patients who have sickle cell disease or insulin-dependent diabetes. However, in certain circumstances ECT might be safer than drug treatment, for example, in all three trimesters of pregnancy (in consultation with the obstetrician), in the elderly and the medically ill. ECT can also be given safely to patients with cardiac pacemakers and a history of epilepsy.

Mechanisms of action and physiological aspects of ECT

The mechanisms of action of ECT are still unknown. Some physiological changes occur during ECT which have implications in at risk patients. If ECT is given without anticholinergic premedication such as atropine, the pulse slows initially and then rises rapidly to up to 190 beats a minute, falling to the original baseline resting rate or below towards the end of the seizure, followed by a less marked tachycardia lasting several minutes. There are corresponding changes in blood pressure when no muscle relaxant is given. Significant hypoxia occurs during ECT with a fall of greater than 5% in oxygen saturation, but this is unlikely to be hazardous, unless associated with myocardial ischaemia or vomiting (Swindells & Simpson, 1987).

Types of stimuli

The first ECT machines produced sine waves in biphasic sinusoidal wave forms and delivered high energy. These machines produced effective clinical response but also marked adverse side-effects such as cognitive impairment. ECT machines manufactured in the last decade deliver brief, high voltage pulses in streams lasting 1.5 to 6 seconds. Brief pulse waves are more efficient stimuli than sine waves and deliver less electrical energy to the brain, with reduced risks of adverse side-effects.

Unilateral versus bilateral ECT

Bilateral ECT is the delivery of the electric current through electrodes placed on opposite sides of the head. The anatomical location is the mid point of each electrode placed approximately 4 cm above the midpoint of a line extending from the tragus of the ear to the external canthus of the eye (Fig. 6.1.1a).

Unilateral ECT is the delivery of the electrical current through an electrode on one side of the head, usually the nondominant cerebral hemisphere. The first electrode is placed in the standard position of 4 cm above the mid-line point between the tragus and canthus, and the second on an arc approximately 18 cm from the first in an ipsilateral position to the vertex (Fig. 6.1.1b). Handedness is a useful guide to cerebral dominance. It may be determined by a series of simple performance tasks, such as asking about the stated preference, which hand is used

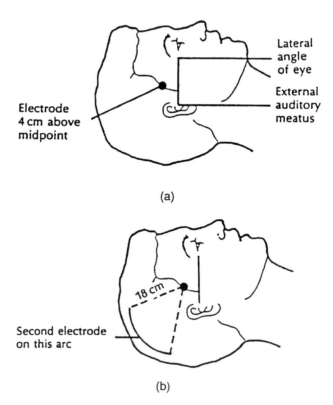

(a)

(b)

Fig 6.1.1. Diagram of electrode positions

to catch and throw and which foot to kick. Right body responses correlate very highly with left brain dominance.

Much debate continues about the relative efficacy of unilateral and bilateral ECT. In most developing countries the bilateral method is used almost exclusively.

Studies published have shown greater advantages for bilateral ECT. These results are summarised by Abrams (1986). The evidence would seem to be that a greater proportion of depressed patients receiving bilateral ECT improve, that the percentage improvement is larger and that fewer treatments are required for melancholic patients (Abrams *et al*, 1983).

However, the choice is not a simple one. Many patients do respond to unilateral ECT.

Guidelines and some ethical considerations on ECT treatment

ECT has been tainted by a historical association with political and medical abuse, and the potential for its misuse remains. In a prospective analysis of symptom complex for ECT treatment in a Nigerian hospital, Sijuwala (1985) raised concerns that ECT was being used for staff's convenience. Anecdotal reports suggest that unprofessional practises of this kind are fairly widespread and not uncommon in developed countries. It could be argued that some level of international monitoring of ECT is warranted. This would probably be most appropriately supervised at the level of the Mental Health Division in the World Health Organization (WHO) with regional monitoring.

Each country should develop within their mental health departments clear guidelines relating to all aspects of ECT, including the minimal acceptable standard of practice. Guidelines should include consent issues, pretreatment evaluation, conditions of the treatment itself, aftercare management, and research work with access to independent ethical committees. Once drawn up, it is equally important that they are implemented and adhered to in local treatment facilities. Appropriate monitoring systems to ensure that procedures are being adhered to and standards being kept should be developed in parallel.

Guidelines on the requirement for consent to ECT are necessary, and are particularly important where formal mental health legislations do not exist and the patient is refusing to consent, or deemed incapable of giving consent to treatment. Important issues to be addressed may include when and by whom should consent be obtained, and the nature and amount of information to be provided. Readers are referred to the guidelines published by the Royal College of Psychiatrists (1995) on this issue.

Morbidity, complications and side-effects

Deaths associated with ECT are very rare, both in developing and developed countries. Most deaths associated with ECT are usually secondary to cardiovascular complications in the setting of previous cardiovascular disease.

Major immediate complications of ECT are also rare; most are associated with unmodified ECT. They include:

1. Cardiovascular: cardiac arrhythmias, myocardial infarction and congestive cardiac failure.
2. Respiratory: pulmonary embolism, aspiration pneumonia and prolonged apnoea.
3. Central nervous system: cerebro-vascular accident and prolonged seizures leading to status epilepticus.
4. Bleeding from peptic ulcers, subconjunctival or nasal haemorrhages. Rupture of the bladder.
5. Orthopaedic: spinal mid-thoracic fractures, fractures of long bones, jaw dislocations and fat embolism secondary to long bone fractures (rarely seen these days).

Orthopaedic complications are virtually never seen; prolonged seizures lasting for more than three minutes or status epilepticus are rare; epilepsy occurring after ECT is also rare, but occasionally tardive grand mal seizures have been reported. Odejide *et al* (1987) reported that despite the use of mainly unmodified ECT in Nigeria since 1952, there have been no reports of tardive seizures, and that the complications linked to this method were relatively few.

Headaches, nausea, vertigo and confusion are common complaints reported after the use of ECT and may last for a few hours after treatment. Complaints of muscle aches and pain usually result from the muscle relaxant.

There is a complex interaction between depression, cognitive impairment and ECT. Temporary memory impairment almost always occurs during a course of ECT treatment, but follow-up data indicate that virtually all cases are back to their previous level of functioning within six months. Short-term retrograde amnesia, that is amnesia for events before the treatment, often occurs and may stretch back for days or weeks. Bilateral ECT is associated with long-term retrograde amnesia, affecting mainly personal memory stores. There is no definite evidence that ECT causes permanent anterograde amnesia, which is impaired retention of information acquired soon after ECT treatment. A study of former patients who complained of permanent memory impairment from previous ECT found that these patients did worse than controls on some memory tests, but they were also found to have residual depressive symptoms, which might have accounted for the memory problems (Freeman *et al*, 1980). In general, when used normally, ECT is unlikely to be followed by permanent memory damage.

Consent to ECT treatment

Informed consent should be obtained from every patient able to give it. This includes the signing of a formal consent document by the patient and the prescribing doctor. New consent should be sought if there is a break of more than three weeks in the series of treatments, and at least every six months in the case of maintenance ECT. The signed form is evidence that consent has been sought, but not of the validity of consent. It could be challenged on the grounds of the patient's competence at the time the form was signed, or that inadequate information had been provided.

In the USA, the consent document is comprehensive and covers nearly all the medico-legal eventualities which may arise because of fears of litigation. In the United Kingdom and most other countries, the document is much less extensive. Except for a minor (child), who is considered incapable of giving informed consent, no relative may consent to the treatment of another person. However, it is good clinical practice when possible to gain the cooperation of relatives or close friends in decisions about ECT treatment. The patient should be informed that such approaches are being made, and if possible be present at the discussion. This is particularly important in patients receiving ECT treatment for the first time when both the patient and family are often apprehensive. Such a discussion would provide the opportunity to allay anxieties and clear up any misconceptions about the treatment with the prescribing doctor.

In situations where relatives and friends are not available, it is advisable to discuss the treatment with the patient in the presence of another member of staff with whom the patient has developed a good therapeutic relationship. In most conditions for which ECT treatment is indicated, the severity and nature of the illness may impair the patient's concentration and retention of information. Many patients find it reassuring to discuss and clarify explanations given by their doctor in a more informal way with nursing staff and their relatives.

Non-consenters to ECT treatment

Patients who do not consent to ECT include those who lack the capacity to give consent and are deemed incapable, those who consent but are deemed incapable and those considered capable who withhold consent. The American Psychiatric Association Task Force on ECT (1990) operationally defines the capacity to provide consent as being able to: 1) comprehend the nature and seriousness of the treatment is being offered; 2) understand the information provided concerning the treatment; and 3) form a rational response based upon the information.

In normal circumstances most patients who lack the capacity to consent include those requiring ECT on a fairly urgent basis to prevent death or serious deterioration in health. When a patient refuses to consent or is thought to be incapable of giving consent to ECT, the procedure followed varies according to national and state governed mental health legislations, and where legislations do not exist according to locally acceptable standards. In the USA, the use of involuntary ECT is now rare: in Alabama state hospitals for example, no less than three specialists and five other medical staff members are required to approve ECT treatment for a non-consenting patient.

In the UK, when ECT is considered essential in a non-consenting patient, the first step is to decide whether there are grounds for invoking the appropriate section of the mental health legislation to establish that the patient is mentally ill and in need of treatment. The opinion of a second consultant psychiatrist appointed by the Mental Health Act Commission is also required. He or she will consult with non-medical members of staff as well as the patient's relatives or next of kin. Merskey (1990), in discussing the ethical aspects of physical manipulation of the brain, argues that the agreement of the nearest relative is not only essential on legal grounds as in some legislations, but also on ethical grounds. He states that "If those who are likely to be most concerned for the patient cannot also approve the treatment there should be doubts as to its justification. The physician should also be satisfied that even if he has the support of the patient's family, that support is given out of love and not as may happen out of antagonism".

In some developing countries the treating psychiatrist may override a patient's lack of consent without any other consultation. There are several reasons for this. Many developing countries do not have enough psychiatrists to provide second opinions, and where they might be available there are no formal requirements to do so.

Also, doctors in general have a more powerful, authoritative and unchallengeable role in developing countries, in comparison to developed countries. Such unquestioned authority, especially in big public mental hospitals with large numbers of involuntary patients, has to be critically weighed against the other extremes in some developed countries, where formal requirements are unduly clinically restrictive, and arguably inappropriately give significant powers of decision-making to people with no medical training or background. However, in many developing countries, nurses and relatives play very active roles in discussions leading up to the prescription of ECT.

Basic equipment and supplies for ECT

Equipment should be available to induce seizure, monitor physiological response, maintain an airway, deliver positive pressure ventilation and provide resuscitation in case of cardiovascular or respiratory difficulties. The American Psychiatric Association Task Force on ECT (1990) has recommended a list for the treatment area, recovery area and the important medications, which can be adapted for local use, to which the reader is referred.

Before a new ECT machine is used, the instruction manual should be carefully read. The machine should be tested and calibrated by local qualified personnel, with documentation of the test results kept for future comparison. Retesting and servicing should be carried out as recommended and malfunctioning machines should not be used until repaired. The ECT equipment should be connected to the same electrical supply circuit as all other electrical devices in contact with the patient. A designated member of the ECT team should regularly check and document all equipment and supplies to ensure that they are functioning, and replaced when used.

Training, needs and future recommendations

Over the past 50 years, the extent of knowledge and skills required to provide safe and acceptable ECT has grown considerably. The old training dictum of 'see one, do one, teach one', no longer applies and a much more comprehensive, educational and training experience is required. Psychiatric training in medical and nursing schools should address the role of ECT in contemporary psychiatry.

ECT is a practical procedure which must be learnt by apprenticeship as well as by reading and application of the knowledge. Recent reports from developed countries suggest that ECT training is inadequate and at times seriously lacking (Pippard, 1992; APA Task Force on ECT, 1990), and there is no evidence to suggest that the situation is better in developing countries. All trainee psychiatrists should have the opportunity to watch a number of treatments *in vivo*, have time to familiarise themselves with ECT machines, and be supervised by a designated trainer before they are allowed to carry out unsupervised treatment.

6.2 Drugs in psychiatry

Psychotropic drugs affect normal and abnormal psychological processes through their action on the brain. The first reference in Western literature to a psychotropic substance is found in the Bible "Noah began to be a husbandman and he planted a vineyard . . . drank of the wine and was drunken . . .". The history of psychiatry as a medical speciality and the use of psychotropics in the treatment of mental illness is comparatively much shorter. It was not until the second half of the twentieth century, following the introduction of chlorpromazine, that drug treatment became a major area of practice and research in mental illness.

Prior to the 1950s most psychotropic substances were naturally occurring and mainly used for recreational purposes. However, the root of the plant *Rauwolfia serpentina*, containing reserpine, has been recommended for psychiatric disturbances for over 3000 years in Indian textbooks. In the 1950s, reserpine became one of the first new psychotropic drugs. In most developing and some developed countries, herbal medicine still plays a major role in the management of medical and psychiatric problems. In China for example, herbal medicine is used by doctors alongside conventional drugs, while in Africa and India herbal medicines are also used extensively, but mainly by traditional healers.

Classification

The World Health Organization (WHO) suggests the following classification of drugs which affect mainly mental symptoms:

1. *Antipsychotics*: control and exert therapeutic effects on the psychotic symptoms in schizophrenia, mania and organic conditions. They have a major calming effect and are also called major tranquillisers and neuroleptics. They frequently produce Parkinsonian-like extrapyramidal side-effects.
2. *Antidepressants*: are effective in the treatment of pathological depressed mood states, and do not normally affect the mood of healthy people.
3. *Anxiolytic/anti-anxiety/hypnotic drugs*: reduce anxiety, tension and agitation. They also have a calming effect and are sometimes called minor tranquillisers. In large doses they produce drowsiness, acting as sedatives while in higher doses they promote sleep, acting as hypnotics.

4. *Psychostimulants*: act as stimulants to increase the level of alertness and motivation. They usually affect the mood of healthy people.
5. *Psychodysleptics*: produce abnormal mental phenomena, and affect cognition and perception in particular.

Two other groups of drugs not mentioned in the WHO classification are:

6. *Anti-Parkinsonian drugs*: commonly used to control the side-effects of the antipsychotics.
7. *Mood stabilisers*: a heterogenous group which includes the anticonvulsants, carbamazepine and sodium valproate, and lithium salts.

Psychodysleptics have no place in contemporary psychiatric practice and psychostimulants have such limited application that they will not be discussed further.

Even with the addition of the above two drugs to the WHO classification, not all the drugs currently used in psychiatry fit into this scheme.

Absorption

Most psychotropic drugs are weak bases. They are mainly absorbed from the alkaline medium of the jejunum when taken orally, and are absorbed faster when the stomach is empty. Many psychotropic drugs, especially those with anticholinergic activity, delay gastric emptying, which in turn delays their own absorption as well as that of other drugs taken simultaneously.

The intramuscular parenteral route is commonly used in psychiatry for rapid onset of action, and for slow release depot injections. During emotional excitement, such as in agitated and overactive patients, the blood flow through muscles may increase up to ten-fold, favouring rapid absorption. The intravenous route is rarely, if ever, indicated in general psychiatric practice and could be hazardous.

Distribution

Most psychotropic drugs are reversibly bound to plasma proteins which affects their distribution. Psychotropic drugs pass easily from the plasma to the brain and fat tissues, and also transplacentally to the foetal circulation during pregnancy. There are important implications of plasma binding. A change in the concentration of plasma proteins, particularly hypoproteinaemic states, can lead to a higher level of unbound drugs in the plasma unless the dose is lowered. In some developing countries, malnutrition and hypoproteinaemia may be a problem in children and adults. Bound psychotropic drugs can be displaced from binding sites by other drugs given simultaneously, which also increases the level of unbound drug in the plasma. In the treatment of overdose, dialysis is least useful in highly bound drugs because the free concentration is low.

Metabolism

Most psychotropic drugs are metabolised in the liver and oxidation is the commonest form of metabolism. A wide variety of reactions are catalysed by the liver microsomal enzymes, including hydroxylation, dealkylation and sulph-oxide formation. The monoamine oxidases (MAOs) are mitochondrial enzymes that oxidate a range of substances, but are not a part of the typical liver microsomal enzymes.

When psychotropic drugs are taken orally, metabolism begins in the gut walls and in the liver before reaching the general circulation, in the so-called 'first pass' metabolism, and individuals vary in their capacity for such a metabolism. For example, up to 75% of chlorpromazine and more than 90% of fluphenazine are metabolised in the 'first pass' when administered orally. The implication is that some patients may benefit from a switch of an oral to a depot administration of these drugs.

Some drugs work by inhibiting metabolism. For example, disulfiram inhibits aldehyde dehydrogenase which causes the accumulation of acetaldehyde after the ingestion of alcohol, while the monoamine oxidase inhibitors (MAOIs) irre-versibly inhibit the MAOs and the drug effects wear off only when new enzymes have been synthesised.

Some psychotropic drugs are known to induce their own metabolism by increasing the synthesis of microsomal metabolising enzymes, which can result in up to 50% reduction in plasma concentrations of the drugs. Some of these drugs include chlorpromazine, imipramine, phenobarbitone (barbiturates), phenytoin and carbamazepine.

Excretion

Most psychotropic drugs or their metabolites are excreted in the urine. Normally urine is slightly acid, which favours the excretion of weakly basic drugs such as amphetamines and tricyclic antidepressants. Psychotropic drugs can also be excreted in the enterohepatic cycle, which is via the liver into the bile, from where they can be reabsorbed from the intestine.

Psychotropic blood levels

For most psychotropic drugs there is no close temporal relationship between plasma concentration and therapeutic effect. Therefore, measuring blood levels is not clinically useful, except for lithium, to avoid toxic levels and clozapine because of the risk of fatal agranulocytosis.

Clinical guidelines

In 1906, Cabot remarked "We educate our patients and their friends to believe that every or almost every symptom and disease can be benefited by a drug, some ignorant practitioners believe this". Developed countries have been described as over-medicated societies where drugs are promoted to deal with all the distresses of living. In the United States and England, 10% of the population take some form of psychotropic medication each day. In developing countries, people are more likely to seek alternative traditional help.

Good clinical psychopharmacology practice requires diagnostic and psycho-logical management skills as well as the ability to plan a drug therapeutic regime

Pharmacodynamics: describes the effects of the drug on the body.

Therapeutic index: a relative measure of a drug's toxicity and safety, which is defined as the ratio of the median toxic dose (TD 50), to the median effective dose (ED 50). Lithium salts have a low therapeutic index, whereas most antipsychotic drugs have a high therapeutic index.

Tolerance: the phenomenon of becoming less responsive to a particular drug as it is administered over time; it is usually associated with physical dependence.

Physical dependence: the need to continue administering a drug in order to prevent the appearance of withdrawal symptoms. Most psychotropic drugs do not produce physical dependence, except the hypnotics, anxiolytics and amphetamines. However, many psychotropics take several days to weeks to produce their therapeutic effect, and there is usually a comparable delay after discontinuation before the effects are reduced.

and to manage available drugs. The psychiatrist should become familiar with two to three drugs from each of the main groups, so that adjusting dosage and recognising side-effects become easier. The goal of drug treatment should be established in terms of target symptoms and length of time that the drug needs to be administered, and there should be a short-term and long-term treatment plan.

After choosing an appropriate drug, it should be prescribed in adequate dose and for long enough on the basis of the type of drug and the particular disorder being treated. A drug should not be changed or others added without good reason, as one recognised obstacle to a patient's compliance and adequate dose increase is intolerable side-effects.

Drug combinations have little value in current psychiatric practice because the flexibility of adjusting the dose of the individual drugs when prescribed separately is lost. However, sometimes there are good reasons to combine individual drugs from different groups, for example adding lithium to antidepressants or to antipsychotics to augment the therapeutic response.

The dose of drug for a given patient should be decided after consideration of severity of symptoms, age, body size, and factors which might affect drug metabolism, such as concurrent medication and poor physical health.

In the oral form, many psychotropic drugs are given three times a day, but most have a long enough half-life to be taken once or twice a day, especially after acute symptoms have subsided. Most patients respond adequately to the recommended dose ranges such as those in the *British National Formulary* (BNF; British Medical Association and the Royal Pharmaceutical Society of Great Britain, 1996). Depot injections should be given once monthly when possible, but some patients may require more frequent administration in the acute phase of the illness.

Patient education

Before patients are given their first drug prescription they should be informed of their diagnosis, the symptoms that the drug should reduce and the time it will take to produce a therapeutic effect, possible side-effects, and the length of time they might need to be on the drug. It is important that a family member or close friend is present when this information is given, to ensure that the patient gets the necessary support.

Patients and their relatives usually have ambivalent attitudes to drug treatment. Some fear that taking drugs means that they are not in control of their lives, that they are being used for experiments and that they may have to take them forever. The psychiatrist should attempt to give a clear, honest and simple explanation of the facts appropriate to the patient's level of education. The time spent in discussing these concerns is often well spent and enhances the therapeutic relationship. In some situations, it is appropriate to give patients and their family increasing responsibility for adjusting the dose of their medication as treatment progresses.

Prescribing for special groups

Most of the core psychiatric disorders such as schizophrenia and affective disorders first present in early adulthood. Children only rarely need to be prescribed psychotropic drugs. They have a higher metabolic rate than adults and may require a higher ratio of milligrams of drug per kilogram body weight. However, in practice it is best to begin with a small dose and to increase until clinical effects are observed.

The elderly tend to be more susceptible to adverse side-effects, drug metabolism may be slowed down and they are often taking other drugs. It is best to start with approximately one-half of the average adult dose and slowly increase it, observing for clinical as well as adverse effects.

In pregnancy the basic rule is to avoid administering any drug, particularly during the first trimester of pregnancy. The two most teratogenic psychotropic drugs are lithium and the anticonvulsants. Lithium taken during pregnancy is associated with a higher incidence of foetal abnormalities, such as Ebstein's abnormalities of the cardiovascular system. Lithium, and if necessary other psychotropics used should be discontinued in patients who become pregnant.

When a patient who becomes pregnant is already receiving a psychotropic drug other than lithium for an established mental illness, the risk of relapse must be weighed against the possible teratogenic effects of the drug. Ideally, a full discussion of the risk factors associated with pregnancy should take place with any female of childbearing age who is on long-term psychotropic medication, and should include reliable methods of contraception.

Antipsychotics

The main indication for antipsychotic drugs is in the treatment of schizophrenia. They are also effective in controlling psychotic symptoms associated with other disorders such as in alleviating anxiety symptoms; calming and sedating patients with toxic delirium, agitated depression, acute behavioural disturbances; treating vomiting and vertigo, and to potentiate the effects of analgesics. The antipsychotic benperidol is used in the treatment of deviant antisocial behaviour, although its value has not been established.

Classification

Antipsychotic drugs can be grouped into eight classes (Fig. 6.2.2):

1. *Phenothiazines*: this group is characterised by a three-ringed phenothiazine nucleus with different side chains attached to the nitrogen atom in the middle ring, which leads to three further sub-groupings:

    Group 1: the aliphatic compounds, such as chlorpromazine (Largactil/ Thorazine) have marked sedative effects with moderate antimuscarinic and extrapyramidal side-effects.

    Group 2: the piperidines are characterised by moderate sedative effects, marked antimuscarinic effects, but fewer extrapyramidal side-effects than either of the other two groups; an example is thioridazine (Melleril).

    Group 3: the piperazines include trifluoperazine (Stelazine) and fluphenazine (Prolixen and Moditen). They are sedative with fewer antimuscarinic effects but more pronounced extrapyramidal side-effects than the first two groups. Drugs from the other chemical classes tend to resemble group 3 phenothiazines.

2. *Thioxanthenes*: these also have a three-ringed nucleus. Examples include flupenthixol (Fluanxol and Depixol) and zuclopenthixol (Clopixol).

3. *Butyrophenones and butylpiperidines*: these drugs are related chemically to the analgesic pethidine. Haloperidol (Serenace, Haldol) and oxypertine (Intergrin) are two examples from this group; they are prone to causing extrapyramidal side-effects. Although chemically quite distinct from phenothiazines, their therapeutic effects are similar, but some patients may do better with one drug than another.

4. *Diphenylbutylpiperidines*: this class is somewhat similar in structure to the butyrophenones. In comparison to other antipsychotics, they have a longer half-life. Pimozide (Orap) and fluspirilene (Redeptin) are examples from this group.

5. *Dihydroindoles*: oxypertine is an example from this group. It is said to produce less weight gain than other antipsychotics.

6. *Dibenzodiazepines and dibenzoxazepines*: these compounds are based on a modification of the three-ringed phenothiazine nucleus and include drugs such as clozapine (Clozaril) and loxapine (Loxapac). Clozapine is presently only indicated in treatment-resistant schizophrenia and is being closely monitored by the manufacturer. It may produce fewer neurological side-effects, but can produce fatal agranulocytosis.

7. *Atypical antipsychotics*: the true atypical neuroleptics will, by definition, lack extrapyramidal side-effects, which not all do at present (Hale, 1993). Sulpiride (Dolmatil and Sulpitil), remoxipride hydrochloride (Roxiam) and risperidone (Risperdal) are examples of the new antipsychotics which

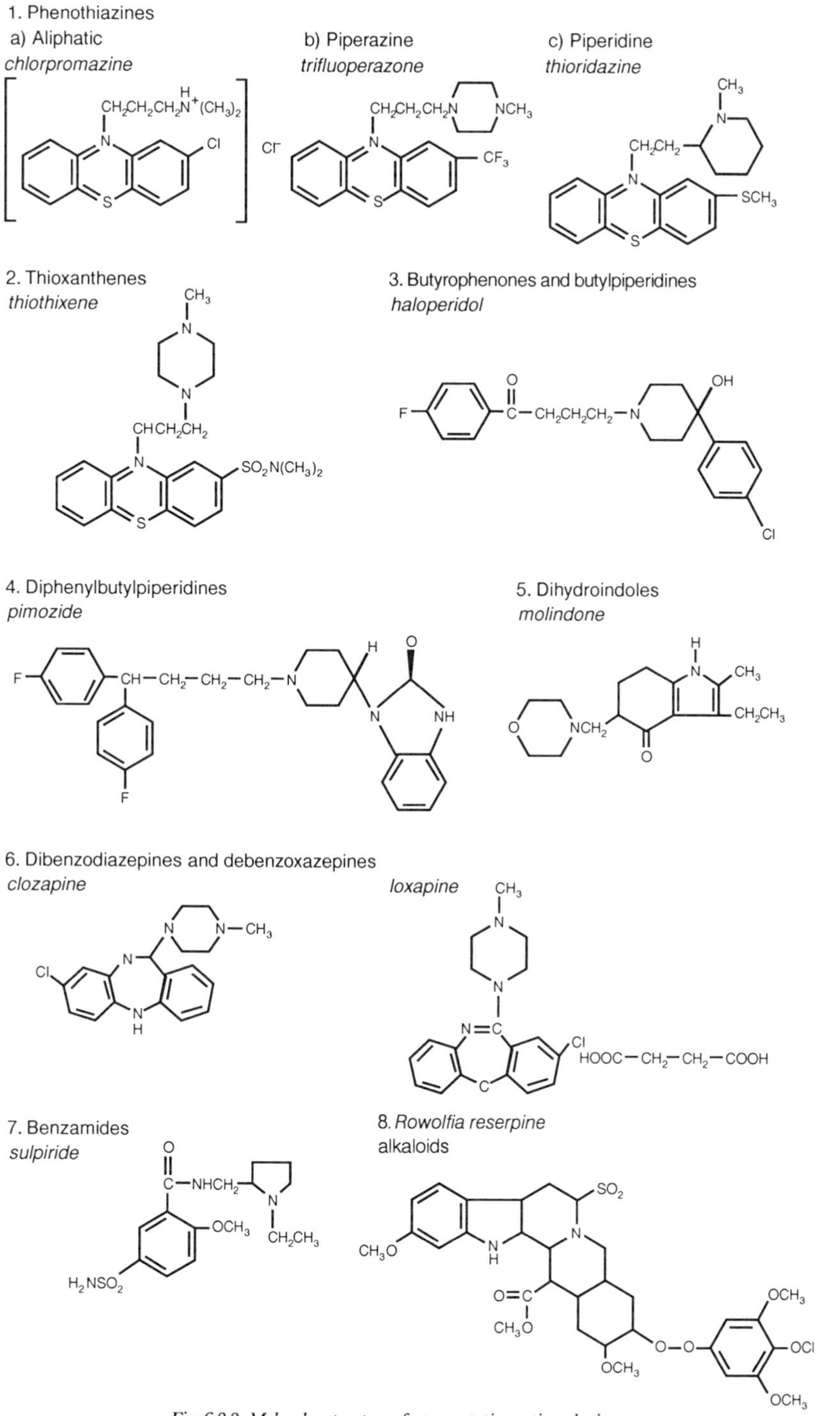
1. Phenothiazines
a) Aliphatic
chlorpromazine
b) Piperazine
trifluoperazone
c) Piperidine
thioridazine
2. Thioxanthenes
thiothixene
3. Butyrophenones and butylpiperidines
haloperidol
4. Diphenylbutylpiperidines
pimozide
5. Dihydroindoles
molindone
6. Dibenzodiazepines and debenzoxazepines
clozapine
loxapine
HOOC—CH2—CH2—COOH
7. Benzamides
sulpiride
8. Rowolfia reserpine
alkaloids

Fig. 6.2.2. Molecular structure of representative antipsychotics.

currently are only available in oral form. They are structurally distinct from other antipsychotics. Risperidone is the newest of the three and was launched in 1993. Sulpiride and risperidone are said to be effective against both the positive and negative symptoms of schizophrenia, while all three are reported to have a low level of extrapyramidal and sedative side-effects. The manufacturers of two other newly developed atypical neuroleptics, raclopride and sertindole are developing depot forms of these drugs.

8. *Rauwolfia alkaloids*: reserpine is the classical example from this group and mentioned because of its historical importance. It is no longer used as an antipsychotic because of its adverse side-effects.

Choice of antipsychotics

There is no significant difference in the clinical efficacy of currently available antipsychotics. Selection should depend primarily on the degree of sedation required, the patient's susceptibility to side-effects, and in developing countries the cost and availability of the drugs. When sedation is required, chlorpromazine is recommended, and when sedation is undesirable, trifluoperazine or haloperidol are recommended. Thioridazine and promazine are frequently prescribed for the elderly because of their more tolerable side-effects. A reasonable starting daily dose for a psychotic adult patient would be 300–400 mg of chlorpromazine orally, or 15–20 mg of haloperidol orally or intramuscularly, in divided doses.

Depot antipsychotics

The introduction of depot antipsychotics has arguably been described as a major advance in the treatment of schizophrenia. Non-compliance with antipsychotic treatment is an obstacle to the success of community care for patients with mental illness such as schizophrenia, and many psychiatrists believe that depot preparations still hold the key to compliance (Hale, 1993). Depot preparations are cheap and widely available in developed and developing countries. Table 6.2.1 shows the approximate equivalent doses of some commonly prescribed depot antipsychotics.

Administration is by deep intramuscular injection usually in the gluteal, thigh or deltoid muscles. A test dose should be given first and the patient observed for a few days for undesirable reactions. In general, the test dose is about a half of the minimum therapeutic dose shown in Table 6.2.1. Most depot preparations come in an oily medium, and no more than 2–3 ml should be administered at any one site. Fluspirilene (Redeptin) comes in an aqueous suspension and is usually prescribed weekly in a maintenance dose of 2–8 mg because of its shorter duration of action.

It has been suggested that depot injections may give rise to a higher incidence of extrapyramidal side-effects and tardive dyskinesia than oral preparations. Johnson (1990), however, noted that whichever route of administration is used the same drug molecules reach the brain, and because antipsychotics are readily stored in fatty tissues creating secondary depot, after several weeks on oral medication they cease to be truly short acting and can remain in the body

TABLE 6.2.1
Equivalent doses of depot antipsychotics

Antipsychotic	Dose (mg)	Interval
Fluphenazine decanoate (Modecate)	25	2 weeks
Fluphenazine enanthate (Moditen)	25	2 weeks
Flupenthixol decanoate (Depixol)	40	2 weeks
Haloperidol decanoate (Haldol)	100	4 weeks
Zuclopenthixol decanoate (Clopixol)	200	2 weeks

for months after oral use is discontinued. Depot antipsychotics such as fluphenazine are controversially associated with depression in schizophrenia, but the aetiology of depression in schizophrenia is complex. Zuclopenthixol depots are said to be useful in agitated and aggressive patients, whereas flupenthixol can cause over-excitement in such patients. Common though not serious effects of depot injections include pain, erythema, swelling and nodule formation at the site of administration.

Acute and maintenance treatment

Undoubtedly antipsychotics have become a mainstay of the acute treatment of schizophrenia since they were first used in the 1950s. Experience shows that they are effective in damping down acute disturbance associated with florid symptoms and in abbreviating episodic exacerbations of florid symptoms. However, some psychiatrists remain doubtful (Bleuler, 1978; Ciompi, 1980*a,b*) whether the use of maintenance treatment alters the final outcome of the illness, whereas most will agree that their use has reduced the risk of relapse into florid illness and of rehospitalisation.

In maintenance treatment the reduction in the risk of relapse has to be set against the side-effects of prolonged treatment such as tardive dyskinesia, which has been called the 'most important public health problem of the decade' (Gardos & Cole, 1980). However, there are no criteria available to predict which patients will not require prolonged antipsychotics. In addition, antipsychotics can only be expected to play a limited role in the treatment of schizophrenia. Preliminary WHO (1979) studies suggest that the prognosis of schizophrenia is better in developing countries, which might reflect the complex roles of such variables as expressed emotion, social support, cultural attitudes and levels of tolerance to mental illness. Tantam & McGrath (1989) have done a critical review of the prolonged use of antipsychotics in schizophrenia and offered some useful suggestions to which the reader is referred. As a general guideline, drug treatment following a first acute episode of schizophrenia may be continued for 1 to 2 years, and in chronic cases for at least five years.

Oral v. depot antipsychotic drugs in maintenance treatment

The main advantage of oral medication is its greater flexibility because of shorter duration of action, but this may become less important after long-term administration for reasons mentioned previously. The disadvantages are increased risks of poor compliance and the potential for misuse. Depot antipsychotics provide a more predictable and consistent blood level of drugs as initial biotransformation processes in the gut and liver are bypassed. They may reduce defaulting from treatment because patient monitoring is easier and may be more cost-effective as they reduce the frequency of hospital readmissions. In many developing countries the main psychiatric hospitals are usually centralised and not readily accessible to patients in rural areas. Depot antipsychotics may also provide the opportunity for consistent regular supportive input by local mental health workers.

Pharmacokinetics

The pharmacokinetics of the antipsychotics vary considerably. For example, the first pass metabolism of chlorpromazine is about 75% whereas haloperidol is negligible; also, the non-aliphatic phenothiazines and butyrophenones have very few metabolites whereas chlorpromazine has over 75. They have a half-life range of 10–20 hours.

Pharmacodynamics

The potency of antipsychotic drugs is said to be closely correlated with their affinity for dopamine receptors. Most of the neurological and endocrinological side-effects arise from dopamine receptor blockade. They also differentially block noradrenergic, cholinergic and histaminergic receptors. Patients tend to develop tolerance to most of the side-effects, but not to the antipsychotic effect.

Side-effects

The unwanted effects of antipsychotic drugs can be divided into neurological and non-neurological. Low potency drugs such as chlorpromazine tend to cause more non-neurological side-effects, whereas high potency drugs such as haloperidol tend to cause more neurological ones.

Extrapyramidal symptoms

These can be divided into groups: acute dystonia, akathisia and Parkinson's syndrome. Symptoms occur usually within a few days to weeks of starting treatment. They are dose dependent and usually disappear when the drug is discontinued. Tardive dyskinesia occurs later, does not always recover when the drug is stopped and may even get worse. Extrapyramidal symptoms occur in up to 40% of patients treated with antipsychotics.

Acute dystonia

Acute dystonia presents as involuntary contraction of skeletal muscles. The clinical presentation can be bizarre. Characteristic features include protrusions and twisting movements of the tongue; grimacing; spasmodic torticollis of the neck; oculogyri crisis in which there is an initial fixed stare followed by a turning upwards of the eye; trismus and grotesque writhing and posturing involving the whole body. The attack may last several hours or fluctuate before subsiding spontaneously. It is particularly common in young men and often quite distressing. It usually appears within the first two days of treatment and is most often seen with the butyrophenones and piperazine compounds. The treatment is an anti-Parkinsonian drug such as benztropine (Cogentin) 1–2 mg intramuscularly or intravenously, repeating the dose if necessary, or diazepam 10 mg intravenously.

Parkinson's syndrome (pseudo-Parkinsonism)

The clinical picture resembles idiopathic Parkinsonism and even more Parkinsonian symptoms following encephalitis. The main features include stiffness of the limbs, coarse tremors of the hands and feet at rest, rigidity, stooped posture, drooling of saliva, and a mask-like expressionless face. The symptoms are commoner in older women, often take weeks to a few months to appear after the drug is started, and sometimes diminish even though the dose has not been reduced.

The symptoms respond to anti-Parkinsonian drugs, but unlike idiopathic Parkinsonism not to L-dopa, which may exacerbate the psychosis. The antipsychotic drug should be discontinued for a few days, or the dose sharply reduced. Most patients will not deteriorate if the antipsychotic is temporarily discontinued. An anti-Parkinsonian drug should also be given. These include benzhexol (Artane) 2–4 mg; procyclidine (Kemadrin) 5–10 mg; orphenadrine (Dissipal) 50–100 mg; benztropine (Cogentin) 1–2 mg and biperiden (Akineton) 2 mg in single adult doses. They can be given up to three times daily if necessary. However, they should be withdrawn after about 4–6 weeks to assess whether the patient has developed tolerance to the Parkinsonian side-effects and if further treatment is indicated. Approximately 50% of patients will need to continue the treatment. Parkinsonian symptoms may last up to two weeks after the antipsychotic is completely withdrawn, and up to three months in the elderly. In such cases the anti-Parkinsonian drug should be continued until the symptoms subside. Routine administration of anti-Parkinsonian drugs is not recommended except as a precaution against acute dystonia in a young person who has not previously received antipsychotics. Their anticholinergic effects may add to those of the antipsychotics and be implicated in the pathogenesis of tardive dyskinesia. Benzhexol is sometimes misused because of its euphoric effects.

Akathisia

This is an inner feeling of unpleasant agitation and inability to tolerate inactivity, presenting as restlessness and relentless pacing. Milder cases may present as a subjective feeling of restlessness confined to the legs. Akathisia is probably underdiagnosed as the symptoms are usually attributed to a worsening of the psychosis or lack of cooperation. It may appear at any time during treatment, but usually starts within the first two weeks. The acute form usually improves with a reduction in the dose of medication, but not the occasional late form which sometimes co-exists with tardive dyskinesia. Propranolol and the benzodiazepines have been shown in some studies to be effective.

Tardive dyskinesia

The syndrome consists of abnormal, irregular, involuntary choreoathetoid movement of muscles of the head, limbs and trunk. The symptoms range from minimal, often missed by patients and their family, to grossly incapacitating ones. The most common sub-type is the 'bucco-linguo-masticatory' (BLM) syndrome. BLM symptoms range from infrequent lateral jaw movements with puckering and pouting of the lips and slight tongue movements which distend the cheeks, to a presentation dominated by unceasing movements of the lower face, associated with mouth opening and protrusion of the tongue. Other sub-types may present with body rocking, shoulder shrugging, back arching, pelvic thrusting, torticollis and choreiform movements with myoclonic jerks in the limbs. The symptoms are exacerbated by stress and disappear during sleep.

Tardive dyskinesia is associated with long-term treatment on antipsychotic drugs, is rarely seen before six months of treatment, and is uncommon before 4–5 years. Long exposure to medication, being female, being elderly and having brain damage are factors increasing risk. The syndrome has been observed in up to 60% of chronic institutionalised patients and interestingly, in 1–5% of schizophrenic patients before the introduction of antipsychotics. In drug-related cases, the cause is thought to be dopamine super-sensitivity resulting from prolonged dopaminergic blockade.

There is no effective treatment for tardive dyskinesia, therefore prevention is very important. This is best achieved by using antipsychotic drugs only when clearly indicated, and in the lowest effective doses for long-term treatment. When the syndrome is recognised, consideration should be given to reducing or stopping the medication if at all possible. Between 5–40% of all cases will eventually remit after stopping the antipsychotic. This may take up to four years, but the condition may also worsen. If dyskinesia persists after several months of stopping the drug, or it is essential to continue treatment, then a cautious trial of one of the following recommended drug treatments should be made: tetrabenazine, sodium valproate, carbamazepine or the benzodiazepines.

Convulsant effects

Low potency antipsychotics such as chlorpromazines are more epileptogenic than high potency ones such as haloperidol. Patients with a previous history of epilepsy and organic brain disease are at increased risk.

Sedation

Patients should be warned about driving or operating machinery when first treated with antipsychotics. However, tolerance often occurs and taking the full dose at bedtime usually eliminates day time sedation.

Anti-adrenergic effects

The main anti-adrenergic effect is severe postural (orthostatic) hypotension which usually occurs during the first few days of treatment on high doses of chlorpromazine and thioridazine. It can usually be managed conservatively by getting the patient to lie down with the feet elevated; but in rare, extreme cases a vasopressor such as norepinephrine (no adrenaline) may be necessary. Epinephrine (adrenaline) is contraindicated in phenothiazine-induced hypotension. This effect limits the maximum parenteral dose of low potency antipsychotics. For example no more than 50 mg of chlorpromazine should be given intramuscularly and even this dose may cause fainting in physically unwell people.

Anticholinergic effects

Peripheral anticholinergic effects are quite common and include dry mouth, blurred vision, constipation, urinary hesitancy and retention, reduced sweating and in rare cases the precipitation of glaucoma.

Central anticholinergic symptoms are uncommon except at toxic levels, but may include severe agitation, disorientation, hallucination, seizures, high fever, dilated pupils, stupor and coma. Treatment includes discontinuing the drug, close medical supervision and physostigmine (2 mg by slow intravenous infusion) to reverse the effect.

Cardiac effects

The cardiac effects of the phenothiazines include dysrhythmias with electrocardiogram changes such as prolongation of the QT interval and T-wave blunting. They are secondary to the quinidine-like action and most marked with thioridazine.

Sudden deaths

There are a few reports of sudden deaths of patients usually occurring following the intramuscular administration of antipsychotic drugs. These deaths have been mainly associated with the use of above recommended doses of low potency antipsychotics. The cause of death in these cases is likely to be related to the antiadrenergic and cardiac effects of the drugs and possibly its accidental injection into a vein rather than into muscle.

Metabolic effects

Antipsychotics can result in breast enlargement, galactorrhoea, amenorrhoea, and false pregnancy tests in females. Decreased libido has been reported in both sexes and impotence in males. Other effects include the inappropriate secretion of anti-diuretic hormones and a diabetic shift in some patients' glucose tolerance test.

Weight gain

This is common and is particularly associated with chlorpromazine and long-term depot antipsychotics. Depot haloperidol, and oral pimozide and oxypertine are less prone to cause excess weight gain. Local advice on diet is recommended, as well as the use of the minimum amount of antipsychotic medication in patients.

Pigmentation

Thioridazine taken in doses of over 800 mg per day can produce irreversible pigmentary retinopathy, which can progress to blindness even after it has been discontinued. Chlorpromazine may produce granular deposits in the posterior cornea, anterior lens and occasionally brownish discolouration of the conjunctiva of the eyes in patients who have taken an accumulated dose of 1–3 kg over many years. However, retinal damage is not seen in these patients and their vision is almost never impaired.

Hypersensitivity reactions

Cholestatic jaundice

Chlorpromazine is associated with the development of cholestatic jaundice, which usually occurs within the first month of treatment. When jaundice occurs the drug should be stopped immediately, and the symptoms nearly always subside spontaneously within a few weeks. After the liver function tests return to normal another antipsychotic should be used. However, drug-induced hepatitis may occur with all antipsychotics.

Haematological effects

Leukopenia with white blood cell counts of about 3500 is a common but not a serious problem. In a minority of patients there is a fall in the total white cell count progressing to fatal agranulocytosis. The onset is usually rapid and tends to occur within the first three months of treatment. Commonly associated antipsychotics include chlorpromazine and clozapine. Patients on these drugs who complain of fever or sore throat should have a full blood count as soon as possible, and if significant leukopenia is found the drug should be stopped and antibiotic treatment started. The patient should be transferred to the nearest medical facility as the mortality rate may be as high as 30–50% even with aggressive treatment. Rarer complications include thrombocytopenia, haemolytic anaemias and pancytopenia.

Skin reactions

Chlorpromazine is associated with allergic dermatitis and photosensitivity in fair skinned and Caucasian patients, but other skin rashes may occur early in treatment and remit spontaneously.

Neuroleptic malignant syndrome

This is a life-threatening idiosyncratic reaction with onset usually within ten days or so after starting treatment. It is commoner in young female patients.

The symptoms include severe motor, mental and autonomic dysfunction. There is generalised muscle hypertonicity, which may cause dysphagia and dyspnoea. Akinesia, mutism, stupor and impaired consciousness are the main mental symptoms. Hyperpyrexia develops with unstable blood pressure, excessive sweating, salivation and urinary incontinence. The symptoms usually evolve over 24–72 hours and the untreated syndrome may last 10–14 days. Laboratory findings usually include raised creatinine phosphokinase and white blood cell count. Myoglobin in the plasma can result in renal shutdown. The mortality rate is between 15–20%, but survivors are usually without residual disability. The drugs most frequently associated with the syndrome are haloperidol and fluphenazine.

Treatment is symptomatic. All antipsychotic drugs should be stopped and the patient transferred to a medical bed as soon as possible. They should be cooled and adequate fluid balance maintained, preferably intravenously. A trial of diazepam for muscle stiffness, dantrolene used in the treatment of malignant hyperthermia or a centrally acting dopamine agonist such as bromocriptine may be useful. If an antipsychotic has to be used again, a low potency drug such as thioridazine is recommended.

Overdoses

Unless a patient has also taken other central nervous system depressants such as alcohol, the outcome of high potency antipsychotic overdose is favourable. However, low potency thioridazine is the most cardiotoxic antipsychotic. The symptoms of overdose include hypotension, mydriatic pupils, and drowsiness which may progress to delirium, coma and seizures. Treatment is symptomatic, which may include gastric lavage and activated charcoal, diazepam for convulsions, and norepinephrine or dopamine for hypotension.

Antidepressants: monoamine reuptake inhibitors (MARIs)

This group comprises the bicyclic, tricyclic and tetracyclic ring structured compounds with similar efficacy but different side-effect profiles. Figure 6.2.3 shows the molecular structures of selected MARIs. The tricyclics are the most established and longest in clinical use. More recently, the serotonin specific reuptake inhibitors (SSRIs) were introduced.

The first generation antidepressants (heterocyclic antidepressants) can be divided into tertiary and secondary amines. Tertiary amines include imipramine and amitriptyline; whereas secondary amines include nortriptyline (see Fig. 6.2.3). Second generation tricyclic antidepressants, for example lofepramine, refer to drugs with a similar but less marked side-effect profile compared to first generation compounds. Tetracyclic antidepressants include maprotiline and mianserin.

Pharmacokinetics

MARIs have an average half-life of between 10–70 hours. However, many have active metabolites which prolong the half-lives of the active compounds. Tertiary

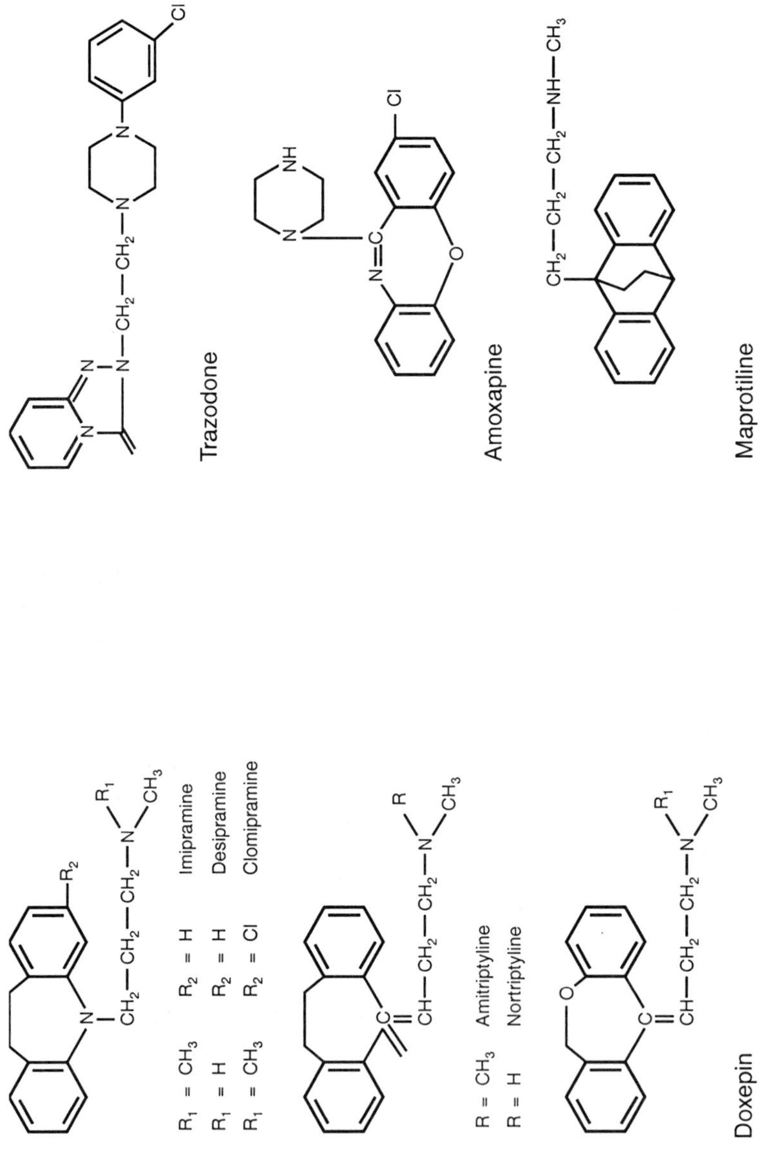

Trazodone

Amoxapine

Maprotiline

Imipramine $R_1 = CH_3$ $R_2 = H$
Desipramine $R_1 = H$ $R_2 = H$
Clomipramine $R_1 = CH_3$ $R_2 = Cl$

Amitriptyline $R = CH_3$
Nortriptyline $R = H$

Doxepin

Fig. 6.2.3 Formulae of some antidepressants.

amines are demethylated to secondary amines, and the tricyclic nucleus is oxidised in the liver, then conjugated and excreted in the urine.

Pharmacodynamics

MARIs increase the availability of noradrenaline and/or serotonin at post-synaptic neurone receptors by blocking their reuptake into pre-synaptic nerve terminals. The first generation tricyclics also block muscarinic and histamine receptors.

Side-effects

Anticholinergic effects

These side-effects are quite common. First generation tricyclic antidepressants such as amitriptyline and imipramine have potent anticholinergic effects, whereas trazodone, mianserin and lofepramine have significantly less. By contrast, the SSRIs have no anticholinergic effects.

Cardiovascular effects

Tricyclic antidepressants, like the antipsychotics have a quinidine-like effect, and at therapeutic doses may cause similar electrocardiogram changes. Tachycardia and hypotension are common. Mianserin, trazodone and lofepramine are less cardiotoxic while the SSRIs have a minimal to absent cardiovascular effect.

Sedation

Antidepressants such as amitriptyline, trimipramine, and trazodone tend to be sedative. Drugs with significantly less to minimal sedative effects include imipramine, lofepramine and the SSRIs. Tiredness and daytime drowsiness may occur with the more sedative drugs, but insomnia is a common depressive symptom and night-time sedation is welcomed by most depressed patients.

Psychiatric effects

Insomnia may occur with the less sedative antidepressants. A manic episode may be precipitated in manic–depressive patients and even in those without a previous history. When there is a past history of drug-induced mania, lower doses of antidepressants should be used while observing for signs of emergent mania.

Neurological effects

A fine tremor of the hands is common. Less common effects include incoordination, headache, muscle twitching and seizures in predisposed patients.

Other effects

Gastrointestinal symptoms such as nausea, vomiting and diarrhoea are common side-effects of the SSRIs. They may also cause restlessness and anxiety. However, unlike the tricyclics, the SSRIs do not cause weight gain. Less common side-effects of antidepressants include allergic skin rashes, mild cholestatic jaundice, inappropriate secretion of anti-diuretic hormone and agranulocytosis. The sudden cessation of antidepressants may be followed by nausea, anxiety, sweating and insomnia.

Overdose and toxic effects

An overdose of the tricyclics can produce serious and sometimes fatal effects. Urgent medical management in hospital is usually required. The toxic dose range is 1–4 mg per kilogram body weight and the fatal range is 15–20 mg per kilogram. Symptoms include hypotension, ventricular fibrillation, respiratory depression with hypoxia, agitation, convulsions, hallucinations, delirium and coma. Anticholinergic effects such as dry mouth, dilated pupils, urinary retention, bowel paralysis and temperature dysregulation are common. Death is usually due to cardiac arrhythmia and hypotension.

Cardiac monitoring is important, but most patients only require supportive care. The tricyclic antidepressants delay gastric emptying and gastric lavage is valuable for about four hours after an overdose, as well as activated charcoal orally. Tricyclics are radio-opaque and an abdominal X-ray might be useful in a patient presenting with an uncertain history. Maintaining the acid base balance is important because of the ensuing metabolic acidosis which tends to complicate any severe poisoning. Anticonvulsants such as diazepam, or phenytoin which is also an antiarrhythmic drug, may be necessary. Prolonged resuscitation is advisable in tricyclic overdose and if possible cardiac monitoring should be continued for 3–4 days after the acute episode has subsided.

Notes on the SSRIs

There are four SSRIs currently available: fluvoxamine maleate (Faverin), fluoxetine hydrochloride (Prozac), paroxetine (Seroxat) and sertraline (Lustral).

They are said to be of comparable efficacy to the tricyclics and to have good safety records in overdose. However, more information is required on the use of the SSRIs with lithium and ECT. In comparison to the older tricyclics, the SSRIs are very expensive and currently cost up to 10–15 times more.

Interaction with other drugs

The plasma levels of both the heterocyclic antidepressants and antipsychotics are increased by their co-administration. Their anticholinergic and sedative effects are also potentiated. Other central nervous system depressant drugs such as alcohol, anxiolytics, hypnotics and the opioids will have additive sedative effects when taken with these drugs. The tricyclics potentiate the effects of adrenaline and related drugs found in local anaesthetics, and the anti-hypertensive effects of clonidine and guanethidine. Mianserin or the SSRIs can be used to treat depressed patients on antihypertensives. The birth-control pill may decrease plasma levels of antidepressants.

Management

Patients presenting with depressive symptoms should be assessed to rule out underlying physical causes, to determine the severity of the symptoms, the role of psychosocial factors, the amount of support available, and whether in-patient or out-patient treatment is indicated (see Chapter 10). Familiarity with at least three drugs is important. One should be sedating such as amitriptyline for agitated, anxious and depressed patients; a less sedating one such as imipramine for retarded, depressed patients; and the other with minimum anticholinergic and cardiotoxic side-effects such as lofepramine or an SSRI.

Only one antidepressant drug should be given at a time. Once a suitable antidepressant is chosen, it should be explained to the patient that full therapeutic benefit is likely to be delayed for up to three weeks, and that improvement is usually gradual. They should also be told that the common side-effects will appear earlier than therapeutic effects, but reassured that most of these effects tend to diminish as the treatment progresses. The patient's mental state must be checked frequently, especially in the early weeks of treatment to detect suicidal ideas and to monitor progress.

An average adult starting dose of antidepressant is 75 mg of amitriptyline per day or of imipramine in divided doses. This should be increased by 25–50 mg weekly to 150 mg daily, or to a maximum of about 200 mg of amitriptyline and 300 mg of imipramine in hospital patients. The dose increase should be titrated against side-effects and the patient's response. Paroxetine and fluoxetine both start at 20 mg per day, which is also the therapeutic dose, but the dose of paroxetine can be increased in 10 mg increments up to 50 mg per day if necessary, and up to 60 mg per day of fluoxetine is recommended in bulimia nervosa.

Treatment should continue for at least a month at the dose at which full symptom control was achieved, after which it can be gradually reduced to the minimum dose (usually not less than 75 mg of amitryptiline per day or the equivalent of other antidepressants) tolerated without depressive symptoms re-emerging. The drug should be continued for at least 6–9 months before an attempt is made to decrease and discontinue it completely, if the patient's clinical history and response permits it. If relapse occurs when the dose is being reduced, the former dose should be reinstated for at least another three months before lowering it cautiously a second time. Relapse is less likely if the full dose is maintained for the first six months after remission, but all patients should be given a trial of cautious reduction, especially those presenting with a first episode of depression. Patients who do not respond to adequate treatment should have a review of the diagnosis, compliance and possible psychosocial and physical maintaining factors.

Antidepressants: monoamine oxidase inhibitors (MAOIs)

The MAOIs have been in use in psychiatry for many years, but there is still controversy about the nature of their therapeutic actions and whether they are as effective as the heterocyclic antidepressants in treating depression. They have anxiolytic properties and are effective in phobic anxiety states and in atypical depressed patients with hypochondriacal symptoms. The main limitation of the MAOIs is their dangerous interactions with certain common foods and other drugs. In many developing countries, the MAOIs will probably have very little place in the treatment of depression because of the dietary restrictions and hazardous risks involved.

A new group of reversible inhibitors of monoamine oxidase (RIMAs) is currently being tried in Europe. RIMAs include moclobemide (Manerix) and brofaromine. They are said to have the advantages of reduced potential for dangerous dietary interactions, as well as a rapid reversal of inhibitory effects at the end of treatment. Moclobemide is said to be as effective as tricyclics and has a low risk in overdose. If the RIMAs prove to be effective and safe, the older MAOIs may soon become obsolete.

Lithium

Indications

Lithium has both antimanic and antidepressant effects. In acute mania, lithium can be started concurrently with most antipsychotics. When the florid symptoms have subsided after about 2–3 weeks, the antipsychotic can then be gradually withdrawn. In acute depression lithium can be used in combination with standard antidepressants. Lithium is said to be effective in treating aggressive, impulsive disorders in the mentally retarded and in prisoners. It is also sometimes used as an adjunctive treatment in schizophrenia and a few studies have reported its effectiveness in the treatment of premenstrual syndrome, borderline personality disorder and alcohol binge drinking.

Lithium is the prophylactic treatment of choice in recurrent affective disorders. In 1989 the WHO issued a consensus statement and guidelines for initiating lithium treatment. It recommended that if a patient has had more than one severe episode of depressive illness, especially if there has been one or several other episodes apart from the present one in the last five years, then long-term prophylactic therapy should be considered. This treatment can either be with antidepressants, in particular one to which the patient has shown response, or a lithium salt. Prien & Kupfer (1986) showed that continuation treatment with lithium is as effective as imipramine in preventing further depressive disorder and more effective in preventing manic recurrences. When mania is the index illness, lithium reduces both relapses and recurrences. A clinically useful guideline is to start lithium prophylaxis when a patient has had three episodes of manic depression (bipolar affective disorder) or of depression in five years or two episodes in two years.

Pharmacokinetics

Lithium is absorbed from the gut within 6–8 hours after ingestion. The serum level peaks in 0.5–2 hours, and in about four hours for slow release preparations.

The half-life is approximately 20 hours, reaching equilibrium after 5–7 days of regular intake. Lithium is eliminated by the kidneys, and like sodium is filtered and partly reabsorbed. When the renal proximal tubule absorbs more water, lithium absorption is increased and vice versa. Increased sodium intake decreases reabsorption of lithium, whilst restricted sodium intake increases plasma lithium levels. Lithium is also excreted in small amounts in faeces, sweat and saliva.

Pharmacodynamics

The mechanism of action of lithium remains unclear, but the following effects are noted:

1. Lithium stimulates the exit of sodium ions (Na) from cells and may interact with both calcium (Ca) and magnesium (Mg) to increase cell membrane permeability.
2. Lithium is thought to have the following action on neurotransmitters:
   a. inhibits the synthesis and release of acetylcholine;
   b. increases presynaptic destruction of catecholamines;
   c. decreases the sensitivity of postsynaptic receptors and increases the reuptake of neurotransmitters, thereby overall decreasing the amount of neurotransmitters in the synaptic cleft.
3. Other biological actions of lithium include the restoration of diurnal rhythm of corticosteroids to normal in diurnal mania and restoration of normal slow-wave EEG rhythm during sleep in depressed patients.

Side-effects

Common early side-effects of lithium include nausea, vomiting, diarrhoea, slight thirst, dry mouth, metallic taste in the mouth, muscular weakness, fine tremor of the hands and fatigue. A mild diuresis may occur shortly after treatment is started. Gastrointestinal symptoms can be reduced by giving lithium in divided doses, or taking it with food.

Later effects of lithium include polyuria and polydipsia, which can occur at therapeutic plasma lithium concentrations if renal concentrating ability is poor. However, in some cases reversible nephrogenic diabetes insipidus develops which may take several weeks to remit and does not respond to the standard medical treatment. There have been controversial reports of longer-term chronic renal impairment. Enlargement of the thyroid gland occurs in up to 5% of patients taking lithium and hypothyroidism in up to 20% of female patients. If hypothyroidism develops during treatment and there are strong indications to continue lithium, thyroxine replacement should be added. Reversible electrocardiogram changes occur with T-wave flattening and widening of the QRS complex. Oedema, weight gain and papular rash may also occur, whereas neurological effects such as ataxia, dysarthria, choreoathetosis and tardive dyskinesia rarely occur.

Toxic effects

The toxic effects of lithium are dose-related. Symptoms usually appear at serum levels greater than 2.0 mmol/l. They are mainly neurological and include coarse tremor, ataxia, slurred speech, muscle twitching, nystagmus, disorientation, convulsion, and coma progressing to death. Urgent medical intervention is required. Lithium should be stopped immediately and a high intake of oral and/or intravenous fluid provided to stimulate osmotic diuresis. In several cases (serum levels above 3 mmol/l), forced alkaline diuresis or dialysis may be necessary. Lithium is rapidly cleared if renal functions are normal and most people recover completely. In overdoses, early management should include gastric lavage with a wide bore tube. Activated charcoal is not beneficial.

Management of patients

Patients on lithium should be carefully managed because of the narrow therapeutic to toxic dose ratio. In developing countries, lithium should only be prescribed where there are facilities for blood investigations to be done on a 3–6 monthly basis.

Before the start of treatment, patients should have a physical examination with recorded weight, and a urine check for proteins and sugar. Full blood count, thyroid function tests, serum levels of electrolytes, urea, creatinine and/or a 24-hour urine creatinine level are the basic investigations required. Oral, and when possible written information should be given to patients and their carers about lithium. Information should include symptoms of early toxic effects and the circumstances in which they commonly arise, such as during periods of excess fluid loss from gastroenteritis, infections and heavy sweating.

The most commonly prescribed salt is lithium carbonate, but it is also available as the citrate. An average adult starting dose is 750–1000 mg per day. The serum lithium level should be checked at least weekly in the initial stabilising period and the dose adjusted to achieve a therapeutic level of 0.4–0.8 mmol/l, in a sample taken 12 hours after the last dose. In judging clinical response, it should be remembered that it may take several months before lithium achieves full therapeutic effect. The normal dose range is 800–2000 mg per day.

The monitoring of lithium prophylaxis can be arranged in primary care settings. The advantage of special lithium clinics lies in the ease of handling samples and administrative matters as well as the social support that can be provided. This might not be practicable in some developing countries, but achievable in many. Once serum lithium levels are stable, a three-monthly review is adequate with a six-monthly repeat blood profile which should include renal and thyroid function tests. Lithium is usually continued for at least a year and often much longer. It should not be abruptly withdrawn as patients may become irritable and emotionally labile.

Interaction with other drugs

There have been reports of toxic interaction between lithium at higher serum levels, with doses of haloperidol greater than 40 mg per day. This may present as confusion, with signs of extrapyramidal and cerebellar dysfunction. Thiazide diuretics can also precipitate lithium toxicity. Patients requiring surgery involving a muscle relaxant should stop lithium 48–72 hours before surgery as it can potentiate the effects of the muscle relaxant.

Anxiolytics and hypnotics

Severe anxiety symptoms and insomnia are usually symptomatic of an underlying medical or psychiatric disorder. Anxiety is a natural response to stressful events and usually resolves within days or weeks, however, it may last much longer and interfere with normal daily activities. Psychological treatments such as counselling, behavioural and cognitive therapies, and/or drug treatment may be indicated. Benzodiazepines, MARIs, MAOIs, phenothiazines, zopiclone (Zimovane), buspirone (Buspar) and propranolol (Inderal) are examples of drugs used in the treatment of anxiety and insomnia. Anxiolytics and hypnotics are most useful when given for a short time to tide the patient over a crisis, or to help in tackling a specific problem.

General uses and indications

Many anxiolytics and hypnotics are prescribed for a wide spectrum of conditions. Commonly used hypnotics include nitrazepam, flurazepam and temazepam. Chloral hydrate is sometimes prescribed for children and the elderly. Chlormethiazole (Heminevrin) is a commonly prescribed hypnotic which has anticonvulsant properties and can be used for alcohol withdrawal symptoms in a reducing dose regime over a 7–10 days period. However, chlormethiazole can interact dangerously if taken with alcohol, resulting in death from respiratory failure. Chlordiazepoxide and diazepam are equally effective in a similar reducing dose regime for the treatment of alcohol withdrawal symptoms.

Diazepam is also used as an anticonvulsant, a muscle relaxant, in abreactive technique, for premedication, in minor operative procedures and for drug-induced agitated psychotic states.

Benzodiazepines

The benzodiazepines are still widely prescribed despite their recognised dependence problems and will be discussed in some detail.

Classification

The benzodiazepines are usefully classified as 2-keto, 3-hydroxy and the triazalo compounds, which are based on modifications of a benzene ring fused to a seven-sided diazepine ring (Fig. 6.2.4). The 2-keto compounds include diazepam (Valium), flurazepam (Dalmane), and chlordiazepoxide (Librium). The 3-hydroxy compounds include temazepam, lorazepam (Ativan) and oxazepam.

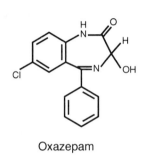
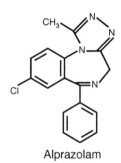

Benzodiazepine nucleus:

2-keto benzodiazepine:

Diazepam

3-hydroxy benzodiazepine:

Triazalo benzodiazepine:

Oxazepam

Alprazolam

Fig. 6.2.4. Representative benzodiazepine structures.

Triazolam and alprazolam (Xanax) are examples of the triazalo benzodiazepines.

Pharmacokinetics

The benzodiazepines are rapidly absorbed from the gut and most reach peak plasma level in 1–3 hours. Lorazepam is reliably absorbed when given intramuscularly, unlike diazepam which should be given intravenously as a non-irritant emulsion, or as a rectal suppository when rapid onset of action is necessary. The benzodiazepines are highly bound to plasma proteins.

Metabolism takes place in the liver, but differs between the subclasses, resulting in half-lives ranging from 30–100 hours in the keto drugs, and to 2–3 hours in the triazalo ones. Patients who have hepatic disease and the elderly may therefore develop toxicity on the longer half-life drugs after 7–10 days, even at therapeutic dose.

Side-effects

The benzodiazepines are generally well tolerated. At anxiolytic dose the main side-effects are sedative, while at higher doses ataxia, drowsiness and dizziness may occur. The elderly may also get uncommon side-effects such as confused thinking and leg pains. Minor degrees of drowsiness, impaired coordination and judgement can affect driving skills and the operation of dangerous machinery. Benzodiazepines resemble alcohol in that in some circumstances they may produce a paradoxical release of aggression.

Toxic effects

These drugs have few toxic effects and are very safe in overdose. After an overdose, the patient usually falls asleep and wakes up after 24–48 hours with rebound insomnia over the next few days.

Tolerance dependence and withdrawal

When benzodiazepines are taken for short periods of time, that is 1–4 weeks in moderate doses, there are usually no dependence or withdrawal effects. But there is now general agreement that, if continued, psychological and physical dependence can develop any time after this period. It has been estimated that between 5–50% of people who take the drugs for more than six months will become dependent (Hallstrom, 1985). Shorter acting compounds produce dependency and withdrawal symptoms much more quickly than longer acting ones.

The withdrawal syndrome is characterised by somatic and psychic anxiety symptoms and includes apprehensive feelings, insomnia, nausea, tremor, restlessness, sweating, and heightened sensitivity to perceptual stimuli. Consequently, it may be difficult at times to decide whether the patient is experiencing withdrawal symptoms or a recrudescence of anxiety symptoms (Rodrigo & Williams, 1986). At very high doses of greater than 60 mg per day equivalent of diazepam, more severe withdrawal symptoms such as convulsion, psychosis and amnesia may occur.

Withdrawal regime

After a prolonged period on benzodiazepines, it is best to gradually reduce the dose and withdraw the drugs to avoid or reduce the withdrawal symptoms. Psychological support is an important part of the treatment. The suggested regime from the *British National Formulary* (1996) is a good guide. The patient can be transferred to the equivalent daily dose of diazepam, or remain on the same drug and have it withdrawn in steps of about 1/8 (range 1/10 to 1/4) of the daily dose fortnightly. The approximate equivalent dose of 5 mg of diazepam for other commonly prescribed benzodiazepines are:

> 15 mg chlordiazepoxide
> 500 micrograms lorazepam
> 5 mg nitrazepam
> 15 mg oxazepam
> 10 mg temazepam
> 125–250 micrograms triazolam

If withdrawal symptoms occur, the present dose should be maintained until the symptoms improve. The withdrawal time can vary from four weeks to a year or more. Antidepressants should only be prescribed if there are clinical symptoms of depression and antipsychotics should be avoided as they tend to aggravate the withdrawal symptoms.

Other drugs

Zopiclone is a new non-benzodiazepine hypnotic which is a cyclopyrrolone-group compound, but it is thought to act on the same receptors as the benzodiazepines. Its half-life is 5–8 hours and like other hypnotics it should not be used for long-term treatment despite its reported advantages over the benzodiazepines. For example, the standard adult dose is 7.5 mg, with no need to increase the dosage or to taper it when stopping treatment. Rebound effects are said to be minimal.

Buspirone is a new drug for the treatment of anxiety. It belongs to the azaspirodecanedione class of compounds and is said to act at specific serotonin receptors (5-HT-1A). Buspirone does not alleviate benzodiazepine withdrawal symptoms and does not have the sedative, hypnotic or anticonvulsant effects of the benzodiazepines. Its anti-anxiety effects may take 1–3 weeks to appear. The adult starting dose is 5 mg twice to three times daily which can be gradually increased to 45 mg daily in divided doses.

Zopiclone and buspirone are thought to have low dependence and abuse potential, but because they are new drugs this has not yet been established in practice.

Beta-blockers such as propranolol which have well-established indications in the treatment of many cardiovascular problems may also be used to alleviate the somatic symptoms of anxiety such as palpitations, sweating and tremor. They do not directly affect psychological symptoms of anxiety such as worry and fear, or non-autonomic symptoms such as muscle tension.

Minimal drug cupboard

There has not been any significant improvement in the efficacy of psychotropic drugs since their inception and most of the newer drugs are being marketed on the basis of less or safer side-effect profiles in comparison to their predecessors. However, as with any relatively new drugs, further clinical experience may eventually uncover unknown adverse effects. They are also invariably more expensive. It is therefore advisable when considering what to include in a minimal psychotropic drug cupboard to have well-established drugs whose efficacy and side-effects are known, and which are also available in generic preparations to reduce the cost. Some developing countries can manufacture generic formulations which further reduce the cost price of the drugs.

The drugs recommended for the management of psychosis are depot fluphenazine, oral and parenteral preparations of chlorpromazine and haloperidol. Benztropine mesylate (Cogentin) may be used in oral parenteral form for drug-induced Parkinson's side-effects. Oral preparations of lithium carbonate, amitriptyline and imipramine are recommended for the mood disorders. Diazepam in oral, suppository and parenteral forms is a useful drug for the short-term management of a range of psychiatric and medical conditions and it is recommended for completion of the minimum drug cupboard. This list of drugs is affordable and would enable adequate management of most psychiatric disorders. Given the right financial backing, more drugs from each group can be added to the basic list to provide a wider choice of side-effects' profile.

References

ABRAMS, R., TAYLOR, M. A., *et al* (1983) Bilateral versus unilateral electroconvulsive therapy: efficacy in melancholia. *American Journal of Psychiatry,* **140**, 463–490.

—— (1986) Is unilateral electroconvulsive therapy really the treatment of choice in endogenous depression? In *Electroconvulsive Therapy: Clinical and Basic Research Issues* (eds S. Malitz & H. A. Sackeim). *Annals of the New York Academy of Sciences,* **462**, 50–55.

AMERICAN PSYCHIATRIC ASSOCIATION TASK FORCE ON ECT (1990) The practice of ECT: recommendations for treatment, training and privileging. *Convulsive Therapy,* **6**, 85–120.

—— (1978) *Electroconvulsive Therapy.* Report No. 14. Washington, DC: APA.

BLEULER, M. (1978) *The Schizophrenic Disorders: Long-term Patient and Family Studies.* London: Yale University Press.

BRITISH MEDICAL ASSOCIATION AND ROYAL PHARMACEUTICAL SOCIETY OF GREAT BRITAIN (1996) No. 31. *British National Formulary.* Avon: Bath Press.

CIOMPI, L. (1980*a*) The natural history of schizophrenia in the long-term. *British Journal of Psychiatry,* **136**, 413–420.

—— (1980*b*) Catamnestic long-term study on the course of life and aging of schizophrenics. *Schizophrenia Bulletin,* **6**, 606–618.

COMAS-DIAZ, L. & GRIFFITH, E. H. (1988) *Clinical Issues in Cross-Cultural Mental Health.* New York: John Wiley.

FREEMAN, C. P. L., WEEKS, D. & KENDELL, R. E. (1980) ECT: patients who complain. *British Journal of Psychiatry,* **137**, 17–25.

GARDOS, G. & COLE, J. O. (1980) Overview: public health issues in tardive dyskinesia. *American Journal of Psychiatry,* **137**, 776–781.

GELDER, M., GATH, D. & MAYOU, R. (1989) Drugs and other physical treatments. In *Oxford Textbook of Psychiatry* (2nd edn), pp. 624–693. Oxford: Oxford University Press.

HALE, T. (1993) Will the new antipsychotics improve the treatment of schizophrenia? *British Medical Journal,* **307**, 749–750.

HALLSTROM, C. (1985) Benzodiazepines: clinical practice and central mechanisms. In *Recent Advances in Psychiatry,* Vol. 5 (ed. K. Granville-Grossman). Edinburgh: Churchill Livingstone.

HICKLING, F. W. (1988) *Clinical Guidelines and Cross Cultural Mental Health* (eds L. Lomas-Diaz & E. Griffiths). New York: John Wiley.

IHEZUE, U. H. (1983) Psychiatric in-patients in Anambra State, Nigeria: a psychosocial study. *Acta Psychiatrica Scandinavica,* **68**, 277–286.

JOHNSON, D. A. W. (1990) Depot therapy – advantages, disadvantages and issues of dose. In *Depot Antipsychotics in Chronic Schizophrenia* (Proceedings of a Symposium, Copenhagen November 1990) (eds B. Wistedt & J. Gerlach), pp. 4–16. Amsterdam: Excerpta Medica.

KAPLAN, H. I. & SADOCK, B. J. (1988) Biological therapies. In *Synopsis of Psychiatry – Behavioural Sciences Clinical Psychiatry* (5th edn) (eds R. Cancro & J. Grebb), pp. 492–531. Baltimore: Williams and Wilkins.

MERSKEY, H. (1990) Ethical aspects of physical manipulation of the brain. In *Psychiatric Ethics* (2nd edn) (eds S. Bloch & P. Chodoff), pp. 185–214. New York: Oxford University Press.

ODEJIDE, A. O., OHAERI, J. U. & IKUESAN, B. A. (1987) Electroconvulsive therapy in Nigeria. *Convulsive Therapy,* **3**, 31–39.

PIPPARD, J. (1992) Auditing the administration of ECT. *Psychiatric Bulletin,* **16**, 59–62.

PRIEN, R. F. & KUPFER, D. J. (1986) Continuation drug therapy for major depressive episodes: how long should it be maintained? *American Journal of Psychiatry*, **143**, 18–23.

RODRIGO, E. K. & WILLIAMS, P. (1986) Frequency of self-reported 'anxiolitic withdrawal' symptoms in a group of female students experimenting anxiety. *Psychological Medicine*, **16**, 467–472.

ROYAL COLLEGE OF PSYCHIATRISTS (1995) *ECT Handbook. The Second Report of the Royal College of Psychiatrists Special Committee on ECT.* CR38. London: Royal College of Psychiatrists.

SIJUWALA, O. A. (1985) Use of electroconvulsive therapy in a Nigerian hospital. *East African Medical Journal*, **62**, 60–64.

SMALL, J. G., MILSTEIN, V., *et al* (1986) Electroconvulsive therapy in the treatment of manic episodes. In *Electroconvulsive Issues* (eds S. Malitz & H. A. Sackheim). *Annals of the New York Academy of Science*, **462**, 33–49.

SWINDELLS, S. R. & SIMPSON, K. H. (1987) Oxygen saturation during ECT. *British Journal of Psychiatry*, **150**, 695.

TANTAM, D. & MCGRATH, G. (1989) Prolonged use of neuroleptics in schizophrenia: a review for the practitioner. *International Clinical Psychopharmacology*, **4**, 167–194.

WORLD HEALTH ORGANIZATION (1973) *Report of the International Pilot Study of Schizophrenia*, Vol. 1. Geneva: WHO.

WORLD HEALTH ORGANIZATION MENTAL HEALTH COLLABORATION CENTRES (1989) Pharmacotherapy of depressive disorders, a consensus statement. *Journal of Affective Disorders*, **17**, 197–198.

3. Section III. Symptoms

7. Schizophrenia

O. GUREJE

Prevalence

Schizophrenia has a worldwide distribution and its prevalence appears to be just under 1%. However, this rate reflects the results of epidemiological studies conducted principally in developed countries of Europe and America. Systematic, large-scale epidemiological studies addressing the question of the community prevalence of schizophrenia in developing countries are generally lacking. An exception is a World Health Organization (1973) multi-site, international study, which was conducted in ten countries, three of them developing (Sartorius *et al*, 1986). The results suggest that the incidence of schizophrenia, measured as the annual rate of first-in-lifetime contacts with any type of care-giving service, is fairly similar throughout the world. This uniformity of incidence has been contested by Stevens (1987), who argued that the criteria for inclusion in the WHO study might have lumped together clinically heterogeneous groups of patients with some suffering from illnesses other than schizophrenia. In addition, similar incidence rates in different parts of the world do not necessarily lead to similar prevalence rates since differential recovery rates would affect the accumulation of affected individuals. It is also of interest that there appear to be pockets of high prevalence in places such as northern Sweden, western Ireland, and Finland (Torrey, 1987).

The incidence of schizophrenia may also be falling, at least in developed countries. There is accumulating evidence that the number of admitted cases in these countries is on the decline (Eagles, 1991). Whether this observation reflects the changing criteria for the clinical diagnosis or a genuine fall in incidence is yet to be determined. However, the evidence that the clinical picture of the illness has changed in these countries appears to be stronger. For example, fewer cases are registered among patients from developed countries (Mann *et al*, 1986). This contrasts with the picture in many developing countries where a catatonic presentation is still relatively common. It is not known what role, if any, underlying organic factors such as sub-nutritional states play in this differential clinical picture.

Schizophrenia commonly has its onset in late adolescence or young adulthood and this feature may have a bearing on comparative community prevalence figures in developed and developing societies, as the age distribution pyramids of these two societies tend to be markedly different. There is, however, a strong gender effect on the age at onset. Most studies have found a mean age at onset of about 24 years for men while it is about two years later for women. Also, while most male patients have developed the illness before the age of 30, a substantial proportion of females have the first episode of illness after 30 years of age (Gureje, 1991).

Clinical features

Schizophrenia is a syndrome composed of abnormal clinical signs and symptoms in the areas of behaviour, volition, attention, cognition, and motor activities. While a number of these features are suggestive of the illness, none is pathognomonic of it. Also, while many patients manifest some or a combination of these abnormalities, few patients manifest all. Indeed, a substantial proportion of the patients have just one or two of the characteristic symptoms. This, coupled with the fact that the diagnosis of schizophrenia in a patient carries considerable social implications, requires the clinician to be careful to exclude other possible causes of schizophrenia-like symptoms.

The diagnosis of schizophrenia has undergone considerable variation in recent years, partly because of the need to foster cross-national reliability and also in an attempt to define a clinically homogeneous disorder. While the former goal has been realised by the use of widely accepted diagnostic criteria, the latter is still far from being achieved. In the present state of psychiatric nosology, any group of clinical patients with the disorder will most likely show biological, familial, and prognostic heterogeneity. The reason for this may be that we are dealing with a group of disorders rather than one disorder but are unable to identify the component parts because of present limitations in our knowledge.

Historically, schizophrenia has tended to be diagnosed according to the dictates of the particular school of psychiatric phenomenology that is in vogue among practising clinicians. Originally, Kraepelin had described an illness with early onset and progressive deterioration, characterised by cognitive impairment, giving it the name 'dementia praecox'. Most early workers adopted this narrow definition and required of their patients a uniformly deteriorating course. However, later workers adopted symptom-based definitions of the illness, to allow a cross-sectional diagnosis of schizophrenia.

Up to the 1970s, the diagnosis of schizophrenia in North America was based on the features which Eugen Bleuler had described as being pathognomonic of it. Bleuler, in introducing the term 'schizophrenia', had expressed the view that the distinguishing characteristics of the illness were the fragmenting of the thinking processes, a symptom he referred to as 'associative loosening', along with features such as affective blunting, ambivalence, and disordered attention (autism). On the other hand, European psychiatrists relied mainly on the set of clinical features described by Kurt Schneider. According to Schneider, eleven symptoms were pathognomonic of schizophrenia in the absence of organic causation. These First Rank Symptoms, as they were called, can be broadly grouped into three sections:

1. Hallucinations (false sensory perception occurring in the absence of any relevant external stimulation of the sensory modality involved):
    a. Voice commenting on the patient's actions

   b. Two or more voices arguing or discussing the patient in the third person
   c. Thought echo or the patient hearing his own thought being said aloud.
2. Passivity experiences (experiences that seem neither willed nor directed by
   the patient):
   a. Somatic passivity (bodily experiences)
   b. Thought insertion (cognitive experience/foreign thoughts in one's mind)
   c. Thought withdrawal (thoughts missing)
   d. Thought broadcasting (thoughts not being silent)
   e. 'Made' impulses (foreign wishes or decisions)
   f. 'Made' volition (foreign plans or goals)
   g. 'Made' affect (foreign emotions).
3. Special type of delusion:
   a. Delusional perception (an illumination in which an experience is seen as
       having an everyday and an esoteric meaning, the latter being as much
       intended as the former).

It can be difficult to determine reliably the boundaries between Bleulerian
symptoms and normal experience. Affective flattening, autistic behaviour, and
thought disorder are not all-or-none phenomena that could only be present in
illness, since some normal people display mild forms of these features. The
distinctive quality of Schneiderian symptoms is more reliably recognised.

Reliance on these two conceptually different sets of features led to the diagnosis of schizophrenia as a widely divergent clinical entity in North America
and in Europe up to the 1970s. Differences confirmed by the United States/
United Kingdom study showed that many patients diagnosed as schizophrenic
in the US would not have been so in Britain (Cooper *et al*, 1972). The concept of
schizophrenia in the US included many patients who would be regarded as
suffering from affective, or personality disorders in the UK.

Since the practice of psychiatry in most developing countries was (and still is)
influenced by the prevailing practice in the centres in which most of their
psychiatrists received training, the European tradition of heavy reliance on
Schneiderian symptoms prevailed in most of these countries, particularly in
many African countries. The findings of the US/UK study suggested that no
cross-national consensus was present that could encourage comparisons of
research findings. It was in an effort to rectify this that the first set of diagnostic
criteria for schizophrenia, together with a number of other psychiatric disorders,
in which both inclusion and exclusion criteria were explicitly itemised, was
formulated by workers at the University of Washington (Feighner *et al*, 1972).
Subsequent refinements led to the Research Diagnostic Criteria (Spitzer *et al*,
1978) and, later, to the criteria specified in the third edition of the *Diagnostic and
Statistical Manual of Mental Disorders* (DSM–III; American Psychiatric Association, 1980) which is the official classification system in the United States. The
revised edition of this, the DSM–III–R, has been in use in many centres across
the world and experience gained with its use has helped to develop DSM–IV
(APA, 1994). The World Health Organization has also revised the definition of
schizophrenia as contained in the ninth edition of the *International Classification of
Diseases* (ICD–9; WHO, 1978). The tenth edition (ICD–10; WHO, 1992), which
has become the official classification system of most member states, incorporates
inclusion and exclusion criteria. However, while the DSM–III–R specifies a

minimum duration of six months disturbance which should include the presence of at least one month of active phase symptoms of schizophrenia, the ICD–10 requires only one month. On the other hand, both DSM–IV and ICD–10 are in agreement that a diagnosis of schizophrenia can be made in cases of presenting for the first time over the age of 45 years. While such criteria commonly determine the selection of patients for research, most clinicians tend to be flexible in their application when conducting purely clinical assessments.

The clinical presentation of schizophrenia is protean. The illness can start acutely or manifest insidiously. Two fairly typical ways that patients with this disorder can present are illustrated by the following examples.

1.   A young man of about 27 years of age was noticed by friends and relatives to have become suddenly very argumentative and irritable. Ordinary statements by others now seemed to have a special meaning for him and he took offence at the most innocuous utterances. He lived in the large family compound and had his farm close to those of his uncles. In the previous two weeks, he stopped greeting his father's senior wife and hinted to one or two people that he was sure the woman was sucking his blood. The main entrance to his farm was now protected with a small fetish gourd and he had taken to searching for footsteps in this farm first thing in the morning before starting to work. He had been forcibly brought to the hospital after relatives became terrified of his intentions, as he had for the previous two days been continuously honing a cutlass in the middle of the family compound and looking menacingly at relatives as they came in and went out. When he was seen in the clinic, the doctor could not do a thorough mental state examination because the patient was verbally aggressive, and threatening to kill all those who he said were in league to murder him. He was particularly eager to deal with his father's senior wife. He accused her of turning into a bed bug at night to suck and poison his blood. The doctor was eager to loosen the rope with which relatives had tied his wrists as he could see that both hands had become swollen. He prescribed an intramuscular injection of chlorpromazine which sedated him after a few minutes and permitted his wrists to be untied. The diagnosis of schizophrenia was confirmed the following day when the patient gave further details of his persecutory beliefs. He said that he had been hearing voices of 'witches' talking about him among themselves for over three weeks and that his thoughts had often been taken away by these people who had planted their own in his mind.

2.   A 30-year-old married woman was brought to the clinic by her mother and two brothers. She had been receiving treatment at a traditional healer's home for the past four months. Prior to that, she had spent about three months within the premises of a syncretic church receiving treatment from the church leader. The relatives gave a history of gradual deterioration in self care, neglect of her four young children, murmuring and giggling to herself, and hoarding rubbish. None of them could indicate precisely when these changes in her behaviour were first noticed. She had been married for eleven years and was living with her husband in another town until seven months before, when her mother was informed by her husband that she was unwell. Her husband had not been seen for two months prior to hospital consultation, apparently discouraged by her lack of response to the treatment so far. The children were with her husband and had not been seen by the patient for over four months. In the clinic she looked gaunt, weak and poorly nourished. She had a productive cough which her mother said had worsened since appearing more than four weeks ago. Her

hair was dishevelled and she had scarification marks on her arms and back – evidence of the flogging she had received as part of the traditional treatment. She continually looked around the consulting room as if she could see or hear things that others could not. She smiled fatuously to herself and occasionally looked amused by what the doctor said or what he asked the relatives. However, she herself could give no understandable response to any of the doctor's questions to her. For example, when asked what her name was, she replied, looking at no one in particular: 'Tomi is going to school. Her orange is white for the table of God. Beautify them. Will you not beautify them?'

The first patient exemplifies an acute onset of the illness with rapidly emerging psychotic symptoms: persecutory delusions, thought withdrawal and third-person auditory hallucinations. Anger manifesting in irritability or aggression may be signs that a patient is labouring under tormenting hallucinations or delusions. There is a risk of violence, or even homicide, if the patient acts in response to these abnormal experiences.

The second patient demonstrates the insidious evolution of the disorder with gradual drifting away from her usual social contacts and from reality. Unaccustomed neglect of self-care and strange episodes of what may appear as absent-mindedness or being lost in thought may be the first signs noticed by relatives. Sometimes it may be vague digressions in speech or what may appear to be increasing difficulty of the listener to understand the patient. By the time the patient is brought to the clinic, he or she may be totally lost in his or her own world with completely unintelligible speech or using new words (neologisms). At this stage, the degree of thought disorder may be such that other aspects of the mental status examination cannot be conducted as it is impossible to communicate effectively with the patient.

The special circumstances of patients presenting in some developing countries are also shown by these examples. It is not uncommon to find that patients have suffered severe injuries during attempts to bring them to hospital by relatives. Severe cuts and lacerations are among the commonest of such injuries. Occasionally, urgent steps have to be taken to salvage a hand that has been severely deprived of its blood supply by tightly applied manacles. Also, 'iatrogenic' injuries sustained from flogging which is still commonly practised by certain traditional healers, ostensibly to drive evil spirits out of the patient, can lead to body ulcers.

In many developing countries, men are commonly brought to hospital much earlier than women. While this could be because of their greater liability to violence, it may also reflect the cultural attitude that the welfare of males is more important than that of females, mainly because of the male bread-winning role. Married women may be at a greater disadvantage because of the frequent practice of husbands leaving their wife to be cared for by her own family. Indeed, it is not uncommon for such women to be abandoned by their husband if their recovery is delayed. Patients who are brought to hospital very late may, along with a much worse mental condition, have evidence of malnutrition, infection, or both.

In clinical practice, it is still useful to try to establish the presence of one or more first rank symptoms before a diagnosis of schizophrenia is made. While the symptoms are not specific to the illness, being present in about 10% to 15% of patients with affective or organic psychosis, they have been reported in diverse cultural settings and are often demonstrable in about 70% to 80% of patients with the disorder. Also, as earlier pointed out, they could, with sufficient clinical skill, be elicited reliably. In the absence of first rank symptoms, the presence of a syndrome lasting several weeks, of systematised delusions along with hallucinations, or the presence of marked formal thought disorder with evidence of decline in social functioning could be sufficient ground for making the diagnosis once a prominent disturbance of mood is excluded and if there is no evidence of organicity.

Subtypes

Since Kraepelin and Bleuler, schizophrenia has commonly been subtyped into:

1. *Paranoid*: the clinical picture is dominated by the patient's delusions
2. *Hebephrenic or disorganised*: disorders of affect, such as incongruity, together with grossly disorganised thought, and severe loss of social judgement (such as indecent exposure of self) may predominate
3. *Catatonic*: the clinical presentation is characterised by motor abnormalities such as excitement or retardation (slowing of movement), posturing (prolonged maintenance of an unvarying, often abnormal, posture), negativism (doing the opposite of a requested action), catalepsy, and waxy flexibility (a characteristic tone to a limb which can be pliantly moved to a new shape which is then held)
4. *Mixed or undifferentiated*: the patient cannot be fitted into any of the above subtypes.

Simple schizophrenia is often added to these four subtypes. This is characterised by eccentricity and, occasionally, some mild thought disorder but without active psychotic symptoms such as delusions and hallucinations. It is a less reliable diagnosis, particularly as it overlaps with schizotypal personality disorder.

A new way of subtyping the illness has focused on the grouping together of positive or florid symptoms and negative or defect symptoms. According to this, schizophrenia can be divided into two groups: one in which the clinical picture is characterised by delusions, hallucinations and incongruity of affect (discrepancy between emotional display and the content of speech) (Type 1 schizophrenia), and another, characterised by social withdrawal, poverty of speech, affective blunting (diminished non-verbal expressiveness), and loss of volition (Type 2 schizophrenia) (Crow, 1980). This new approach at subtyping the illness has received encouraging research support. Patients with Type 2 illness are more likely to have poor premorbid functioning, cognitive impairment, and to show evidence of structural brain abnormality as demonstrated by enlarged ventricles on computerised tomographic (CT) scans. Such patients also do not respond as quickly or as well to drug treatment. On the other hand, patients with the Type 1 subtype are less likely to have poor premorbid adjustment, and to show cognitive impairment, and usually have normal ventricle volumes. The positive symptoms may reflect excessive dopaminergic transmission in the brain as they tend to respond to drug treatment.

The problems with the negative–positive sub-division of schizophrenia include the fact that many patients cannot be fitted neatly into either of these categories as they have a mixture of both groups of symptoms. There is also evidence that patients who have been ill for a considerable length of time have more negative symptoms, suggesting that these subtypes may not be stable over time.

Schizoaffective disorder

Many patients presenting with symptoms suggestive of schizophrenia have prominent affective symptoms, especially depression. When both groups of symptoms are equally salient, many clinicians make a diagnosis of schizoaffective psychosis (originally a term developed for brief psychoses of good prognosis, but rarely used in this way now). The nosologic status of schizoaffective disorder has been contentious mainly because it depends so much on the clinical boundary of schizophrenia. When schizophrenia is defined narrowly, as is now done in DSM–III–R, it is relatively straightforward to regard patients with prominent affective symptoms at the onset of their illness as having another type of disorder. On the other hand, a broad definition of schizophrenia emphasises the presence of psychotic symptoms and pays less regard to co-existing affective symptoms, thus leaving little room for a schizoaffective category.

Cumulative evidence from various sources suggests that the clinical status of schizoaffective disorder lies somewhere between schizophrenia and affective disorder. Thus, there is evidence that patients with the disorder respond to a combination of neuroleptics and lithium, which is otherwise known as having no significant therapeutic value in schizophrenia. The course of schizoaffective disorder is better than that of schizophrenia but worse than that of affective disorder. The picture is, however, complicated by family studies which suggest that the pattern of the affective component of the illness has some bearing on risks of illness to the family. Thus, schizoaffectives who manifest manic symptoms have similarities with patients suffering from affective disorder while schizoaffectives with depression have a familiar distribution of illness that is close to that of schizophrenics.

Schizotypal personality disorder

Both DSM–III–R and ICD–10 have a diagnostic category by this name. Its phenomenologic similarity to schizophrenia is emphasised by the fact that five of the eight diagnostic criteria listed in DSM–III–R for its diagnosis are very similar to those listed for the prodromal stage of schizophrenia.

Patients with the disorder show a life-long pattern of eccentricity of behaviour, formal thought disorder characterised by woolliness, circumstantiality and over-elaboration, blunted affect, and social aloofness. They may also have paranoid ideas, ideas of reference, and illusions. The clinical picture is, therefore, similar to that observed in patients with negative symptoms of schizophrenia. The presence of active psychotic symptoms at any period in the patient's history precludes this diagnosis and suggests that of schizophrenia.

Differential diagnosis

Symptomatic psychosis

Various infective, neurological, or nutritional deficiency conditions can present with psychosis that may not be readily distinguishable from schizophrenia. The need to exclude such conditions in the differential diagnosis of schizophrenia is of more importance in developing countries where organic causes of psychotic presentation may still be common. Thus, a history of fever, gastrointestinal symptoms, and general malaise must sensitise the clinician to exclude the possibility of psychotic presentation of typhoid fever.

Compared with most developed countries, some developing countries may have as much as a ten-fold prevalence rate of epilepsy, often of the temporal lobe type. It is not uncommon for psychotic experiences of all sorts to form part of the peri-ictal manifestations of temporal lobe epilepsy (see also Chapter 11). A history of episodic psychotic disorder, usually lasting less than a day and of which the patient has no or only vague recollection, is suggestive. It is essential to remember that complex partial seizures do not always become generalised and lead to a loss of consciousness, and that the inter-ictal electro-encephalogram may be normal.

It is also always necessary to exclude the possibility of a drug-induced psychosis (see Chapter 9) as abuse of drugs such as alcohol, khat, amphetamine or arguably cannabis, may lead to acute psychotic episodes mimicking schizophrenia. Many such episodes tend to clear completely within a few days although persistent psychotic states may be triggered in vulnerable individuals.

Acute undifferentiated psychosis

This is a short-lasting psychotic episode commonly precipitated by a stressful event. It has been reported by a number of authors to be particularly common in developing African countries (German, 1972). Patients present with a dramatic psychotic breakdown with no evidence of a prodromal disturbance. Any of the characteristic symptoms of schizophrenia could be present, along with affective symptoms and, commonly, those of disorientation and perplexity. The disorder has been given different names in the past such as bouffée delirante, and acute transient psychosis.

Apart from the sudden onset of this disorder and its rather polymorphous clinical presentation, the only other possible differentiating feature from schizophrenia is its self-limiting course. It is not known what proportion of these patients later develop clearly-defined schizophrenic illness.

Paranoid (delusional) disorder

This is a disorder in which the central psychopathology is the presence of a systematised delusional belief which is commonly persecutory but could also be hypochondriacal or grandiose. It is differentiated from schizophrenia by the lack of auditory hallucinations and typical Schneiderian first rank symptoms.

Affective psychosis

Although affective psychoses may have many symptoms in common with schizophrenia, including the course of the disorder, catatonia and in some cases first rank symptoms, previous history, predominance of the mood disorder, and the presence of biological symptoms usually enable the correct diagnosis to be made. Affective psychoses are discussed further in Chapter 10.

Aetiology

Genetic factors

The most robust aetiological factor associated with schizophrenia is heredity. The observation that schizophrenia sometimes clusters in families is an old one and systematic epidemiological studies conducted in the past three decades or so have confirmed this observation. Thus, the risk of an individual developing the illness is now known to increase with greater consanguinity with a schizophrenic patient. While the lifetime risk for the general population is just under 1%, the risks to relatives increase from about 2% for second degree relatives, 8% for full siblings, 36% for children with both parents affected, to just over 50% for mono-zygotic twins (Tsuang & Vandermey, 1980). Indeed, the genetic contribution to the causation of the illness is firmly established by twin studies. Data from such studies show that while the liability to developing the illness for a co-twin of an affected individual is about 12%, that is, just about the same as that for any other sibling, that for the co-twin of a monozygotic twin pair is much higher. The question as to whether this observation is due to nature or to nurture has been examined by comparing the risk of developing the illness between children who were adopted away from a schizophrenic biological mother with adopted children whose biological mothers were not schizophrenic. The results consistently show a higher risk for the children of schizophrenic mothers (Heston, 1966; Kety *et al*, 1975).

Even though we know that genetic factors contribute a significant proportion of the variance in the liability to schizophrenia, we do not at the present time know the nature of any genetic anomalies. However, the new technologies of molecular genetics and of linkage studies may provide the answer.

Dopamine hypothesis

There are many studies in which the neurobiological features associated with the illness have been investigated. While the number of such features is legion, a few of them stand out for having been replicated by independent workers and also for being present in a substantial proportion of patients with the disorder.

The dopamine hypothesis of schizophrenia posits that the disorder reflects hyperactivity of dopaminergic transmission in the mesolimbic, mesocortical, and nigrostriatal areas of the brain of patients. The hypothesis provides the most robust neurochemical explanation of the illness. Support for it was, however, largely inferential until recently. The hypothesis was based on the observation that patients with the illness benefit from anti-dopaminergic drugs and also that abuse of drugs that stimulate dopamine transmission, such as amphetamine, produce schizophrenia-like psychosis. The new brain imaging technique of positron emission tomography has now been used to provide direct evidence of increased dopamine receptors in parts of the brain of some patients with the illness. Post-mortem neurochemical studies have provided further evidence of increased dopamine receptors (D_2 receptors) in the caudate, putamen, and nucleus accumbens of patients when compared with controls (Mita *et al*, 1986; Hess *et al*, 1987).

The dopamine hypothesis has been less successful in emphasising the efficacy of the newer neuroleptics, and other neurotransmitters such as 5HT may also play a role.

Structural brain damage

Recent neuroimaging techniques have also provided evidence of structural abnormalities in the brains of schizophrenic patients as compared with normal controls. There is now a large number of studies showing that such abnormalities include large cerebral ventricles (both lateral and third), wider sulci, and decreased size of some parts of the brain (Johnstone *et al*, 1976; Weinberger *et al*, 1980; Andreasen *et al*, 1986).

Neuropathological studies of schizophrenia suggest that a substantial proportion of patients with the illness show reduction in the sizes of the amygdala and the hippocampus, thinning of the parahippocampal gyrus, and abnormalities in the distribution of neurons in the frontal and cingulate cortex (Brown *et al*, 1986; Falkai & Bogerts, 1986; Benes & Bird, 1987).

Given the pattern of the risks to family members of affected persons as previously noted, it is obvious that while genetic inheritance is of importance in the causation of the illness, it is by no means the only important factor. This is demonstrated by the concordance rate of about 50% in monozygotic twins. For a totally inheritable disease, we would of course expect this concordance to be 100%, since monozygotic twins have the same genes. It is also the experience of many clinicians treating schizophrenic patients that large numbers of such patients have no identifiable family members with the illness. Consequently, the inference is that certain environmental factors must also be significant.

Viral hypothesis

One influential aetiological hypothesis of schizophrenia suggests that it may be a result of viral infections (Hare, 1979). In effect, a number of studies have shown the link between births of patients with schizophrenia and periods of viral epidemics (Torrey *et al*, 1988; Barr *et al*, 1990). Specifically, a relationship has been noted between the reported cases of diphtheria, pneumonia, measles, polio, zoster varicella, and influenza and the births of schizophrenic patients.

Perinatal brain damage

Another group of environmental factors that have been implicated in the aetiology of schizophrenia relate to pregnancy and birth complications. The observation that a sizeable proportion of patients with schizophrenia have cytoarchitectural abnormalities and reduced cortical thickness without gliosis, both of which could be produced by early brain damage (Kolb *et al*, 1983), is one indication that obstetric complications could be important in the aetiology of the illness. Even more suggestive are the reports of some observers (e.g. Lewis, 1989) that, compared with matched controls, schizophrenics had experienced more frequent and more severe pregnancy and birth complications. Such complications include pre-eclampsia, prolonged labour, and malpresentation. Their association with the disorder cannot be accounted for by differences in social class.

A legitimate question that could be asked about this link is if perinatal injuries are partly responsible for schizophrenia, why do the clinical manifestations begin two decades or so after birth? There are two possible answers. First, there is evidence that some individuals who develop schizophrenia in adult life have commonly shown eccentricity, attentional problems, and other behavioural anomalies in their childhood. That is, schizophrenia may be the end result of a clinical diathesis, the adult manifestation of a disorder that may have shown other atypical manifestations in childhood. Secondly, damage to a specific area in the brain may manifest as different syndromes depending on the age of the victim, i.e. the stage of maturity attained by the brain. So it is possible for the same brain damage to present as an attentional problem in childhood and as schizophrenia in adulthood.

Is the evidence strong enough to regard obstetric complications as a major cause of schizophrenia? Possibly not. First, the link between these complications and the illness is rather weak. The evidence to date suggests an increase in absolute risk of less than 1% for individuals with the worst histories of obstetric complications. Secondly, if these complications were of major significance in the aetiology of the disorder, one would expect countries with a poor obstetric record to have a much higher prevalence of schizophrenia than those with good obstetric care. Present evidence does not provide support for this (Goodman, 1988).

Social and family factors

In the past, the cause of the illness was sought within the context of family and social interactions. The notion that abnormal maternal rearing practices could lead to the later development of schizophrenia, the so-called schizophrenogenic mother hypothesis was put forward by Fromm-Reichman (1948). Another aetiological hypothesis linked the development of the illness to a 'skewed' pattern of relationship in the home such that mothers were the dominant figures while fathers were submissive, or the presence of 'marital schism' in the home where both parents held and expressed contrary views (Lidz & Lidz, 1949). Bateson *et al* (1956) proposed a double-bind theory suggesting that children who were reared in situations in which, for example, they were consistently given conflicting verbal and other cues were more likely to develop the illness. The hypothesis proposed by Wynne & Singer (1963) was probably more susceptible to empirical validation. Using projective tests, these authors described a pattern of communication deviance in the parents of schizophrenic patients characterised by vagueness, looseness, fragmentation, and a lack of closure, and suggested that these abnormalities might in some ways be related to the genesis of the disorder. This observation was later partly replicated by other authors using similar research designs (Hirsch & Leff, 1975). However, rather than being a cause, the observed speech abnormalities appeared to be the effects of having these ill subjects in the families.

These early theories are now largely only of historical significance, not merely because of serious problems with replication and difficulties associated with drawing causal inferences from them, but also because they cannot accommodate some of the features that are commonly associated with schizophrenia. Any aetiological hypothesis of the illness must, for example, be able to accommodate such commonly observed phenomena as the usual age of onset in adolescence or early adulthood, the empirical evidence for an abnormality in dopaminergic transmission in the brains of the patients with the illness, and the association of stress with the onset and course of illness (Weinberger, 1987). Also, such theories must not contradict the well-known clinical and prognostic heterogeneity of the illness.

Expressed emotion

Although it seems unlikely that schizophrenia can be caused by the psychological stress of family life, it is clear that the emotional aspects of relationships between schizophrenic patients and their relatives have important effects on the course of the illness. One of the most influential measures of these family factors, expressed emotion, incorporates hostility, critical comments, and emotional over-involvement by other family members toward the patient. It has been shown that patients are at greater risks of frequent relapse if they live with relatives who are hostile, make critical comments about the patients or are too emotionally involved in the lives of the patients (Vaughn *et al*, 1982). It seems that while identical relationships may exist in developing and developed countries with regard to the overall influence of expressed emotion on relapse (Leff *et al*, 1987), the features of the phenomenon may differ. Thus, a WHO collaborative study showed that even though relatives of Danish and of Indian patients displayed identical levels of hostility, critical comments and emotional over-involvement were less common among Indian relatives (Wig *et al*, 1987).

Life events

It has long been suggested that stress plays a part in the precipitation of the illness. In recent years, this link has been studied by determining the rate of specific adverse life events just before the onset of the illness and comparing the incidence of such events among normal controls. Such studies are bedevilled by serious methodological problems, especially those relating to accurate dating of onset of the illness and deciding whether any life event is a cause or an effect. Possibly as a result of these problems, the results of even the more sophisticated studies are inconsistent (Brown & Birley, 1968; Day *et al*, 1987; Gureje & Adewunmi, 1988). An important observation is that even when investigators have found an increase in the incidence of life events prior to the onset of the illness, such events have often been rather insignificant, ordinary events that would not be regarded as particularly stressful (Brown *et al*, 1978). The implication of this observation is that rather trivial and ordinary life events may be enough to trigger the illness in vulnerable individuals. There is no evidence that life events on their own accord can bring about schizophrenia in individuals who are otherwise not vulnerable.

Drugs

It has already been noted that intoxicated states may mimic schizophrenia, but such episodes resolve as the drug effects wear off. In fact there is surprisingly little by way of empirical studies to suggest that schizophrenia, as it is currently defined, can be caused by abuse of drugs. In particular, the notion that cannabis causes schizophrenia is more anecdotal than supported by hard data (Andreasen *et al*, 1987).

Assessment and treatment of acute episodes

The diagnosis of schizophrenia requires information both about the presenting clinical characteristics of the patient and the previous course of the illness. Complete information can rarely be obtained from the acutely ill patient. Close relatives and friends, especially those who may have had frequent contact with the patient and may therefore be knowledgeable about the beginning of the illness, are important sources of such information. It is necessary to get this information at the first consultation as those accompanying the patient may have to return to distant villages after the patient has been admitted. Questions should be asked about recent changes in behaviour, social interactions, and speech. It is essential to obtain a detailed and objective description of these changes and not to be satisfied with general statements. It is not uncommon to find that insistence on details conflicts with relatives' expectations since, often, they have had no need to provide more than generalities to traditional healers who they may already have consulted. Indeed, there are some linguistic groups that would expect the doctor to be satisfied with their use of euphemisms such as "he has suddenly developed a fever".

While the more obvious manifestations of illness such as aimless wandering, talking to self, dressing inappropriately or bizarrely may be more easily volunteered by relatives, it is more difficult to get them to remember more subtle behavioural changes that may have set in many months before the acute signs. In order to make the clinical diagnosis of schizophrenia, as opposed to that of ill-defined and commonly short-lived acute psychotic episodes, the clinician may have to pose a series of direct questions to the relatives to identify a period of social or occupational decline lasting several weeks or months before the onset of active symptoms. Whenever possible, every item of the history obtained from relatives should be checked with the patient. Even if a denial is the only response of the patient, it is still useful to obtain his or her reaction to these details. Information about what previous remedies, including traditional and religious healing, have been sought should next be obtained. This should be done without any hint of disapproval.

In general, assessment should proceed from a listing of the presenting complaints through an elaboration of these complaints, to past medical history (physical and mental), family history, personal history of the patient (including social and occupational adjustment), details of the premorbid personality, a mental state examination and, finally, a physical examination.

The examination of the mental state should begin with a general description of the patient's appearance and behaviour in the consulting room, including the state of personal hygiene, the appropriateness of dressing and grooming, the general nutritional state, and the patient's acceptance of or hostility to the clinical contact. Evidence of aloofness, social withdrawal, or posturing should be noted. Patients should be asked to describe their subjective mood and the clinician should note their affect. Schizophrenic patients may sometimes show blunted or flat affect, a narrowing or restriction of emotional display, including movement of facial muscles, gesticulations, and inflections in the voice. The speech will also provide clues to the thinking process of the patient. Disorders of the content of thought, especially persecutory or grandiose, and delusions should be sought; disorders of the form of thought should be noted, and examples recorded. Abnormal experiences must be elicited. The commonest of these are auditory hallucinations. Their presence may be suggested by the patient's behaviour but direct questions should also be put to the patient to determine the presence of hallucinatory experience that has not been spontaneously reported. In testing the cognitive functioning of the patient, the clinician should be sensitive to the limitations imposed by illiteracy and the local language. For example, certain languages have no words for months of the year. Also, in testing for the long-term memory of a poorly educated patient, it is more appropriate to ask for the names of five large towns in the region than to ask for dates of historical events.

Workers manning primary health care facilities who are not medically trained would not be expected to conduct this detailed form of examination on patients. For such workers, it is enough to be able to recognise or elicit a few psychotic features and to limit their impression to this. They should be competent and equipped to administer oral or intramuscular sedating neuroleptic when necessary and thereafter make a referral.

A common clinical observation which is supported by some research evidence is that more patients are brought to treatment in developing than in developed countries on the basis of fears or actual threats of violence, attempted suicide and self-injury (Sartorius *et al*, 1986). Many such patients are brought to the clinic with their hands and feet tied by relatives. It is to be expected that such patients will be hostile and aggressive when so physically restrained even if they were not before such treatment. Patients may have been subjected to various forms of physical abuse while undergoing traditional treatment. Apart from the medical urgency of relieving a pair of swollen and painful wrists or ankles that could be in danger of necrosis, there is also the need to gain the cooperation and confidence of the patient if any meaningful assessment is to take place.

In deciding on how to proceed in unchaining a manacled patient, the clinician should also be mindful of his own safety. It is best to ensure that the patient has no access to dangerous weapons, that means of self-defence are available (for example, the presence of male clinical assistants), and that, if need be, rapid parenteral sedative can be administered. Engaging patients in discussion allows the clinician to reassure them and ascertain how likely they are to remain calm once unchained. Simply removing the physical restraints without taking these precautions is dangerous. The clinician should appear calm and confident, listen to his patients, and try to reassure them that they are now in a place where no harm can come to them. Relatives about whom the patient is suspicious should be politely asked to leave the immediate vicinity. If discussion is totally impossible and the patient is persistently verbally threatening, he should be sedated immediately and then set free. In this case, interview may only be possible much later, possibly after a day or two following admission, although a physical examination should be conducted as soon as possible.

Treatment

Physical treatment (see also Chapter 6)

The treatment of an acute episode of schizophrenia may have to commence with the sedation of the aggressive or agitated patient. Depending on the urgency of the situation, it may be necessary to administer such sedating drugs parenterally. Chlorpromazine is the drug of choice for achieving this end. It is given in initial doses of about 25 mg or 50 mg, depending on the weight of the patient, every 6 to 8 hours. However, chlorpromazine given parenterally may cause acute hypotension and the patient's blood pressure should be checked before repeat doses are given. It is sometimes necessary to combine it with a benzodiazepine in order to bring about rapid sedation. Lorazepam is an effective sedating anxiolytic and an intramuscular injection of 2 mg will normally be enough to sedate an adult patient. Diazepam can also be used; however, it takes longer to act except when given intravenously and in doses of 0.1 to 0.2 mg per kilogram body weight. It is also an irritant.

Patients who are very disturbed, aggressive or hostile to relatives will often have to be admitted to hospital. However, the clinician working in a developing country is sometimes restricted by limited admission facilities or inability of relations to afford the costs of admission. When patients cannot be admitted, it is essential that arrangements be made to see them frequently, especially at the beginning of treatment with neuroleptic drugs and when they are still disturbed by active psychotic symptoms. Compliance with treatment is also more likely if patient and relatives are warned at the beginning about possible side-effects of medication and that recovery is likely to be gradual.

Whether the patient is admitted or not, regular treatment should be instituted with any available neuroleptic. Chlorpromazine or thioridazine are available in most drug cupboards and either of these is a useful drug to start with. The patient should be commenced on 75 mg per day of either drug in divided doses. This should be increased as necessary, to a maximum of 600 mg per day. Only very few patients will need more than this level of medication and, for such patients, it could be that a more potent but less sedating neuroleptic will be needed. Trifluoperazine and haloperidol are two such drugs commonly available.

In order to avoid unnecessary polypharmacy, most clinicians would not prescribe anti-Parkinsonian drugs routinely for admitted patients but would rather treat any drug reactions as they emerge. This good clinical practice may however be impractical when patients are not admitted and have to return to places where immediate recourse to medical personnel may be impossible. The usual anti-Parkinsonian drugs are benzhexol, biperiden, orphenadine, procyclidine or benztropine. Oral benzhexol at a dose of 5 mg per day may be necessary as prophylaxis against the more frightening drug reactions such as acute dystonia and akinesia. Patients who are not on prophylaxis and who develop such reactions will gain rapid relief with parenteral benztropine, biperiden, or procyclidine.

Once the patient has recovered from the acute episode, the clinician should begin a gradual, progressive reduction of medication. The dosage of the maintenance medication will have to be decided on the basis of the clinical history, the rapidity of the recovery from active psychosis, and the degree of recovery. However, it is common to maintain patients on about one-third to one-half of the dosage necessary for the treatment of the acute phase. While all schizophrenic patients should have this initial maintenance medication, possibly about 15–20% can expect to be completely weaned off medication within six to twelve months of recovery. While there are some features that are associated with good prognosis, it is rarely possible to make an *a priori* decision about who is not in need of long-term drug treatment. The clinician often has to make the decision about drug discontinuation as time goes on. It is, however, essential that patients who are not in need of prolonged medication should be recognised early so as to minimise the risks of developing tardive dyskinesia.

Compliance with maintenance medication will be enhanced if patients do not have to travel long distances for follow-up assessments. It is thus best that primary health care facilities at village level be manned by personnel who have received some training in the follow-up assessment and can make appropriate decisions about referral when signs of imminent relapse are detected or patients begin to show evidence of drug reactions. It is not necessary that such facilities stock every drug that may be prescribed for patients. It is enough for them to be able to accept patients' supplies for safe keeping and monitor compliance. The personnel at such centres should also be able to administer intramuscular depot injections.

Depot injections of neuroleptics provide another way of improving compliance with maintenance medication. Many patients prefer this method because it takes away the necessity for daily oral drugs. While depot injections are very useful in the long-term treatment of the schizophrenic patient, high costs sometimes preclude their widespread use in developing countries. This, and their tendency to cause tardive dyskinesia make it essential that only patients who are poorly compliant should be placed on depot drugs. The two commonly available depot drugs are fluphenazine decanoate and flupenthixol decanoate.

Adverse drug reactions, particularly tardive dyskinesia, should be continually monitored in the follow-up clinic. Even though tardive dyskinesia affects a minority of patients after prolonged use of neuroleptics, it is important to bear in mind that, in a few patients, it can develop after a relatively short period on medication (Gureje, 1989). Patients who develop the more severe forms of the disorder may suffer serious social handicap in developing countries where supernatural explanations may be proffered for the disability. Detection of the problem during its early stages should lead to immediate review of the clinical need for neuroleptic medication. Even if a permanent withdrawal is not feasible, a dose reduction or a temporary drug holiday may provide some benefit. While there is no cure for established tardive dyskinesia, there is some evidence that early signs may be reversible.

Electroconvulsive therapy (ECT) remains a useful form of treatment of the acute forms of schizophrenia (Taylor & Fleminger, 1980; Abraham & Kulhara, 1987). It certainly is a handy and effective intervention in settings where admission facilities are very limited and the acutely ill patients cannot be relied on to comply with regular medication use. There is some evidence that it has a slight advantage over neuroleptic drugs in the control of the illness in the first few weeks of an acute episode even though, after this early stage of the illness, there is no demonstrable difference between the two treatment approaches. ECT is particularly useful in the management of the catatonic form of the illness which is still relatively common in many developing countries. Many patients for whom this form of treatment is indicated will need an average of six exposures even though improvement is often apparent after the first two or so, particularly in the more severe cases of catatonia. Other than those side-effects relating to the mode of administration, and a short-lived memory impairment, ECT is a safe form of treatment. In particular, there is no evidence linking it with structural brain damage or with the development of epilepsy.

Psychosocial treatment

It is now fairly well established that the course of the illness is influenced significantly by the emotional reactions of relatives or carers with whom the patient lives (Leff *et al*, 1987). Family interventions which reduce relatives' expressed emotion also reduce the relapse rate (Leff *et al*, 1982). It is, therefore, good practice for the clinician to conduct a few educational sessions with the family as soon as the patient begins to recover. Such sessions should be geared towards demystifying the illness by explaining to relatives that it is an illness just like any other, removing any suspicion they may hold that certain people are responsible for the patient's illness, and educating them about how their interactions with the patient may affect the course of the illness. In many traditional societies in the developing world, mental illness is regarded as resulting from a curse or poisoning by enemies, especially if no one in the patient's immediate family suffers from a similar illness. Such beliefs may sometimes discourage compliance with medical treatment.

A substantial minority of schizophrenic patients will derive little or no benefit from regular maintenance medication. Such patients tend to acquire negative symptoms and to deteriorate in personality and intellect. Many of these patients are abandoned by relatives and, in developing countries with no social policies designed to take care of them, they become vagrants.

Vagrants are also seen in developed countries. Vagrant psychotics are commonly poorly clad, malnourished, and suffering from debilitating medical illnesses. They are also frequently physically abused or ridiculed either for amusement or because they behave inappropriately to members of the public. In general, they are perceived by the public as evidence that mental illness is incurable. Their care requires an enlightened political leadership informed by those trained in the care of the mentally ill. The social and moral benefits of providing decent long-stay wards for individuals who may never be economically productive again are often difficult for policy makers to see. Helping them to appreciate such benefits can lead to dramatic improvement in the condition of these patients.

Outcome

Schizophrenia is a disorder with widely varying evolution and outcome (Ciompi, 1988). The old view regarding it as an illness with uniformly deteriorating prognosis has now been shown to be incorrect by the results of a number of follow-up investigations. These studies have shown that, whichever set of criteria is used for the selection of the patients and whatever sort of outcome is investigated, any large group of schizophrenic patients will show heterogeneous outcome (Kulhara & Chandiramani, 1988).

There is some evidence that the illness may have a better short-term outcome in developing than in developed industrialised countries. This evidence has come principally from the results of a WHO collaborative study in which the two-year outcome of the illness was compared in ten countries, three of them developing (Sartorius *et al*, 1986). The investigators studied unselected patient samples from all the centres but analysed the outcome data for seven developed and two developing countries. They reported a significantly higher proportion of patients with a mild two-year clinical outcome in the developing countries as compared with the developed countries, while the reverse was true for the proportion of patients with severe outcome characterised by unremitting psychotic illness, or incomplete remissions during which conspicuous personality changes had occurred. Identical proportions of patients fell in the intermediate outcome groups from both settings.

The WHO diagnosis was made using the Present State Examination (Wing *et al*, 1974) and derived from the computer-based (CATEGO) and ICD–9 classifications. Since these classifications do not take duration of illness into consideration, it has been argued that the results reported might have been influenced by the inclusion of commonly-occurring brief psychoses in the patient samples in the developing countries (Stevens, 1987). Thus, it remains to be seen whether this differential outcome between developing and developed countries will also be observed if patients are selected using DSM–III–R, DSM–IV or ICD–10 criteria.

The long-term outcome of the illness, even though rather complex and highly varied, could be simplified thus: 25% will recover completely; 30% will have minor residual symptoms or infrequent relapses and be able to achieve a career and raise families; 35% will have moderate symptoms or frequent relapses and, even though able to live in the community and be economically productive, will be unable to function at anything near their premorbid capability; while 10% will deteriorate into severe chronicity with seriously incapacitating disorders of thinking, speaking, and volition.

While it is often difficult to predict accurately how the illness of a particular patient will evolve, there are nevertheless a few generally accepted statistical predictors for a better outcome. Better recovery is more likely among patients who have more stable premorbid personality, acute onset of illness, positive symptoms, and a quick response to initial treatment. There is strong evidence that stress affects the course of the illness. In particular, patients who live with supportive and accepting relations do better than those living with relations given to critical and hostile comments about them (Leff *et al*, 1987).

References

ABRAHAM, K. R. & KULHARA, P. (1987) The efficacy of electroconvulsive therapy in the treatment of schizophrenia: a comparative study. *British Journal of Psychiatry*, **151**, 152–155.

AMERICAN PSYCHIATRIC ASSOCIATION (1980) *Diagnostic and Statistical Manual of Mental Disorders* (3rd edn). Washington, DC: American Psychiatric Association.

—— (1987) *Diagnostic and Statistical Manual of Mental Disorders* (3rd edn, revised) (DSM–III–R). Washington, DC: APA.

—— (1994) *Diagnostic and Statistical Manual of Mental Disorders* (4th edn) (DSM–IV). Washington, DC: APA.

ANDREASEN, N. C., NASRALLAH, H. A., DUNN, V., *et al* (1986) Structural abnormalities in the frontal system in schizophrenia: a magnetic resonance imaging study. *Archives of General Psychiatry*, **43**, 136–144.

——, ALLEBECK, P., ENGSTROM, A., *et al* (1987) Cannabis and schizophrenia: a longitudinal study of Swedish conscripts. *Lancet*, **2**, 1483–1486.

BARR, C. E., MWNDNICK, S. A. & MUNK-JORGENSEN, P. (1990) Exposure to influenza epidemics during gestation and adult schizophrenia: a 40-year study. *Archives of General Psychiatry*, **47**, 869–874.

BATESON, G., JACKSON, D., HALEY, J., *et al* (1956) Towards a theory of schizophrenia. *Behavioral Science*, **1**, 251–264.

BENES, F. M. & BIRD, E. D. (1987) An analysis of the arrangement of neurons in the cingulate cortex of schizophrenic patients. *Archives of General Psychiatry*, **44**, 608–615.

BROWN, G. W. & BIRLEY, J. L. T. (1968) Crises and life changes and the onset of schizophrenia. *Journal of Health and Social Behaviour*, **9**, 203–214.

——, SKAIR, F., HARRIS, T., *et al* (1978) Life events and psychiatric disorders. I: some methodological issues. *Psychological Medicine*, **3**, 74–87.

BROWN, R., COLTER, N., CORSELLIS, J. A. N., *et al* (1986) Postmortem evidence of structural brain changes in schizophrenia. *Archives of General Psychiatry*, **43**, 36–42.

CIOMPI, L. (1988) Learning from outcome studies: towards a comprehensive biological-psychosocial understanding of schizophrenia. *Schizophrenia Research*, **1**, 373–384.

COOPER, J. E., KENDELL, R. E., GURLAND, B. J., *et al* (1972) *Psychiatric Diagnosis in New York and London.* Maudsley Monograph No. 20. London: Oxford University Press.

CROW, T. J. (1980) Molecular pathology of schizophrenia: more than one disease process? *British Medical Journal*, **280**, 66–68.

DAY, R., NIELSEN, J. A., KORTEN, A., *et al* (1987) Stressful life events preceding the acute onset of schizophrenia: a cross-national study from the World Health Organization. *Culture, Medicine and Psychiatry*, **11**, 123–205.

EAGLES, J. M. (1991) Is schizophrenia disappearing? *British Journal of Psychiatry*, **158**, 834–835.

FALKAI, P. & BOGERTS, B. (1986) Cell loss in the hippocampus of schizophrenics. *European Archives of Psychiatry and Neurological Sciences*, **236**, 154–161.

FEIGHNER, J. P., ROBINS, E., GUZE, S. B., *et al* (1972) Diagnostic criteria for use in psychiatric research. *Archives of General Psychiatry*, **26**, 57–63.

FROMM-REICHMAN, F. (1948) Notes on the development of treatment of schizophrenia by psycho-analytic psychotherapy. *Psychiatry*, **11**, 263–273.

GERMAN, G. A. (1972) Aspects of clinical psychiatry in sub-Saharan Africa. *British Journal of Psychiatry*, **121**, 461–479.

GOODMAN, R. (1988) Are complications of pregnancy and birth causes of schizophrenia? *Developmental Medicine and Child Neurology,* **30,** 391–406.

GUREJE, O. (1989) The significance of subtyping tardive dyskinesia: a study of prevalence and associated factors. *Psychological Medicine,* **19,** 121–128.

—— (1991) Gender and schizophrenia: age at onset and sociodemographic attributes. *Acta Psychiatrica Scandinavica,* **83,** 402–405.

—— & ADEWUNMI, A. (1988) Life events and schizophrenia in Nigerians: a controlled investigation. *British Journal of Psychiatry,* **153,** 367–375.

HARE, E. H. (1979) (Comments) Schizophrenia as an infectious disease. *British Journal of Psychiatry,* **135,** 468–470.

HESS, E. J., BRACHA, H. S., KLEINMAN, J. E. & CREESE, I. (1987) Dopamine receptor subtype imbalance in schizophrenia. *Life Sciences,* **40,** 1487–1497.

HESTON, L. L. (1966) Psychiatric disorders in foster home reared children of schizophrenic mothers. *British Journal of Psychiatry,* **112,** 819–825.

HIRSCH, S. R. & LEFF, J. (1975) *Abnormalities in Parents of Schizophrenics.* Maudsley Monograph No. 22. London: Oxford University Press.

JOHNSTONE, E. C., CROW, T. J., FRITH, C. D., *et al* (1976) Cerebral ventricular size and cognitive impairment in chronic schizophrenia. *Lancet,* **ii,** 924–926.

KETY, S. S., ROSENTHAL, D., WENDER, P. H., *et al* (1975) Mental illness in the biological and adoptive families of adopted individuals who have become schizophrenic. In *Genetic Research in Psychiatry* (eds R. Fieve, D. Rosenthal & H. Brill), pp. 147–165. Baltimore: Johns Hopkins University Press.

KOLB, B., SUTHERLAND, R. J. & WHISHAW, I. Q. (1983) Abnormalities in cortical and subcortical morphology after neonatal lesions in rats. *Experimental Neurology,* **79,** 223–244.

KULHARA, P. & CHANDIRAMANI, K. (1988) Outcome of schizophrenia in India using various diagnostic systems. *Schizophrenia Research,* **1,** 339–349.

LEFF, J. P., KUIPERS, L., BERKOWITZ, R., *et al* (1982) A controlled trial of social intervention in families of schizophrenic patients. *British Journal of Psychiatry,* **141,** 121–134.

——, WIG, N. N., GHOSH, A., *et al* (1987) Expressed emotion and schizophrenia in North India III. Influenza of relatives' expressed emotion on the course of schizophrenia in Chandigarh. *British Journal of Psychiatry,* **151,** 166–173.

LEWIS, S. W. (1989) Congenital risk factors for schizophrenia. *Psychological Medicine,* **19,** 5–13.

LIDZ, R. W. & LIDZ, T. (1949) The family environment of schizophrenic patients. *American Journal of Psychiatry,* **106,** 332–345.

MANN, S., CAROFF, S. & BLEIER, H., *et al* (1986) Lethal catatonia. *American Journal of Psychiatry,* **143,** 1374–1381.

MITA, T., HANADA, S., NISHINO, N., *et al* (1986) Decreased serotonin S2 and increased dopamine D2 receptors in chronic schizophrenics. *Biological Psychiatry,* **21,** 1407–1414.

SARTORIUS, N., JABLENSKY, A., KAORTEN, A., *et al* (1986) Early manifestations and first-contact incidence of schizophrenia in different cultures. *Psychological Medicine,* **16,** 909–928.

SPITZER, R. L., ENDICOTT, J. & ROBINS, E. (1978) Research diagnostic criteria: rationale and reliability. *Archives of General Psychiatry,* **35,** 773–782.

STEVENS, J. (1987) Brief psychoses: do they contribute to the good prognosis and equal prevalence of schizophrenia in developing countries? *British Journal of Psychiatry,* **151,** 393–396.

TAYLOR, P. J. & FLEMINGER, J. J. (1980) ECT for schizophrenia. *Lancet,* **i,** 1380–1382.

TORREY, E. F. (1987) Prevalence studies of schizophrenia. *British Journal of Psychiatry,* **150,** 598–608.

——, RAWLINGS, R. & WALDMAN, I. N. (1988) Schizophrenic births and viral diseases in two states. *Schizophrenia Research,* **1,** 73–77.

TSUANG, M. T. & VANDERMEY, R. (1980) *Genes and the Mind.* Oxford: Oxford University Press.

VAUGHN, C. E., SNYDER, K. P. & FREEMAN, W. B. (1982) Family factors in schizophrenic relapse: a replication. *Schizophrenia Bulletin,* **8,** 425–426.

WEINBERGER, D. R. (1987) Implications of normal brain development for the pathogenesis of schizophrenia. *Archives of General Psychiatry,* **44,** 660–669.

——, BIGELOW, L. B., KLEINMAN, J. E., *et al* (1980) Cerebral ventricular enlargement in chronic schizophrenia: an association with poor response to therapy. *Archives of General Psychiatry,* **37,** 11–13.

WIG, N. N., MENON, D. K., BEDI, H., *et al* (1987) Expressed emotion and schizophrenia in North India II. Distribution of expressed emotion components among relatives of schizophrenia in Aarhus and Chandigarh. *British Journal of Psychiatry,* **151,** 156–173.

WING, J. K., COOPER, J. E. & SARTORIUS, N. (1974) *Measurement and Classification of Psychiatric Symptoms.* Cambridge: Cambridge University Press.

WORLD HEALTH ORGANIZATION (1973) *Report of the International Pilot Study of Schizophrenia*, Vol. 1. Geneva: WHO.
——— (1978) *Mental Disorders: Glossary and Guide to their Classification in Accordance with the Ninth Revision of the International Classification of Diseases* (ICD–9). Geneva: WHO.
——— (1992) *The Tenth Revision of the International Classification of Diseases and Related Health Problems* (ICD–10). Geneva: WHO.
WYNNE, L. C. & SINGER, M. T. (1963) Thought disorder and family relationships of schizophrenics II. A classification of forms of thinking. *Archives of General Psychiatry,* **9**, 199–206.

8 Organic brain syndrome

S. K. KHANDELWAL

Mental disorders are no less common in the developing world than in the so-called developed world yet mental health still occupies a position of low priority. Although there are reasons to believe that this picture is changing, research into organic psychiatry or organic mental disorders is still limited, with publications usually confined to the local journals and unavailable outside their country of origin.

Organic brain syndrome (OBS), or mental disorder, includes those psychiatric disorders that are caused by cerebral disorder or dysfunction. In the context of the *Tenth Revision of the International Classification of Diseases and Related Health Problems* (ICD–10; WHO, 1992), the term 'organic' simply means that a syndrome so classified can be attributed to an independently diagnosable cerebral or systemic disease. ICD–10 has also used the term 'symptomatic' to refer to those organic mental disorders in which cerebral involvement is secondary to a systemic, extracerebral disease (see Table 8.1).

Classification of organic brain syndrome

The modern period of descriptive psychiatry for organic brain disorders started with the French school (Horvath *et al*, 1989). Pinel and Esquirol described senile dementia in the 19th century and Bayle described dementia paralytica and its association with inflammation of the meninges, leading to a full patho-physiological description of neurosyphilis. The French school also described the mental state of confusion characterised by disorganisation of thought processes, memory and perception, and disorientation. It became a widely held belief that all psychiatric diseases were brain diseases and that every physical disease produced a characteristic mental picture.

In 1910, the German psychiatrist Bonhoeffer proposed the modern views that all acute medical and brain diseases may present with overlapping and non-specific mental syndromes: delirium, excitement, twilight states, hallucinosis and incoherent thinking. Eugen Bleuler (1924) described chronic organic psycho-syndrome characterised by impaired intellectual skills, emotional lability and

TABLE 8.1
Classification of organic, including symptomatic, mental disorders according to ICD–10 (WHO, 1992)

F00	Dementia in Alzheimer's disease
F01	Vascular dementia
F02	Dementia in other diseases classified elsewhere
F02.0	Dementia in Pick's disease
F02.1	Dementia in Creutzfeldt–Jakob disease
F02.2	Dementia in Huntington's disease
F02.3	Dementia in Parkinson's disease
F02.4	Dementia in HIV disease
F03	Dementia not otherwise specified
F04	Organic amnesic syndrome, not induced by alcohol and other psychotic substances
F05	Delirium, other than by drugs or alcohol
F06	Mental disorders, not involving cognitive impairment due to brain disease, damage or dysfunction, or to physical disease
F06.0	Organic hallucinosis
F06.1	Organic catatonic disorder
F06.2	Organic delusional disorder
F06.3	Organic affective disorders
F06.4	Organic anxiety disorder
F06.5	Organic dissociative disorder
F06.6	Organic emotionally labile (asthenic) disorder
F07	Personality and behavioural disorders due to brain disease, damage or dysfunction
F07.0	Organic personality disorder
F07.1	Postencephalitic syndrome
F07.2	Postconcussional syndrome

Adapted from ICD–10. Copyright with World Health Organization (1992). Reproduced with permission.

poor impulse control and associated it with generalised cortical damage. Manfred Bleuler (1951) described focal psychosyndromes, associating local brain lesions, for example brain tumours, with changes in emotional responses and impulse controls.

However, it was following the introduction of DSM–III (American Psychiatric Association, 1980) that the classification of organic psychiatric syndromes recorded a revolutionary change with clear and operationally defined diagnostic criteria (Lipowski, 1980a, 1984).

ICD–10 has adopted a modified version of DSM–IV (APA, 1994) to extend the concepts of organic disorders to include disorders with cognitive impairment but with other psychological symptoms (Table 8.1).

In developing countries where malnutrition, infectious disease and epilepsy are widely prevalent, it is quite common to see different kinds of acute and chronic mental disorders without clear disorientation or confusion (Wig, 1983). These cases often received labels like 'typhoid psychosis' or 'malaria psychosis' rather than the symptomatic diagnosis of schizophrenia (Wig, 1990). With the new classifications of organic psychiatric conditions, it is now possible to classify such mental and behavioural disorders associated with a wide range of physical conditions.

Epidemiology of organic psychiatric syndromes in the developing countries

A large number of epidemiological studies have appeared from the developing countries in the last 30 years (see Giel & Harding, 1976; Orley & Wing, 1979; Wig, 1981; German, 1987*a,b*) to highlight the prevalence of mental health problems in these countries. However, there are a number of methodological issues which need a brief consideration before specifics of epidemiology of organic syndromes are considered. First, many of these studies were conducted on specific population groups (mental hospital in-patients, patients attending general hospital psychiatric units, urban or rural communities, specific religious or ethnic groups). Second, a large number of such studies have addressed chiefly the overall prevalence of mental disorders in the community or paid special attention to more common disorders like schizophrenia or depression for whose detection clear criteria were used, while scant attention was paid to the detection of organic disorders. In fact, many of the studies have not even mentioned these disorders nor made explicit the criteria used for their detection. Third, there is often inconsistency in the terms used to describe organic disorders: e.g. 'organic brain syndrome', 'organic psychosis', or 'organic reactions'. Fourth, cases of epilepsy have been included in the prevalence figures of some studies and excluded in others. Finally, since the earlier concept of OBS was identified mainly with a psychotic picture, mild or non-psychotic cases were excluded. In addition, many studies have appeared in local journals often in a language other than English, as in the case of studies from Latin America. Various epidemiological studies from India have found prevalence rates of organic conditions in the range of 0.85 to 5.5 per 1000 population (Dube, 1970; Verghese *et al*, 1973; Sethi *et al*, 1974; Thacore *et al*, 1975), while others (Sethi *et al*, 1967; Elnagar *et al*, 1971) do not report even a single case. Hospital- or community-based studies from Africa have also paid little attention to the rate of OBS.

Delirium

The syndrome of delirium, as we understand it now, is referred to by a number of different names in textbooks of medicine and psychiatry, e.g. acute brain syndrome, acute confusional state, acute OBS, acute organic psychosis, acute psycho-organic syndrome. Though still used very commonly, these terms are unsatisfactory for the reasons discussed earlier.

The term 'delirium' has been used in many different ways since its first appearance as early as the first century AD. During the 19th century, delirium was described as a clinical syndrome associated with organic pathology (delirium tremens and alcoholism; Wernicke's encephalopathy), disturbed consciousness and other psychological symptoms (Berrios, 1981). Bonhoeffer described five clinical varieties of acute exogenous reactions associated with physical illness: delirium, epileptic excitement, twilight state, hallucinosis and amentia (Berrios, 1981). Wolff & Curran (1935) studied these phenomena in detail and noted that impaired consciousness and cognition were cardinal features of the syndrome.

They also pointed to a wide variety of accompanying mood and behavioural disturbances. Engel & Romano (1959) validated their work emphasising the presence of cognitive impairment and diffusely slow electroencephalogram as the universal features of delirium.

The present day classifications use and define delirium much more specifically and broadly. ICD–10 defines it as an aetiologically non-specific syndrome, characterised by concurrent disturbances of consciousness and attention, perception, thinking, memory, psychomotor behaviour, emotion and the sleep-wake cycle.

Epidemiology

The precise estimates of prevalence of delirium are difficult to obtain owing to its varied manifestations and severity, poor recognition by clinicians and psychiatrists, its association with a physical disorder whose severity determines the priority for management, and its variable course which may rapidly lead to stupor, coma, or to complete resolution of symptoms. Still, delirium is probably the most commonly occurring mental disorder. The prevalence in the community is likely to be dependent on the medical epidemiology of the community. In developing countries with high rates of infectious diseases and a large proportion of young population (as much as 40% below the age of 15 years), the incidence of delirium is likely to be very high since the very young are especially susceptible to delirium precipitated by even minor physical illnesses. Similarly, the elderly are susceptible to episodes of delirium. It is estimated that 10–15% of medical-surgical patients and up to 50% of geriatric patients meet the criteria for delirium at some time during hospitalisation (Beresin, 1983). The onset of delirium during the course of a medical illness is likely to double the rate of morbidity and mortality (Rabins & Folstein, 1982; Horvath *et al*, 1989).

Clinical features

The clinical picture of delirium follows a fairly constant pattern despite varied aetiology. Brain function is disrupted by biochemical, metabolic, electrical or mechanical disturbances. Some variability, though small in relative terms, is seen in symptomatology depending upon the rate of progression, the intensity and nature of the noxious agent, and the personality and background of the patient (Lishman, 1987).

Impairment of consciousness is the primary change in delirium and it is important to recognise it even when it is mild, when it may not be the most obvious symptom. It may vary from a barely perceptible dulling of consciousness to profound coma. When mild, cognitive processes (attention, concentration, thoughts, perception and memory) are impaired in association with reduced awareness of the environment. The patient is easily distracted and responses are slow and indiscriminate. With more severe degrees of impairment, attention is hard to arouse, ill-sustained and poorly focused (Lishman, 1987). The patient is drowsy and sleeps excessively, which in extreme cases may progress to profound coma. Impairment of consciousness and its associated features are usually worse at night or may fluctuate from day to day.

The patient's spontaneous and purposeful activities show gradual decline and may become slow, purposeless and perseverative. Responses to external stimuli become apathetic or simply automatic. At times there may be restlessness, hyperactivity and excitement with excessive tendency towards startle reactions. In such cases, the behaviour may be directed by delusions and hallucinations. Thus, the patient's behaviour may show two types of presentation: overactivity with psychotic features, or lethargy and somnolence (Lipowski, 1980b). Thinking becomes slow, less logical and incoherent. Excessive talking and rambling, irrelevant or incoherent speech may indicate disorganised thinking. Ideas of reference and persecution are common, fragmentary and transient.

Quite commonly it is the more florid perceptual abnormalities which draw attention to the presence of delirium in patients suffering from some physical disease (Lishman, 1987). In delirium the visual modality is most affected. Misinterpretations, illusions and hallucinations are very common but are usually fleeting and changeable. Abnormal visual perceptions combined with faulty thinking and memory lead to disorientation in place. Tactile and auditory hallucinations also occur, though less commonly.

The stress of physical illness, cognitive impairments and the patient's premorbid personality may bring affective changes. Mood is usually labile, and depression, anxiety, irritability, fear, hostility and suspiciousness are frequent. Some patients may be euphoric or perplexed. Gradually the affect becomes shallow and apathetic.

Orientation and memory disturbances are common and may be among the earlier manifestations of delirium to attract attention. Due to defects in attention, comprehension, new learning and perception, there are disturbances of registration, retention and recall. All this results in disturbances such as disorientation in time and place, misidentification, confabulation and amnesia on recovery.

Abnormal signs in physical and neurological examinations are common, though gross neurological abnormalities are rarely encountered in patients with diffuse cerebral impairment. Thus abnormal involuntary movements such as tremors, impaired coordination, dysphasia, urinary incontinence, focal neurological signs, autonomic nervous system dysfunction and seizures are frequently encountered on careful examination. These associated features tend to be seen more commonly in elderly patients with delirium than in younger patients (Liston, 1982).

Aetiology

Virtually any illness or disease may be causally associated with the development of delirium, although in many instances the specific aetiology is never elucidated (Wells, 1985). Some of the common causes of delirium are presented in Table 8.2. Predisposing factors include chronic illness, extremes of age, structural brain disease, multiple medications, drug and alcohol abuse, loss of sensory modalities, sleep deprivation, fatigue, weakened psychological defence mechanisms, social isolation and unfamiliar environment (Liston, 1982, 1984). In developing countries, infectious and communicable diseases may be among the front-line illnesses as the potential causes for organic psychiatric conditions. Jilek &

TABLE 8.2
Common causes of delirium

1. Central nervous system disorders
    Head injury
    Tumours and subdural haematoma, cerebral abscess
    Degenerative diseases
    Vascular diseases: subarachnoid haemorrhage, thrombosis embolism
    Infections: meningitis, encephalitis, AIDS encephalopathy
    Epilepsy
2. Metabolic disorders
    Uraemia
    Hepatic failure
    Pulmonary failure
    Cardiac failure
    Electrolyte imbalance
3. Endocrine disorders
    Thyrotoxicosis
    Cushing's disease, Addison's disease
    Hypoglycaemia
4. Nutritional and vitamin deficiencies
    Anaemia
    Thiamine deficiency
    Nicotinic acid deficiency
    B_{12} deficiency
5. Systemic infections
    Pneumonia
    Septicaemia
    Exanthemata
6. Toxic causes
    Drug intoxications: anticholinergics, hypno-sedatives
    Alcohol
    Heavy metals

Jilek-Aall (1970), on reviewing many studies from Africa, list the following conditions in order of their relative aetiological importance: trypanosomiasis, cerebral malaria, syphilis, pulmonary infections, bilharziasis, amoebic dysentery, general malnutrition, drug intoxication, helminthic infestations, and climatic effects (heat stroke, rapid dehydration). Often multiple pathologies are present. The resulting clinical picture does not appear to differ in any essential way from the classical description of acute brain syndromes OBS.

Differential diagnosis

The most crucial aspect of the differential diagnosis of delirium is to differentiate it from functional mental disorders. The essential features of delirium (reduced ability to maintain attention to external stimuli and to shift attention appropriately to new external stimuli; disorganised thinking as manifested by rambling; irrelevant and incoherent speech) should be helpful in this differentiation, yet at times, psychotic disorders like schizophrenia may present a diagnostic problem. In delirium, symptoms like hallucinations and delusions are random and haphazard, without evidence of systematisation (American Psychiatric Association, 1994).

Occasionally, depressive symptoms, common in both depressive as well as organic disorders, may pose a problem. Dementia, a major predisposing factor for delirium, is also one of the most important conditions to be differentiated from it. Often the two conditions coexist and it may be difficult to assess the contribution of each disorder to the overall clinical picture. Normally, in dementia the patient remains alert, while delirium produces more florid symptoms.

Careful evaluation of the history, mental status and cognitive functions, and physical examination will usually uncover evidence of delirium. In doubtful cases, serial electroencephalograms showing slowing and disorganisation of alpha-frequency activity may point towards a diagnosis of delirium. Other investigations as listed in Table 8.5 may prove useful in detecting underlying causes of delirium.

Treatment

A patient with confirmed or suspected delirium is best treated in a hospital setting. The fundamental principle in the treatment remains the identification and correction of the underlying physical cause. However, a life-threatening delirium may require therapeutic intervention even before the diagnosis of the underlying cause is established. Maintenance of vital functions and good nursing care can largely reduce morbidity and mortality. The patient's anxiety and agitation must be properly handled by providing rational explanations of his condition to him as well as his family members. The patient should be nursed in a quiet, well lit room without extremes of sensory stimulation. It is important to reduce misidentification and disorientation by having a relative and familiar objects present and by frequent but not excessive attempts towards reorientation.

Medication

Since the patient may be already receiving drugs for the primary physical disorder, it is important to give as few drugs as possible as all psychotropic drugs may interfere with vital functions and level of consciousness. However, drugs may be essential in excited, agitated, hostile, insomniac or psychotic patients. Chlorpromazine and other phenothiazines are widely used and offer the advantage of being inexpensive and freely available in all developing countries. Chlorpromazine administered in divided doses of 100–300 mg will be effective in a large number of cases, although its usefulness is slightly limited by its side-effects such as day-time sedation and hypotension. It should be avoided in the presence of liver disease. Chlorpromazine also reduces the seizure threshold and is not recommended in the first 72 hours of delirium tremens in alcoholics. Alternatively, haloperidol may be used; it produces its antipsychotic effect without sedation or hypotension in daily doses of 10–30 mg. Short-acting benzodiazepines may prove useful for sleep induction at night. They may also be suitable in the presence of liver disease as they are unlikely to precipitate hepatic coma, or induce seizure in delirium tremens.

Prognosis

Studies have shown that delirious patients have a high rate of mortality. Elderly patients diagnosed as having delirium or confusional states (Post, 1965) and medically hospitalised patients diagnosed as delirious at index admission (Rabins & Folstein, 1982) had higher mortality rates than cognitively intact patients. Clinicians should, therefore, be aware of the need to diagnose delirium in its early stages in high risk groups and to institute proper management (Rabins & Folstein, 1982).

Dementia

Dementia is an organic mental disorder characterised by an acquired and generalised impairment of intellectual abilities, memory, and personality, severely impairing social and occupational functioning. Characteristically, there is no impairment of consciousness. The disorder was earlier described to be progressive and irreversible but it may be static and reversible. Thus earlier terms like chronic brain syndrome or chronic organic psychosis are best avoided.

Historical background

The term dementia was probably first used by Celsus in the first century to denote madness. In 1845, Esquirol defined dementia as a cerebral affection marked by impairment of memory, reasoning and attention, and he distinguished three varieties of dementia: acute, chronic and senile. Prichard (1937) described four stages of progression of dementia: impairment of recent memory, loss of reason, incomprehension, and loss of instinctive action. In 1892, Tuke distinguished four types of dementia: primary, secondary, senile and paralytic. Kraepelin used the term 'organic dementia' to denote a psychosis due to disease of the central nervous system and thus differentiated it from dementia praecox. Binswanger introduced the term 'presenile dementia' in 1898.

By the beginning of the 20th century, the term dementia acquired the connotation of an irreversible mental disorder due to chronic brain disease (Lipowski, 1980*b*). However, through careful descriptive studies on phenomenology, pathology, course and prognosis, it was realised that dementia-related syndromes are not always associated with features like chronicity, irreversibility and hopeless prognosis. Details of current diagnostic criteria may be found in DSM–IV and ICD–10.

Epidemiology

The estimates of prevalence and incidence of dementia in the general population are based on limited epidemiological data which do not cover all age-groups. Estimates are mostly available for elderly populations with the result that dementia is identified chiefly as an illness of the elderly. It is estimated that 5% of people above 65 years of age and 20% above 80 years of age have sufficiently severe impairment to warrant the diagnosis of dementia (Mortimer & Schuman, 1981; Gurland & Cross, 1982; Hasegawa *et al*, 1984; Copeland *et al*, 1987; O'Connor *et al*, 1989). It is further estimated in these surveys that Alzheimer's dementia accounts for nearly 65% of all cases of dementia in old age. Studies also suggest that 10–30% of dementia cases have potentially reversible causes (Wells, 1978; Smith & Kiloh, 1981; Clarfield, 1988).

There is a paucity of data from the developing countries. Ramachandran *et al* (1979) and Venkoba Rao & Madhavan (1982) from India estimated the

TABLE 8.3
Clinical diagnosis of dementing illnesses from four hospital-based Indian studies [1] (n=173)

Pre-senile dementia (40–59-year-olds)	20
Senile dementia (>60-year-olds)	30
Alzheimer's disease	6
Arteriosclerotic dementia	26
Neurosyphilis	20
Neoplastic causes	11
Normal pressure hydrocephalus	6
Pellagra and nutritional causes	6
Type unknown	27
Others	21

1. Bharucha *et al*, 1964 (*n*=53); Mani & Kishore, 1964 (*n*=20); Kalyanasundaram *et al*, 1979 (*n*=40); Srinivasa *et al*, 1982 (*n*=60).

prevalence of dementia in selected population groups to be around 6% above 60 years of age. However, it is the impression of many workers from countries in the developing world that dementia in the elderly is extremely rare. Osuntokun *et al* (1990) in Nigeria found not a single case of dementia in a recent survey of neurological disorders in a community survey of 20 000 people, 5% of whom were above the age of 65. It is to be kept in mind that case-ascertainment may be different, and the elderly in these countries may, because of their survival, be particularly resistant to any form of dementia (Henderson, 1986). Dube (1970) explained the low rate of organic psychosis in his epidemiological study on the basis of the low rate of senile psychotic patients. Table 8.3 shows the breakdown of clinical diagnosis of dementing illnesses from four hospital-based Indian studies. Zhang *et al* (1990) in a prevalence study of dementia in Shanghai, China found a rate of 4.6% in the population over 65 years of age, which was higher than rates earlier reported for China and Japan.

Aetiology

Dementia is a behavioural manifestation of widespread cerebral dysfunction caused by a variety of cerebral and systemic diseases. Table 8.4 gives a list of diseases which are commonly associated with dementia. As has been said earlier, Alzheimer's disease is by far the commonest cause of dementia in the Western world. However, other causes are more important in the developing world: chronic malnutrition causing anaemia and avitaminosis, perinatal injuries due to poor child and maternal services, widely prevalent infections like cerebral malaria, Japanese encephalitis, tuberculosis and many other conditions as listed by Jilek & Jilek-Aall (1970) constitute important causes of dementia.

Clinical features

The majority of dementias are due to diffuse pathological effects on the brain, and thus the clinical picture is similar in different disease processes. Dementia is a global impairment of the intellect, memory and personality, with no impairment of consciousness. The majority of causes start insidiously although some disorders are brought on acutely, e.g. head trauma, and prolonged anoxia.

TABLE 8.4
Diseases commonly associated with dementia

Central nervous system disorders
    Degenerative diseases
    Senile dementia
    Alzheimer's disease
    Pick's disease
    Huntington's chorea
    Parkinson's disease
    Creutzfeldt–Jakob disease
    Wilson's disease
    Progressive supranuclear palsy
    Normal pressure hydrocephalus
    Space-occupying lesions
    Cerebral tumours
    Subdural haematoma
    Trauma
    Vascular dementia
    Multi-infarct dementia
    Infections
    Meningitis
    Encephalitis
    Neurosyphilis
    Epilepsy
Metabolic disorders
    Uraemia
    Liver failure
Endocrine disorders
    Hypothyroidism
    Addison's disease
    Hypopituitarism
Nutritional disorders
    Deficiency of B_{12} folic acid, thiamine, nicotinic acid
Anoxia
    Anaemia, post-anaesthesia, cardiac arrest
Toxic disorders
    Alcoholism
    Heavy metal poisoning
    Chronic barbiturate abuse

Memory impairment is one of the earliest signs of a dementing illness and is frequently the symptom which attracts the attention of people around the patient. The memory defect is global, affecting registration, retention and recall for all kinds of material. Recent memory is affected much more than remote memory but in later stages both are equally and so badly affected that all traces of memory may be wiped out. The patient is usually unaware of his memory defects but in early stages of forgetfulness may be vaguely aware of his inability to recall names or other significant events; this may prompt compensation by confabulation, especially if there is frontal lobe involvement. Intellectual deterioration is insidious in onset and usually progressive, leading to difficulty in new learning and problem solving. Disorientation in time is an early sign and once dementia is established, disorientation for place and person also sets in. Attention and concentration in activities of daily life become progressively impaired.

Judgement, decision-making, comprehension and responses are all impaired.

Behavioural changes in dementia are a secondary manifestation of cognitive impairment. Early changes are decline in interest, initiative and motivation for routine activities. Gradually the behaviour becomes disorganised and inappropriate to the social context. Very often there is restlessness, agitation and aimless wandering. Eating habits deteriorate; patients may eat excessively and sloppily. They become indifferent to personal hygiene and appearance, and as dementia worsens, urinary and faecal incontinence develop.

Due to progressive memory decline, poor comprehension and concentration, and difficulty in new learning and thinking becomes slow and impoverished. Verbal stereotypies and perseverations replace logic and reason. During initial stages, ideas of reference and paranoid delusions, especially of 'people stealing away things', are common. As a result of faulty memory and orientation a patient may misplace an article and then blame others for its disappearance (Reisberg, 1987). Usually such ideas and delusions are fragmented and poorly systematised. Nominal dysphasia is a common disturbance. With progression of the illness, thinking becomes totally disorganised, incoherent and fragmentary and eventually the patient may become totally mute.

Emotional disturbances progress along with intellectual deterioration. Anxiety, depression, suspiciousness and hypochondriacal features are present from the initial stages and may pose considerable diagnostic difficulty. Irritability and hostile outbursts are also early features. Gradually, emotional lability, affective blunting, shallowness and apathy supervene, making the patient dull and devoid of emotional responses.

Since dementia affects mental functions globally, a host of symptoms may appear during the course of the illness, arising from the premorbid personality of the individual, the nature and severity of the illness and any associated medical illness. Many neurotic symptoms are present during the early stages of the illness. Hallucinations also occur initially in some cases. Though not obvious at first, personality changes may begin much earlier than more dramatic symptoms such as gross behavioural changes and forgetfulness. During the early stages, there is usually exaggeration of premorbid personality traits which may manifest in suspiciousness, irritability and neurotic symptoms. To compensate for declining cognitive abilities, the patient may become rigid in the way he or she carries out routine activities.

Pathology

The syndrome of dementia may result from any widespread damage to the brain, especially involving the cerebral cortex. However, the relationship between the psychopathology of dementia and the observed pathological changes in the brain remains unclear. Some cases of dementia may show no structural change in the brain while many normal elderly people may show areas of cerebral atrophy and ischaemia. Where structural changes are not found, cerebral dysfunction seems to be responsible for the psychopathological manifestations (Tomlinson, 1977). Such cases may be potentially treatable and reversible. The degree of dementia can be correlated with the mass of tissue loss, the density of senile plaques and neurofibrillary tangles, and with the mass of ischaemic softening (Wells, 1978). Specific pathological changes will be described briefly later under specific disorders.

Course and prognosis

Dementia is found predominantly in the elderly, although it can occur at any age. The diagnosis of dementia can be made at any age after four years when the IQ is fairly stable, although an individual with onset at such a young age would be considered to have both dementia and mental retardation according to DSM–IV. Generally, the onset of dementia is infrequent before the age of 40, but rises steeply after the age of 60.

The mode of onset and subsequent course of the illness depend upon the underlying aetiology. In certain well defined neurological diseases, such as cerebral hypoxia, encephalitis or head trauma, the onset may be sudden but the course may remain relatively stationary for a long time. Primary degenerative dementias and multi-infarct dementia are insidious in onset with a gradually deteriorating course over a period of several years and death following usually 2–8 years after onset. In many other instances where dementia is secondary to diseases such as Parkinson's disease, normal pressure hydrocephalus, metabolic and endocrine disorders, vitamin deficiencies, neurosyphilis, benign neoplasm, or subdural haematoma, the onset of dementia is usually gradual, and its progress can be arrested or even reversed. The stages of the illness can be defined by its severity.

The course of the illness is often complicated by the patient's inability to look after himself. Because of poor memory and orientation, such patients often wander away from home and become lost or meet with an accident. Infections often prove fatal. Delirium is a frequent complication due to infection or metabolic or electrolyte disturbances. The onset of delirium further worsens morbidity and mortality.

Diagnosis

An early diagnosis of dementia is of vital importance to plan proper investigation and therapeutic intervention. It is during the mild stage of secondary dementias that maximum restoration of cognitive abilities can be achieved, and even in primary dementias necessary supportive measures, relief from distressing behavioural symptoms, and rehabilitative measures can go a long way if instituted early. Below is a brief account to assist in the recognition of the syndrome and in the identification of its cause.

The diagnosis of dementia is made on clinical grounds, while psychological tests are used only as a diagnostic aid, and laboratory tests are required to identify treatable causes.

A detailed and careful history-taking is of utmost importance to appreciate early changes in behaviour, memory and personality. The patient's denial of symptoms or difficulty in giving a detailed and accurate account of symptoms makes it essential to obtain a history from family members. A major life event or a physical illness may bring to their notice a patient's cognitive impairment, but a careful history may reveal the presence of altered behaviour before such an event.

Leads obtained from the history must be carefully evaluated during mental state examination, which may reveal the presence of the essential features of the disorder. Signs of impairment of behaviour, memory, orientation, thinking, intelligence, attention and concentration will confirm the diagnosis.

Psychological testing as a diagnostic aid may help in differential diagnosis, and in documenting the damage for future reference in monitoring progress. Psychological tests may also help in localising a focal lesion. Certain scales (e.g. Brief Cognitive Rating Scale; Global Deterioration Scale) consisting of several tests are available to provide information about a patient's current functioning in all important areas and thus reveal the pattern of deficit (Reisberg, 1983).

A thorough physical and neurological examination is mandatory to reveal any underlying systemic or brain disease that may be responsible for dementia (Liu *et al*, 1991). Further specific laboratory tests depend upon the findings of the psychiatric, physical, and neurological examinations. Table 8.5 lists common tests which are likely to identify most of the treatable causes of dementia. This list may, however, be modified depending on the specific findings of physical examination.

Differential diagnosis

The differential diagnosis of dementia consists of two steps. First, the clinician must distinguish dementia from other organic and non-organic psychiatric conditions. Second, once the diagnosis of dementia has been established, efforts should be made to identify treatable causes.

Age-associated deficits in recent and remote memory, also referred to as benign senescent forgetfulness, must be differentiated from the forgetfulness of dementia in the elderly. People with this deficit have difficulty in giving details of past experiences but are able to recall the essence of experiences (Kral, 1978; Weinberg, 1980).

Delirium and dementia both result from widespread cerebral dysfunction, leading to global cognitive impairment. Distinction between the two syndromes can be blurred. One difference is that the patient remains alert in dementia. Delirium is further characterised by abrupt onset, short duration, impairment of alertness, attention and perception, and nocturnal exacerbation. The symptoms also tend to fluctuate rapidly in delirium while they are relatively stable in dementia. Not infrequently, dementia and delirium may coexist and both

TABLE 8.5
Laboratory screening for dementia

Complete haemogram
   Serum electrolytes and proteins
   Blood urea and sugar
Serum vitamin B_{12} and folic acid
Serum thyroxine and thyroid stimulating hormone
Serological tests for syphilis
Cerebrospinal fluid analysis
Electrocardiography
Electroencephalography
   X-rays of chest and skull
CT scan of head
Psychometry

syndromes may result from the same cause. If the cause is identified but cognitive deficits persist in spite of adequate treatment, dementia is the likely primary condition.

Schizophrenia, especially when chronic, may lead to some degree of intellectual deterioration. However, age of onset, course, associated symptoms, and absence of a systemic disease and brain pathology rule out dementia.

Depression during old age frequently presents considerable diagnostic problems. It is rarely confused with dementia in young adults. Nearly 10% of elderly patients diagnosed with dementia are suffering from depression only (Ron *et al*, 1979; Caine, 1981; McAllister, 1983). Elderly people with a depressive episode may complain of memory impairment, difficulty in thinking and concentration, and an overall reduction in intellectual abilities. They may also perform poorly on mental state examination and neuropsychological testing (Rabins & Pearlson, 1994). These features may suggest a possible diagnosis of dementia in 25% of elderly depressive patients, and this phenomenon has been called 'pseudodementia'.

The onset of depressive pseudodementia can be dated with more precision, and symptoms usually progress more rapidly than in true dementia. The complaints of memory loss tend to exceed the actual memory impairment observed on psychological testing. Abnormalities of mood in dementia are less frequent and less pervasive than in depression. However, dementia and depression may coexist as recent investigations suggest that 20–30% of patients with dementia have concurrent depression (Ron *et al*, 1979; Burns *et al*, 1990).

Management

All cases of dementia must be thoroughly evaluated to identify the underlying causes of secondary dementias so that specific treatment can begin promptly. It may not be possible to reverse the dementing process entirely, but timely intervention may arrest the process and alleviate some of the symptoms. Potentially remediable disorders (depression, drug toxicity, hydrocephalus, benign intracranial tumours, metabolic and endocrine disorders) may be expected in nearly 15% of cases, and in another 20–25% cases some useful intervention may be possible (Wells, 1978; Smith & Kiloh, 1981; Clarfield, 1988).

Unfortunately, the overall prognosis of dementia remains poor since for a large number of patients with primary degenerative dementia no specific treatment is available. However, supportive measures and symptomatic treatment of behavioural symptoms can go a long way in improving the daily functioning of these patients.

Once the diagnosis of dementia has been established, management issues have to be decided, keeping the patient and his family, environment, occupation, and resources in mind.

Immediate family members must be included in any management plan from the early stages. It is necessary to frankly and honestly appraise them of the nature and likely course of the problem since the family may have to take many short-term and long-term decisions. However, it is also wise to remain humane and not paint an entirely pessimistic outcome. As the disease progresses the family is exposed to severe stress and needs emotional support. The patient may not appreciate much from a detailed explanation of his disease process owing to poor registration and forgetfulness. It may still be appropriate to explain in simpler terms the need for environmental adjustments and therapeutic intervention. During the early stages of dementia many patients may continue to work, especially in developing countries with large populations engaged in agriculture and unskilled jobs which make little demand on the intellect. However, some change in the nature of an occupation or even its termination may need to be brought about depending upon the decision-making and responsibility it requires. One should be careful, though, to avoid introducing sudden and abrupt changes.

The patient's environment and surroundings require careful attention and optimal stimulation. Extremes of stimulation may result in withdrawal or agitation. Patients are best managed in familiar surroundings with familiar routines and frequent family contact, if they are in an institutional environment.

Nearly 80% of elderly people, especially in the rural areas of India continue to live in joint or extended families during their illnesses (Ramachandran *et al*, 1981; Venkoba Rao & Madhavan, 1982; Venkoba Rao, 1987). This is likely to be true for many other developing countries. However, even in the developed countries, families provide an estimated 70% of the care for people with dementing illnesses (Mace, 1986).

Sociocultural factors in many of the developing countries may play a very significant role in the family care of the elderly. For example, ageing in Indian culture does not carry the connotation of a 'useless mouth to be fed' and the elderly are given a fairly high rank in the family hierarchy. They are usually highly respected for the perceived wisdom that ageing bestows and their blessings and advice on important matters are frequently sought (Venkoba Rao, 1981). They are a main part of the family and social network. As part of the cultural value system an individual is expected to 'repay the debt' to his parents by looking after them in their old age. There are suggestions that a higher level of tolerance, acceptance and social support network may account for the more favourable outcome of people with chronic mental illnesses and perhaps the same is true for people with dementia (Sartorius *et al*, 1987; Verghese *et al*, 1989, 1990).

However, rapid industrialisation and urbanisation in developing countries, breaking up of the extended family network system due to migration, and erosion of prevalent cultural values may soon adversely affect the care of patients with dementia in such countries where a parallel system of state sponsored social care is negligible or absent.

Psychological intervention

In the early stages, supportive psychological measures can be very helpful in managing some of the disturbing psychological and behavioural problems of dementia. The aim of psychological intervention is to enable the patient to accept the illness and its handicaps and to utilise maximally his residual functions to maintain an active life. Regular psychotherapeutic contact is highly desirable as the clinician can help the patient to maintain his self-esteem and may also determine from time to time the need for further intervention whenever there is a deterioration in any of the physical, social or cognitive activities. Although regular psychotherapeutic contact may be impractical in many developing countries, intervention could be carried out at the primary care level in most rural communities, with some basic training and support of nursing and auxiliary primary care workers.

Since intellectual impairment cannot be reversed in a large number of cases of dementia, the intervention is aimed at making the daily living less complicated yet active and meaningful. It may involve some changes in the lifestyle and occupational activities of the individual but such changes should focus on providing proper stimulation and additional help so that the patient remains in touch with his surroundings and is not too handicapped by poor orientation. Tasks should be broken into simple steps with frequent repetition of instructions. The patient and the family must be encouraged to maintain social activities as much as possible. Regular physical exercise is recommended to fight inactivity, lethargy and the physical complications of underactivity and immobilisation to which older people are prone.

A number of psychological interventions have been tried in patients with dementia. Comparative evaluations of such procedures like milieu therapy, reality orientation, or recreational therapy have been published. In a review of such studies Whitehead (1984) concludes that psychological interventions have been found to be of help in bringing about improvements in intellectual impairment, behavioural disturbances and general activities, but the standard of many of these studies is low and the results are inconsistent.

Pharmacotherapy of behavioural symptoms

Non-cognitive behavioural symptoms in dementia may be present from the beginning of the disease process or may appear during its course. Behavioural symptoms may produce personality changes, affective symptoms and even psychotic symptoms like delusions and hallucinations. Such symptoms are a major cause of anxiety and concern for caregivers and are a frequent cause of hospital admission (Gustafson, 1975; Reisberg *et al*, 1987). Many investigators have attempted to study the pharmacological treatability of these symptoms with variable results (Raskind *et al*, 1987; Schneider & Sobin, 1994).

Randomised double-blind trials by Sugerman *et al* (1964) (haloperidol), Petrie *et al* (1982) (haloperidol and loxapine), Barnes *et al* (1982) (thioridazine and loxapine) and Cocarro *et al* (1990) (haloperidol, oxazepam, diphenhydramine), have found these drugs to demonstrate modest but significant efficacy in controlling agitated behaviour and promoting the activities of daily life. However, only 35–40% of patients can be globally rated as moderately or markedly improved. It appears that target symptoms such as agitation, hyperactivity, hallucinations, delusions and paranoid ideas must be present if antipsychotic drugs are to be effective.

It is important to be aware of the short-term and long-term sensitivity to psychotropic drugs in the elderly, who may be more prone to develop conventional side-effects. Drugs with potent anticholinergic action may adversely affect their already compromised cognitive state. Akathisia and its dysphoric effects are very common and yet may remain unrecognised. Development of tardive dyskinesia is a major concern when using neuroleptics in the elderly. Thus, the choice of drugs should be based on the side-effects, and low doses must be used, with regular monitoring of therapeutic benefits and adverse consequences (Khandelwal *et al*, 1992).

Symptoms of depression may be present in nearly 30% of demented patients (Reifler *et al*, 1982; Cummings *et al*, 1987; Burns *et al*, 1990). Though there are no double-blind clinical trials using antidepressants in these patients, empirically antidepressants have been used in patients with coexisting dementia and depression with some success. Antidepressants are certainly indicated in depressive pseudodementia. Caution must be exercised while using tricyclic antidepressants in the elderly as they are prone to orthostatic hypotension and anticholinergic side-effects. Treatment must begin with small doses, which should be increased very gradually, keeping a close watch on side-effects and cognitive functions.

Insomnia and nonspecific anxiety and agitation may accompany dementia during its course. Before any trial of pharmacotherapy, medical and environmental causes for such symptoms must be carefully evaluated. Side-effects of psychotropic drugs, chronic obstructive airway diseases, increased urinary frequency, gastric discomfort, and uncomfortable living conditions can all produce insomnia and anxiety symptoms. If drugs are to be used, short-acting drugs like lorazepam or alprazolam are preferable to long-acting drugs like diazepam.

Pharmacotherapy of the disease process

Advances in the understanding of neurochemistry and pathophysiology of memory functions and many degenerative dementias have provided hope that suitable drug intervention may reverse or at least arrest the process of such dementias. Over the years a large number of drugs have been used in experimental and clinical trials with variable results. So far, efforts to increase intellectual functioning in dementia by drugs have been disappointing. Some drugs have been found useful in case-reports but not in replication and double-blind studies. Short-term improvement has been noticed in the functioning of daily life but not in cognition, and significant sustained clinical improvement remains doubtful (Jarvik, 1981; Hollister & Yesavage, 1984).

In conclusion, a large number of pharmacological treatment strategies have been employed with ambiguous results. Future research will focus on identifying neurochemical subtypes and possible chemical correlates.

Summary of management guidelines

From the preceding account, the following practical guidelines can be kept in mind by clinicians from developing countries in the event of dementia. While there are no treatments available that can reverse or stop the progression of degenerative dementia, a number of interventions can be instituted to bring about significant relief. Prognosis and outcome are better in secondary dementias on early detection and treatment.

1. Early detection of dementia is important. The clinician must be sensitive about the possibility of dementia while looking after elderly people.
2. The clinician must familiarise herself thoroughly with the diagnostic criteria of dementias in DSM–IV and ICD–10. These can help her to diagnose a case

with reasonable accuracy without resorting to sophisticated and expensive investigations. However, a small proportion of cases may still require some advanced investigations as warranted by neurological examinations. CT scan is now available in most of the Asian and many African countries.

3. Treatable causes like depression, hypertension, metabolic and endocrine disorders should be looked for and treated effectively.

4. Behavioural symptoms compound the course of illness and produce disability. These should be alleviated with adequate pharmacotherapy and environmental manipulation. It will improve patients' coping and reduce family burden.

5. Severely demented persons are at an increased risk of injuries (falls and fractures), aspiration pneumonia, urinary tract infections and bed-sores. These should be identified and treated appropriately.

6. Risks of inadequate nutrition, dehydration, extremes of climatic conditions and forgetfulness with the patient wandering away from home must be appreciated and explained to the family.

7. Adequate support must be provided to the family members and care-giver of the patient since looking after such patients can be very stressful.

8. Institutional care in the form of day care centres, nursing homes and old age homes is available in most of the developed countries. However, such care is available in only a few of the developing countries and in a limited manner, and cost-effectiveness of long-term care in such facilities is yet to be ascertained. Short-term care of a patient with dementia in such facilities can provide much needed respite to the family, in addition to managing the psychiatric or physical crisis.

Primary degenerative dementia: Alzheimer's disease

Alzheimer's disease is a common clinicopathological condition producing a progressive dementia in middle to late life. It is the most common cause of dementia in the over 65 years age group and hence is frequently termed senile dementia of Alzheimer type (SDAT). It affects 2–5% of the population over the age of 65 and 11–15% of those over 85. Women are affected 2–3 times more than men. The pathological changes in the brain are distinctive and can appear at any time from middle age to very old age.

In Alzheimer's disease the brain gradually atrophies, with nerve cells disappearing from the cortex and elsewhere. Though the atrophy is generalised, it tends to affect frontal and temporal lobes more severely. There is a selective and severe loss of neurons in the base of the brain, septal region, nucleus of diagonal band, and the nucleus basalis of Meynert. At autopsy, on gross examination, the brains of Alzheimer's patients show cortical atrophy, widened sulci and enlarged ventricles. Alois Alzheimer in 1907 described the generalised atrophic changes and the appearance of the remaining neurons as a degenerative alteration of their neurofibrils, by which they lose their filamentous features to become thickened and twisted into 'neurofibrillary tangles'. Another pathologic feature, senile plaques, appears within the cerebral cortex. These are microscopic collections of granular argyrophilic particles that surround an indefinite irregular centre containing fat and amyloid.

Alzheimer's disease defined pathologically is a massive worsening of the ageing process compared to typical pathological changes in mild form which are seen in the brains of all elderly people who are not suffering from cognitive impairment.

Although the cause of Alzheimer's disease is not known, a pattern of polygenic or autosomal dominance is found in some families. Forty per cent of patients have first degree relatives with the disease, and the risk of family members acquiring the disease is three to four times higher than in the general population (Heston *et al*, 1981; Breitner *et al*, 1986a,b). A genetic predisposition is also suggested by the fact that patients with Down's syndrome invariably develop Alzheimer's disease at the age of 25–40 (Jervis, 1948; Rumble *et al*, 1989).

There is some suggestion that Alzheimer's disease is a Western disease. It has been mentioned earlier that dementia is rare in developing countries. Even studies from Japan find multi-infarct dementia to be more common. Whether this reflects a racial characteristic or an environmental influence is not yet clear. Alzheimer's dementia could be a consequence of some exposure to which the species has not adapted, and which is not present in the non-industrialised countries (Henderson, 1986).

The dementia accompanying Alzheimer's disease has most of the symptoms that have been enumerated previously. The onset is insidious and progress is slow, with life expectancy after the onset of dementia varying from two to eight years. Though the cognitive deficits are prominent, the most characteristic features in this type of dementia are the language and neurological disturbances. A clear disorder of language, aphasia of the Wernicke kind, makes an early appearance. The patient has difficulty in naming objects, and grammar is distorted. With further worsening the patient cannot produce useful language and cannot comprehend, read or write. As aphasia progresses, it is associated with apraxia, leading to difficulty in dressing and eventually an inability to use any implements. Agnosia eventually appears, in which the patient no longer recognises objects and even persons. Finally, the patient becomes totally incapacitated, bed-ridden, paretic, and vulnerable to infections.

Since the brains of Alzheimer's patients have decreased acetylcholine transferase, attempts have been made to increase their choline levels. Lecithin, tetrahydroaminoacridine (THA), anticholinesterase and physostigmine have all been tried but none of these approaches has shown any unequivocal promise.

Multi-infarct dementia

If Alzheimer's disease is the prototype of a disease that has a particular pathology that progresses because of insidious degeneration of the brain, then multi-infarct dementia is typical of a condition whose neuropathological lesions are focal, varied and unpredictable, and whose psychopathology depends upon the location, extent, and frequency of these lesions.

Multi-infarct dementia is the outcome of cerebrovascular disease, sometimes associated with diabetes mellitus or hypertension. There are varying numbers of small or large infarcts in the brain produced by occlusive vascular disease.

With diabetes mellitus or hypertension, the occlusion may occur in the smaller cerebral arterial network to produce scattered tiny infarcts, particularly in the basal ganglia and white matter of the brain. The condition so produced with its neuropathologic and psychopathological changes is usually referred to as lacunar state.

The clinical presentation of the patient with multi-infarct dementia is usually a mixture of neurologic and psychological impairment right from the start. The clinical pattern is further characterised by a 'stepwise progression' in which there is an abrupt onset of cognitive dysfunction followed by a gradual recovery. However, with repeated sudden exacerbations, the recovery is less and less complete. This is unlike Alzheimer's disease where onset is insidious, psychological impairments are far advanced, progression is slow, and neurological symptoms appear late. The patients of multi-infarct dementia are typically younger hypertensive men, who are more likely to have focal neurological deficits related to the areas of brain where infarction has occurred, such as hemiplegias, aphasias, and cortical blindness. When ischaemia affects the basal ganglia and periventricular white matter, patients may show the pseudobulbar signs of emotional lability. Besides the usual history of stroke, the patient with multi-infarct dementia may show other evidence of vulnerability to vascular disease, such as evidence of atherosclerotic disease in other organs (e.g. the heart).

Hachinski *et al* (1975) have formulated a simple scale in which characteristic features of multi-infarct dementia can be documented to differentiate it from the degenerative dementias.

Since the dementia is secondary to vascular changes, any intervention to avoid atherosclerosis and to reduce it among those at risk may help to prevent this condition and to stabilise it if established.

Pick's disease

Pick's disease, described in 1892, occurs much less frequently than Alzheimer's disease and is clinically indistinguishable from the latter. Autopsy findings show that unlike Alzheimer's disease, gliosis is prominent and massive cell loss is seen in the frontal and temporal lobes.

Huntington's disease

Huntington's disease is a clinical disorder with a recognisable neuropathology inherited as an autosomal dominant trait. Neuropathological findings include generalised atrophy, with particular involvement of the frontal lobes, caudate nucleus and putamen. For this reason, the dementia of Huntington's disease may appear before the chorea, and in initial stages manifests only as a loss of the patient's customary skills (McHugh & Folstein, 1975). Recent memory impairment is an early symptom. The patient has more difficulty in recording a new experience than in retrieving an earlier one. Mental apathy is an early symptom which affects most of the patient's cognitive functioning. There is loss of interest in work, appearance and routine activities, and slow but progressive decline in cognitive abilities, but without aphasia, apraxia or cortical blindness.

In the later stages, the patient becomes totally apathetic, bed-ridden, incontinent and mute.

Creutzfeldt–Jakob disease

Originally described by Creutzfeldt and Jakob in the 1920s, Creutzfeldt–Jakob disease (CJD), along with kuru and scrapie, belongs to the group of diseases referred to as 'spongiform encephalopathies'. In spite of being a rare disorder, CJD has been studied extensively because of its aetiology. The aetiological agent still remains controversial. It has been suggested that it is a slow virus with a long incubation period running into years or even decades. The onset of illness is generally between the ages of 40 and 60 years. After the initial non-specific symptoms, there is rapid progression of cognitive impairment, neurological deficits and dementia. Cerebellar and extrapyramidal symptoms are generally present. The course is rapidly downhill and a majority of patients with CJD die within two years of onset.

Amnestic syndrome

Amnestic syndrome is an organic mental disorder where impairment of memory is the predominant cognitive defect and is characterised by retrograde as well as anterograde amnesia. A number of organic factors and conditions can give rise to the amnestic syndrome. However, in the absence of epidemiological data, precise frequency of the various causes cannot be estimated. Thiamine deficiency associated with chronic alcoholism (Wernicke–Korsakoff syndrome) is considered to be the most common cause, while less common causes include head injury, brain tumours, cerebrovascular disorders causing bilateral hippocampal infarction and cerebral anoxia. Reversible or irreversible lesions of specific diencephalic or temporal structures are a necessary condition for the development of amnestic syndrome. The hippocampal formation, mamillary bodies and structures in the walls and floor of the third ventricle and thalamic nuclei are the other sites usually affected in the syndrome.

The term Wernicke–Korsakoff syndrome is commonly used to describe a neuropsychiatric condition caused by thiamine deficiency of any origin. Wernicke's encephalopathy represents the acute organic reaction of which Korsakoff's psychosis represents the residual and sometimes permanent defect (Lishman, 1987). Thiamine deficiency, the common metabolic link between the two, may be caused by chronic alcoholism, gastric carcinoma, intractable vomiting and severe dietary deficiency.

Clinical features

Impairment of the memory remains the most prominent feature of amnestic syndrome. Retrograde amnesia (forgetfulness extending over a period of months or years before the onset of illness) and anterograde amnesia (inability to recall events subsequent to the onset of illness) are both present. However, immediate memory as tested by a digit span test remains relatively intact. There is an inability to learn new information. The patient tends to deny or minimise the presence of memory deficits. Confabulation is a common but not a constant feature. Cognitive functions other than memory are usually well preserved, though disorientation may be present in some cases. The patient is usually alert and to some extent able to manage minor and less complicated daily life activities. The organic amnesic states seen in clinical practice can be classified into discrete episodes and persistent memory impairment (Kopelman, 1987). Toxic confusional state, head injury, epilepsy, alcoholic blackout, hypoglycaemia, transient global amnesia and electroconvulsive therapy produce discrete episodes while specific amnesic syndrome, drug toxicity and severe head injury produce persistent impairment.

Nature of deficits in organic amnesia

Neuropsychologists have devoted considerable attention to trying to identify the nature of the memory deficits in organic amnesia. It appears that the anterograde amnesia produced by structural lesions represents a severe impairment in acquiring new information, and any retrieval deficits arise as a consequence of this (Cutting, 1978). However, the rate of forgetting of new information is not accelerated once adequate learning has been accomplished (Baddeley, 1982; Kopelman, 1985). It seems that the clinical impression of faster forgetting in patients with head injury, Korsakoff's syndrome, and Alzheimer-type dementia arises because information has not been adequately absorbed initially. Retrograde amnesia may result from a failure to use contextual cues (with regard to time, order, place and source) in reconstructing experiences, and from incoherent retrieval of past memories and experiences. Psychological and pathophysiological evidence suggest partial independence of the retrograde and anterograde components of amnesia (Kapur *et al*, 1986).

Diagnosis

The diagnosis of the amnestic syndrome is usually straightforward as the patient's history usually reveals the cause, and because of the progression of characteristic memory deficits in the absence of significant global intellectual impairment. Psychogenic amnesia may pose considerable problems in diagnosis if precipitated by head injury, acute alcohol intoxication or epileptic seizures (Kopelman, 1987). Lishman (1987) has described in detail the clinical assessment and investigation of organic amnesia.

Treatment

Chronic malnutrition and vitamin deficiencies which are likely to be rampant in developing countries must be adequately managed. Regular vitamin supplements should be provided to prevent the onset of encephalopathy in vulnerable individuals with long-standing alcoholism. Once features of encephalopathy or Korsakoff's syndrome have developed, they must be treated with high doses of thiamine and other vitamins. Thiamine 50 mg should be administered intravenously daily until the patient is able to tolerate an oral diet and medication.

A timely intervention may result in reversal of the amnestic process.

Mental disorders due to brain dysfunction or physical disease not involving cognitive impairment

These mental disorders are included in ICD–10 (Table 8.1). They are causally related to brain dysfunction due to a primary cerebral disease, or to a systemic disease affecting the brain secondarily while their clinical manifestations are not traditionally organic in the specific sense. According to ICD–10, the decision to classify a clinical syndrome under this category must be supported by evidence of a cerebral or a systemic physical disease and a temporal relationship between the development of underlying disease and the onset of the mental syndrome. The certainty of diagnostic classification is considerably raised in the absence of evidence for an alternative cause of the syndrome and on recovery of the mental disorder following removal or improvement of the underlying presumed cause. The diagnosis is not made if the disturbance occurs in the context of reduced ability to maintain and shift attention as in delirium.

Organic hallucinosis

Organic hallucinosis is characterised by persistent or recurrent hallucinations, usually visual or auditory, that occur in clear consciousness and are due to a specific organic factor. Use of hallucinogens and prolonged use of alcohol are the most common causes of this syndrome. Delusions are usually not prominent but the patient may have delusional beliefs about the reality of the hallucinations. The course of the illness depends upon the underlying cause. Hallucinogen-induced hallucinosis may last only for a brief period while prolonged sensory deprivation in untreated cataract or otosclerosis may cause a chronic hallucinosis.

Organic delusional syndrome

The essential feature of the syndrome is prominent delusions that are due to a specific organic factor in a state of full wakefulness and alertness. These delusions occur most commonly in toxic metabolic disorders. The syndrome is also associated with certain cerebral lesions, particularly of the right hemisphere, affecting the limbic system and basal ganglia. See Cummings (1985) for a review of organic delusions.

Acting on delusional beliefs is not uncommon. Hallucinations and other symptoms commonly seen in schizophrenia may be present and the syndrome needs to be differentiated from a schizophrenic disorder. The appearance of delusions in a person over the age of 35 years without a known history of schizophrenia should always alert the clinician to the possibility of an organic delusional syndrome. Simple delusions respond best to treatment, while complex delusions are more resistant, but overall management of the underlying organic disorder is essential for the recovery of the patient.

Organic mood syndrome

The essential feature of this syndrome is a prominent and persistent depressed or elevated mood resembling either a major depressive episode or a manic episode, resulting from a specific organic factor. A number of physical disorders and drugs have been implicated as causes of secondary depression. The syndrome is usually caused by toxic and metabolic factors. Central noradrenergic-blocking antihypertensive medications, hypothyroidism, Cushing's syndrome, Addison's syndrome, hypercalcaemia, pellagra, vitamin B12 or folate deficiency, and some viral infections may precipitate depression. Occult carcinoma, especially of the pancreas, and diencephalic tumours are rare causes of depression. Depression may also occur after cerebrovascular accidents. Precipitants of manic episodes are less common and include hyperthyroidism, hypocalcaemia and exogenous steroids.

Clinically, the disturbances of mood closely resemble either a depressive or manic episode and the syndrome may vary in severity from mild to severe. Delusions and hallucinations as seen in affective disorders may also be present.

Management of the affective syndrome involves treatment of the underlying physical disorder and drug treatment of the affective symptoms. The doses of antidepressant or antimanic drugs may have to be carefully adjusted because of the presence of the physical disorder. The course of the illness depends on the treatment of the underlying aetiology but the affective syndrome may persist for some time even after its successful treatment.

Organic anxiety syndrome

This is a disorder characterised by the features of generalised anxiety disorder, panic disorder, or a combination of both, but arising as a consequence of an organic disorder. The syndrome is usually caused by an endocrine disorder such as hypothyroidism, hyperthyroidism, phaeochromocytoma, hypoglycaemia and hypercortisolism, or the use of psychoactive substances such as caffeine, cocaine, and amphetamines. Withdrawal from central nervous system depressants like alcohol and sedatives can precipitate an anxiety disorder. Brain tumours in the vicinity of the third ventricle are also an important cause.

Anxiety symptoms are known to occur in many other systemic diseases but are less likely to occur as the only symptoms. The course of the illness depends upon the underlying aetiology. Though recovery results when the responsible physical disorder is corrected, in some cases residual anxiety symptoms can continue for a long time and may require additional treatment.

Organic personality syndrome

The essential feature of this syndrome is a persistent personality disturbance representing a change or accentuation of the habitual patterns of behaviour displayed by the subject premorbidly. There must be evidence of an organic factor before the onset of syndrome which should be causally related to it.

Change in the personality and behavioural manifestations of impaired control of emotions and impulses are the cardinal features. There is consistently reduced ability to persevere with goal-directed activities, and there is inability to postpone gratification. Emotional behaviour is characterised by emotional lability, shallow and unwarranted cheerfulness and inappropriate jocularity. Easy irritability, short-lived anger and aggression are common. Apathy may be a prominent feature in some instances. The subject may engage in antisocial acts, such as stealing, inappropriate sexual advances, ravenous eating, and poor personal care. Rate and flow of language output are markedly altered by circumstantiality, over-inclusiveness and hypergraphia. Mild cognitive impairment often coexists but does not amount to intellectual deterioration. This mostly manifests in poor attention, motivation and initiative.

Organic personality syndrome is usually due to structural brain damage. Common causes are neoplasm, head injury and cerebrovascular accidents. Temporal lobe epilepsy, Huntington's chorea and multiple sclerosis are also associated with this disorder. Endocrine disorders and psychoactive drug abuse are uncommon causes. Chronic heavy ingestion of cannabis has been said to produce marked loss of interest in usual activities, diminished capacity to carry out complex, long-term plans, reduced concentration, social withdrawal and a pervasive amotivational state. However, in this syndrome cultural and personal factors may be more important than cannabis *per se*.

The cause determines the course and prognosis of an organic personality syndrome. An early intervention such as removal of a brain tumour will result in a short duration of the syndrome. It is likely to be long-standing if it is secondary to significant structural damage to the brain such as head injury or a vascular accident. Progression of unresolved cases may lead to dementia. Management of organic personality syndrome will require long-term psychosocial intervention and rehabilitation.

References

AMERICAN PSYCHIATRIC ASSOCIATION (1980) *Diagnostic and Statistical Manual of Mental Disorders* (3rd edn) (DSM–III). Washington, DC: APA.
—— (1994) *Diagnostic and Statistical Manual of Mental Disorders* (4th edn) (DSM–IV). Washington DC: APA.
BADDELEY, A. D. (1982) Domains of recollection. *Psychological Review,* **89**, 708–729.
BARNES, R. & VEITH, R. (1982) Efficacy of antipsychotic medications in behaviorally disturbed dementia patients. *American Journal of Psychiatry,* **139**, 1170–1174.
BERESIN, E. (1983) Delirium. In *Inpatient Psychiatry: Diagnosis and Treatment* (ed. L. I. Sederer). Baltimore: Williams & Wilkins.
BERRIOS, G. E. (1981) Delirium and confusion in the 19th Century. *British Journal of Psychiatry,* **139**, 439–449.
BHARUCHA, E. P., MONDKAR, V. P. & SESHIA, S. S. (1964) Dementia – a clinical study of 53 cases. *Neurology India,* **12**, 80–91.
BLEULER, E. P. (1924) *Textbook of Psychiatry* (Translated by A. A. Brill). New York: Macmillan. Reissued by International University Press, New York (1971).
BLEULER, M. (1951) Psychiatry of cerebral diseases. *British Medical Journal,* **2**, 1233–1238.
BREITNER, J. C. S., FOLSTEIN, M. F. & MURPHY, E. A. (1986a) Familial aggregation in Alzheimer dementia: I. A model for the age-dependent expression of an autosomal dominant gene. *Journal of Psychiatric Research,* **20**, 31–43.

――――, MURPHY, E. A. & FOLSTEIN, M. F. (1986*b*) Familial aggregation in Alzheimer dementia: II. Clinical genetic implications of age-dependent expression. *Journal of Psychiatric Research*, **20**, 45–55.

BURNS, A., JACOBY, R. & LEVY, R. (1990) Psychiatric phenomena in Alzheimer's disease. III: Disorders of mood. *British Journal of Psychiatry*, **157**, 81–86.

CAINE, E. D. (1981) Pseudodementia. *Archives of General Psychiatry*, **38**, 1359–1364.

CLARFIELD, A. M. (1988) The reversible dementias: do they reverse? *Annals of Internal Medicine*, **109**, 476–486.

COCCARO, E. F. & KARMER, E. (1990) Pharmacologic treatment of noncognitive behavioural disturbances in elderly demented patients. *American Journal of Psychiatry*, **147**, 1640–1645.

COPELAND, J. R. M., DEWEY, M. E., WOOD, N., *et al* (1987) Range of mental illness among elderly in the community: Prevalence in Liverpool using GMS–AGECAT package. *British Journal of Psychiatry*, **150**, 815–823.

CUMMINGS, J. L. (1985) Organic delusions: phenomenology, anatomical correlations, and review. *British Journal of Psychiatry*, **146**, 184–197.

―――― & MILLER, B. (1987) Neuropsychiatric aspects of multi-infarct dementia and dementia of the Alzheimer type. *Archives of Neurology*, **44**, 389–393.

CUTTING, J. (1978) Relationship between Korsakoff's syndrome and 'alcholic dementia'. *British Journal of Psychiatry*, **132**, 240–251.

DUBE, K. C. (1970) A study of prevalence and biosocial variables in mental illness in a rural and an urban community in Uttar Pradesh. *Acta Psychiatrica Scandinavica*, **46**, 327–359.

ELNAGAR, M. N., MAITRE, P. & RAO, M. N. (1971) Mental health in an Indian rural community. *British Journal of Psychiatry*, **118**, 499–504.

ENGEL, G. & ROMANO, J. (1959) Delirium, a syndrome of cerebral insufficiency. *Journal of Chronic Diseases*, **9**, 260–277.

GERMAN, G. A. (1987*a*) Mental Health in Africa, I: the extent of mental health problems in Africa today. *British Journal of Psychiatry*, **151**, 435–439.

―――― (1987*b*) Mental Health in Africa, II: the nature of mental disorders in Africa today. *British Journal of Psychiatry*, **151**, 440–446.

GIEL, R. & HARDING, T. W. (1976) Psychiatric priorities in developing countries. *British Journal of Psychiatry*, **128**, 513–522.

GURLAND, B. J. & CROSS, P. S. (1982) Epidemiology of psychopathology in old age: some implications for clinical services. *Psychiatric Clinics of North America*, **5**, 11–26.

GUSTAFSON, L. (1975) Psychiatric symptoms in dementia with onset in the presenile period. *Acta Psychiatrica Scandinavica*, **257**, 8–35.

HACHINSKI, V. C., ILIFF, L. D. & ZHILKA, E. (1975) Cerebral blood flow in dementia. *Archives of Neurology*, **32**, 632–637.

HASEGAWA, K., HONMA, A., SATO, A., *et al* (1984) The prevalence of age-related dementia in the community. *Geriatric Psychiatry*, **1**, 94–105.

HENDERSON, A. S. (1986) The epidemiology of Alzheimer's disease. *British Medical Bulletin*, **42**, 3–10.

HESTON, L. L., MASTRI, A. R., ANDERSON, V. E., *et al* (1981) Dementia of the Alzheimer type: clinical genetics, natural history and associated conditions. *Archives of General Psychiatry*, **38**, 1085–1090.

HOLLISTER, L. E. & YESAVAGE, J. (1984) Ergoloid mesylates for senile dementias: unanswered questions. *Annals of Internal Medicine*, **100**, 894–898.

HORVATH, T. B., SIEVER, L. J., RICHARD, C. M., *et al* (1989) Organic mental syndromes and disorders. In *Comprehensive Textbook of Psychiatry* (5th edn) (eds H. I. Kaplan & B. J. Sadock), pp. 599–641. Baltimore: Williams & Wilkins.

JARVIK, L. F. (1981) Hydergine as a treatment for organic brain syndrome in late life. *Psychopharmacological Bulletin*, **17**, 40–41.

JERVIS, G. A. (1948) Early senile dementia in mongoloid idiocy. *American Journal of Psychiatry*, **105**, 102–106.

JILEK, W. G. & JILEK-AALL, L. (1970) Transient psychoses in Africans. *Psychiatric Clinics*, **3**, 337–364.

JORM, A. F., KORTEN, A. E. & HENDERSON, A. S. (1987) The prevalence of dementia – A quantitative integration of the literature. *Acta Psychiatrica Scandinavica*, **76**, 465–479.

KALYANASUNDARAM, S., MAHAL, A. S. & MANI, K. S. (1979) Dementia – An analysis of clinical, electroencephalographic and pneumoencephalographic variables. *Indian Journal of Psychiatry*, **21**, 114–126.

KAPUR, N., HEATH, P., MENDELL, P., *et al* (1986) Amnesia can facilitate memory performance: evidence from a patient with dissociated retrograde amnesia. *Neuropsychologia*, **224**, 215–222.

KHANDELWAL, S. K., AHUJA, G. K. & GUPTA, S. (1992) Behavioural symptoms in dementia: nature and treatment. *Indian Journal of Psychiatry*, **34**, 36–40.

KOPELMAN, M. D. (1985) Rates of forgetting in Alzheimer type dementia and Korsakoff's syndrome. *Neuropsychologia*, **23**, 623–638.

—— (1987) Amnesia: organic and psychogenic. *British Journal of Psychiatry*, **150**, 428–442.

KRAL, V. A. (1978) Benign senescent forgetfulness. In *Alzheimer's Disease: Senile Dementia and Related Disorders* (eds R. Katzman, R. D. Terry & K. L. Bick). New York: Raven Press.

LIPOWSKI, Z. J. (1980*a*) A new look at organic brain syndrome. *American Journal of Psychiatry*, **137**, 674–678.

—— (1980*b*) Organic mental disorders: Introduction and review of syndromes. In *Comprehensive Textbook of Psychiatry III* (eds H. I. Kaplan, A. M. Freedman & B. J. Sadock), pp. 1359–1392. Baltimore: Williams & Wilkins.

—— (1984) Organic mental disorders – an American perspective. *British Journal of Psychiatry*, **144**, 542–546.

LISHMAN, W. A. (1987) *Organic Psychiatry. The Psychological Consequences of Cerebral Disorder* (2nd edn). Oxford: Blackwell Scientific.

LISTON, E. H. (1982) Delirium in the aged. *Psychiatric Clinics of North America*, **5**, 49–66.

—— (1984) Diagnosis and management of delirium in the elderly patients. *Psychiatric Annals*, **14**, 109–118.

LIU, H. C., TSOU, H. K., *et al* (1991) Evaluation of 110 consecutive patients with dementias: a prospective study. *Acta Neurologica Scandinavica*, **84**, 421–425.

MACE, N. (1986) Caregiving aspects of Alzheimer's disease. *Business and Health*, **3**, 34–35.

MANI, K. S. & KISHORE, B. (1964) Dementia – A clinical and some pathological aspects. *Neurology India*, **12**, 101–110.

MCALLISTER, T. W. (1983) Overview: pseudodementia. *American Journal of Psychiatry*, **140**, 528–533.

MCHUGH, P. R. & FOLSTEIN, M. F. (1975) Psychiatric symptoms of Huntington's chorea: a clinical and phenomenological study. In *Psychiatric Aspects of Neurologic Disease* (eds D. F. Benson & D. Blumer), pp. 267–286. New York: Grune & Stratton.

MORTIMER, J. A. & SCHUMAN, L. M. (1981) *The Epidemiology of Dementia*. New York: Oxford University Press.

O'CONNOR, D. W., POLLITT, P. A., HYDE, J. B., *et al* (1989) The prevalence of dementia as measured by the Cambridge Mental Disorder of the Elderly examination. *Acta Psychiatrica Scandinavica*, **79**, 190–198.

ORLEY, J. & WING, J. K. (1979) Psychiatric disorders in two African villages. *Archives of General Psychiatry*, **36**, 513–520.

OSUNTOKUN, B. O., OGUNNIYI, L. I. G., LEKWAUMWA, *et al* (1990) Epidemiology of dementia in Nigerian Africans. In *Advances in Neurology* (eds J. S. Chopra, K. Jagannathan & I. M. S. Sawhney), pp. 331–342. Amsterdam: Elsevier.

PETRIE, W. M. & BAN, T. A. (1982) Loxapine in psychogeriatrics: a placebo and standard controlled clinical investigation. *Journal of Clinical Psychopharmacology*, **2**, 122–126.

POST, F. (1965) *The Clinical Psychiatry of Late Life*. Oxford: Pergamon.

RABINS, P. V. & FOLSTEIN, M. F. (1982) Delirium and dementia: diagnostic criteria and fatality rates. *British Journal of Psychiatry*, **140**, 149–153.

—— & PEARLSON, G. D. (1994) Depression induced cognitive impairment. In *Dementia* (eds A. Burns & R. Levy), pp. 667–679. London: Chapman and Hall.

RAMACHANDRAN, V., SARADA MENON, M. & RAMAMURTI, B. (1979) Psychiatric disorders in subjects aged over fifty. *Indian Journal of Psychiatry*, **22**, 193–201.

——, —— (1981) Family structure and mental illness in old age. *Indian Journal of Psychiatry*, **23**, 21–26.

RASKIND, M. A. & RISSE, S. C. (1987) Dementia and antipsychotic drugs. *Journal of Clinical Psychiatry*, **48** (May Suppl), 16–18.

REIFLER, B., LARSON, E. & HARLEY, R. (1982) Co-existence of cognitive impairment and depression in geriatric out-patients. *American Journal of Psychiatry*, **139**, 623–626.

REISBERG, B. (1981) Empirical studies in senile dementia with metabolic enhancers and agents that alter the blood flow and oxygen utilization. In *Strategies for the Development for an Effective Treatment for Senile Dementia* (eds T. Crook & S. Gershon). New Canaan: Mark Powley Associates.

—— (1983) The Brief Cognitive Rating Scale and Global Deterioration Scale. In *Assessment of Geriatric Psychopharmacology* (eds T. Crook, S. Ferris & R. Bartus), pp. 19–36. Connecticut: Mark Powley Associates.

——, BORENSTEIN, J., SALOB, S., *et al* (1987) Behavioural symptoms in Alzheimer's disease. *Journal of Clinical Psychiatry*, **48** (Suppl), 9–15.

RON, M. A., TOONE, B. K., GARRALDA, M. E., *et al* (1979) Diagnostic accuracy in presenile dementia. *British Journal of Psychiatry*, **134**, 161–168.

RUMBLE, B., RETALLACK, R., HILBICH, C., *et al* (1989) Amyloid A4 protein and its precursor in Down's syndrome and Alzheimer's disease. *New England Journal of Medicine*, **320**, 1446–1452.

SARTORIUS, N., JABLENSKY, A., ERNBERG, G., *et al* (1987) Course of schizophrenia in different countries: a WHO international comparative 5-year follow up study. *Search for Course of Schizophrenia*, (eds H. Hafner, W. Gattez & W. Janzarik). Heidelberg: Springer.

SCHNEIDER, L. S. & SOBIN, P. (1994) Treatments for psychiatric symptoms and behavioural manifestations in dementia. In *Dementia* (eds A. Burns & R. Levy), pp. 519–540. London: Chapman and Hall.

SETHI, B. B., GUPTA, S. C. & KUMAR, R. (1967) Three hundred urban families – a psychiatric study. *Indian Journal of Psychiatry*, **9**, 280–287.

———, ———, MAHENDRU, R. K., *et al* (1974) Mental health and urban life: a study of 850 families. *British Journal of Psychiatry*, **124**, 243–246.

SMITH, J. S. & KILOH, L. G. (1981) The investigation of dementia: results in 200 consecutive admissions. *Lancet*, **I**, 824–827.

SRINIVAS, H. V., KALYANASUNDARAM, S., DESHPANDE, D. H., *et al* (1982) Diagnostic categories of dementia in a population of Indian patients. *Neurology India*, **30**, 83–92.

SUGERMAN, A. A., WILLIAMS, B. H. & ADLERSTEIN, A. M. (1964) Haloperidol in psychiatric disorders of old age. *American Journal of Psychiatry*, **120**, 1190–1192.

THACORE, V. R., GUPTA, S. C. & SURAIYA, M. (1975) Psychiatric morbidity in a North Indian Community. *British Journal of Psychiatry*, **126**, 364–368.

TOMLINSON, B. E. (1977) The pathology of dementia. In *Dementia* (2nd edn) (ed. C. E. Wells), pp. 113–121. Philadelphia: F. A. Davis.

VENKOBA RAO, A. (1981) Mental health and aging in India. *Indian Journal of Psychiatry*, **23**, 11–20.

——— & MADHAVAN, T. (1982) Geropsychiatric morbidity survey in a semi-urban area near Madurai. *Indian Journal of Psychiatry*, **24**, 258–267.

——— (1987) Family jointness, family and social integration among the elderly. *Indian Journal of Psychiatry*, **29**, 81–103.

VERGHESE, A., BEIG, A., SENSEMAN, L. A., *et al* (1973) A social and psychiatric study of a representative group of families in Vellore Town. *Indian Journal of Medical Research*, **61**, 608–620.

———, DUBE, K. C., JOHN, J. K., *et al* (1990) Factors associated with the course and outcome of schizophrenia – A multicentred follow-up study: result of a five-year follow-up. *Indian Journal of Psychiatry*, **32**, 211–216.

———, JOHN, J. K., RAJKUMAR, S., *et al* (1989) Factors associated with the course and outcome of schizophrenia in India – A multicentred follow up study: Results of 2 year follow up. *British Journal of Psychiatry*, **154**, 499–503.

WEINBERG, J. (1980) Geriatric psychiatry. In *Comprehensive Textbook of Psychiatry III* (eds H. I. Kaplan, A. M. Freedman & B. J. Sadock), pp. 3024–3042. Baltimore: Williams & Wilkins.

WELLS, C. E. (1978) Chronic brain disease: an overview. *American Journal of Psychiatry*, **135**, 1–12.

——— (1985) Organic syndromes: delirium. In *Comprehensive Textbook of Psychiatry* (4th edn) (eds H. I. Kaplan & B. J. Sadock), pp. 838–850. Baltimore: Williams & Wilkins.

WHITEHEAD, A. (1984) Psychological intervention in old age. In *Handbook of Studies on Psychiatry and Old Age* (eds D. W. K. Kay & G. D. Burrows), pp. 181–200. Amsterdam: Elsevier.

WIG, N. N. (1981) Researches in mental health in South-East Asia. *Bulletin of Neuroinformation Laboratory*, **8**, 91–111.

——— (1983) DSM–III: a perspective from the Third World. In *International Perspective on DSM–III* (eds R. L. Spitzer, J. B. W. Williams & A. E. Skodol), pp. 79–89. Washington, DC: American Psychiatric Press.

——— (1990) The Third-World perspective on psychiatric diagnosis and classification. In *Sources and Traditions of Classifications in Psychiatry* (eds N. Sartorius, A. Jablensky, D. A. Regier, *et al*), pp. 181–210. Toronto: Hans Huber.

WOLFF, H. G. & CURRAN, D. (1935) Nature of delirium and allied states: the dysergastic reaction. *Archives of Neurology and Psychiatry*, **51**, 378–392.

WORLD HEALTH ORGANIZATION (1992) *The Tenth Revision of the International Classification of Diseases and Related Problems* (ICD–10). Geneva: WHO.

ZHANG, M., KATZMAN, R., SALMON, D., *et al* (1990) The prevalence of dementia and Alzheimer's disease in Shanghai, China: impact of age, gender and education. *Annals of Neurology*, **27**, 428–437.

9 Alcohol and drug misuse

9.1 Action on prevention and service development

M. ARGANDOÑA

The use of psychoactive substances has created worldwide social, economic, and health problems. This is true both for licit substances, such as tobacco, alcohol, psychotropic drugs and volatile solvents, and for drugs such as cannabis, cocaine, and opiates that are illicit in most countries. Together with environmental degradation, rapid urbanisation, and economic and demographic changes, substance misuse is modifying epidemiological profiles in the developing world; accurate information, however, is generally lacking and assessment of the real trends of drug-related problems needs to be undertaken.

This chapter is concerned with ways in which health services, particularly in psychiatry and mental health, can respond to the demand for and use of psychoactive substances in the developing world, where a number of countries are today severely disturbed by escalating drug-related problems. Despite the disruptive impact, health and social drug-related problems in developing countries are usually not a high political priority. Political action, when it does occur, is often diverted to combating illicit drug production, trafficking and sales. A greater health priority is, however, the effects of substance use on health.

International efforts to control the illicit traffic in drugs have been significantly strengthened during the past 30 years with the 1961 Single Convention on Narcotic Drugs and the 1971 Convention on Psychotropic Substances, and their amendments. National governments, partly reacting to such international conventions and partly as a result of increasing abuse of drugs, have enacted legislation designed to curb illicit drug traffic. Regional agreements, such as the South American Agreement on Narcotic Drugs and Psychotropic Substances, which came into force in March 1977, have also been drawn up in response to the need for multinational collaboration.

The international conventions and the regional agreements contain provisions on prevention of drug use and the treatment of drug-dependent persons. Prevention, treatment and rehabilitation are seen as the most significant ways of controlling the demand for illicit drugs by reducing the number of people using such substances. Although alcohol and other licit substances liable to abuse are responsible for more damage to health and human wellbeing than the drugs scheduled in the 1961 and 1971 Conventions, they are

162

not the subject of international agreements or conventions, except for a 1919 convention relating to liquor traffic in Africa (Porter, 1986).

Terms and definitions

Due to the wide variety of substances used to bring on subjective changes in mental activity, and also due to the multiple immediate and long-term effects of these substances on physiological functioning and behaviour, ambiguous terms are used which might create some degree of confusion. In order to facilitate the clarity of the present chapter, a few definitions will be given from the *Lexicon of Alcohol and Other Drug Terms* (WHO, 1992a).

Psychoactive substances: products that may be intentionally consumed – with or without medical prescription – for the purpose of producing particular subjective states or calming down psychological distress. Most of these substances are liable to abuse.

Abuse: this term is sometimes criticised because of its moral and legal connotations; it is, however, commonly employed in official UN publications and in everyday usage. *Drug abuse* and *alcohol abuse* are widely utilised to refer to harmful or hazardous use, and often to indicate disapproval of any use at all. In this chapter the word abuse will be defined as repeated or episodic self-administration of a psychoactive substance to the extent of experiencing harm from its effects, or from the social or economic consequences of its use.

Misuse of non-psychoactive substances: describes repeated or episodic self-administration of a substance which, though not having dependence potential, is accompanied by harmful physical or psychological effects or involves unnecessary contact with health professionals. This group includes substances such as laxatives, aspirins, steroids or vitamins.

Illicit drug: a psychoactive substance whose production, sale or use is prohibited. The term is inexact, since no drug is illicit everywhere and under all circumstances. *Illicit drug market,* a more exact term, refers to the production, distribution and sale of any drug outside of legally-sanctioned channels.

Drug: it is sometimes understood that this word refers to the (psychoactive) substances that became illicit after being scheduled under the International Conventions, whereas *substance* would rather mean all other psychoactive products. In order to avoid futile discussions, both words will be used in this chapter as synonymous of psychoactive products, either natural or synthetic.

Narcotic: signifies a chemical agent that induces stupor, coma or insensibility to pain. It includes narcotic analgesics such as the opiates. In common parlance and legal usage the term is, however, often used imprecisely to mean illicit drugs irrespective of their pharmacology, e.g. the United Nations' Single Convention on Narcotic Drugs of 1961 includes cocaine and cannabis as well as opioids. Because of this variation in usage, the term is best replaced by those (e.g. opiates) having a more specific meaning.

Addiction: a term of long-standing and variable usage. It is regarded by many as a discrete disease entity, a debilitating disorder rooted in the pharmacological effects of the drug which is remorselessly progressive. From the 1920s to the

1960s an attempt was made to differentiate between addiction and habituation, a less severe form of psychological adaptation. In 1964, the World Health Organization (WHO) recommended that both terms be abandoned in favour of *dependence*, which can exist in various degrees of severity.

Dependence: means the state of needing repeated doses of a drug to feel good or to avoid feeling bad. The term can be used generally with reference to the whole range of psychoactive drugs (drug dependence, chemical dependence, substance use dependence), or can be used with specific reference to a particular drug or class of drugs (e.g. alcohol dependence, opioid dependence). In unqualified form, dependence may be either physical or psychological. Psychological or psychic dependence refers to the experience of impaired control over drinking or drug use (craving, compulsion), while physiological or physical dependence refers to tolerance and withdrawal symptoms (neuroadaptation).

Dependence syndrome: a core concept in alcohol- and drug-related clinical problems; it refers to a cluster of behavioural, cognitive, and physiological phenomena that may develop after repeated substance use.

The current global situation

During the last three decades law enforcement to control the supply and use of drugs has been considered the ideal approach to tackle drug-related problems. Unfortunately, this approach has made access to care and rehabilitation difficult for substance users and dependent persons, and in some countries, as a result of being punished rather than treated, drug users have reacted by going underground.

Planners expected that repression would increase the social and economic prices of street drugs, and therefore be effective in reducing the demand for drugs; it may also have been thought that harshness would deter people from using illicit substances. In practice, repression has produced the opposite effect: an increase in the demand for drugs, expanding crime, and drug injection triggering the spread of HIV infection and AIDS.

The demand for addictive substances has never been greater. This might be the aftermath of a long drugs 'war' during which little attention was paid to the reduction of the demand and to the health problems stemming from the use of drugs. The consumers, i.e. the demand sector, were considered ancillary actors in the dramatic fight against producers and traffickers. Punishment and detoxification plus some sparse information and prevention activities were believed to be sufficient to solve the puzzle posed by the demand for harmful substances. In view of the dubious results of these approaches, and the recognition that some of the assumptions made 30 years ago no longer hold true, new thinking has been necessary to design innovative systems for the improvement of the current situation and the reversal of ominous trends. However, although there may be some signs of improvement with some drugs, the general trend is still towards an increase in drug abuse. In developing countries the problem has been exacerbated partly because they have been seen mostly as producers and, therefore, a cause of the problem, rather than essential members of a complex interaction involving multiple influences among all nations. Producer and transit countries are not just providing dangerous substances to the rest of the world. They are also consumers. It is now admitted that producer countries have the worst drug-related problems, and countries used as 'transit routes' have, additionally, become mixed up in the consumption of addictive substances coming from all over the world.

In many developing countries drug abuse has spread out from the controlled production and use of natural substances, to the abuse of modern concentrated products for which local cultures neither have suitable social rules nor individual protective behaviours. Thus, while opium-eating, coca-chewing, and even hallu-cinogenic substances were integrated as functional components into traditional cultures, the high purity and potent effect of distilled spirits, heroin or cocaine – which have become easily available commodities – led to the rapid growth of abuse-related problems.

With increased supply and increased use, drug-related problems tend also to increase, as has happened with the spread of HIV infection and AIDS with heroin injection. It would also be a mistake to think that in these countries drug abuse affects only a minority of the population. In regions like the Golden Triangle (Kittelsen & Argandoña, 1992), the Golden Crescent (Argandoña & Haworth, 1991), or South America (OPS, 1990; WHO, 1992a), drug-related problems have expanded to large sections of the population, including the very young.

It is not only that developing countries are the hardest hit, they are also the countries with the weakest defence. They usually have a health sector already starved of resources to deal with the endemic diseases associated with poverty, malnutrition, poor housing and lack of sanitation. Often, there are no sources of official funding to divert towards the health sector, to help it deal with the growth of needs resulting from the problems caused by substance use. A complete societal vulnerability ensues, in which the impotence of the health sector to take effective action is matched by comparable constraints in the social sector generally. In other words, drug abuse and its associated health problems become an integral part of the problem of development. Further damage is caused by the increase in the abuse of *licit* drugs, in particular alcohol and tobacco, as well as psychotropic drugs and volatile inhalants, often in combination with illicit substances.

To further complicate the difficulties, illicit farming has turned into a subsis-tence crop for millions of impoverished farmers in rural areas of the poorest countries, and a growing multitude of destitute urban dwellers have no choice but to earn their living by complicity with criminal traffickers. More than 90% of the cocaine and heroin abused worldwide is produced by 12 countries. In these and other countries where illicit drug production make up the major part of the economy, only substantial financial support, international political back-up and fair trade agreements can make a change possible. Illicit crops can be substituted but only if the international market is there, and only if the trade arrangements are favourable. It is the world's demand for drugs which has stimulated the opium and coca growing in the producer countries; thus, it must be a collective respon-sibility to provide for the elimination of these crops, and to offer decorous and profitable alternatives to the farmers.

Not everyone in developing countries consumes psychoactive substances. Many abstain from alcohol and other drugs, for religious, cultural or economic reasons. Advantage can also be taken of the wisdom accumulated through centuries, of traditional cultures and communities, who have managed to integrate specific substances in their daily life without harmful consequences.

New global strategies and national policies

The failure of the simplistic repressive approach to either explain or control the drug pandemic requires a new approach, recognising that there is a drugs market in which the combined forces of supply and demand determine the availability and use of substances. This conceptual frame calls for vigorous State control on both sides – supply and demand – of the drugs market.

The market control approach to drug abuse has proved successful in the developed world with regard to licit drugs, particularly alcohol and tobacco. A wide range of measures such as price policy, strict control of the distribution system, advertising and promotion, stimulation of alternatives to alcoholic beverages, and public information for awareness raising have proved to be most effective to tackle alcohol-related problems.

Encouraging results from the manipulation of the legal market stimulated some professionals in industrialised societies to discuss the liberalisation of the drug market, assuming that such a measure would enhance the access to and quality of health services for drug-dependent persons, and further facilitate epidemiological surveillance of drug-related problems. This approach may, however, increase supply; in addition it is in opposition to international conventions, and is therefore rejected by most of the governments in the international community.

The International Conference on Drug Abuse and Illicit Trafficking (ICDAIT, 1988) convened in Vienna in 1987, produced a wide-ranging comprehensive multidisciplinary outline of future activities in drug abuse control. The agreement on a balanced approach, i.e. action taken to reduce both the supply of and the demand for drugs, was the fundamental outcome of ICDAIT:

> "Without prejudice to the importance of continuing administrative control of narcotic drugs and psychotropic substances and of international cooperation in the fight against the illicit traffic, counter-offensives of another dimension are now needed at the national and international levels to respond to the threat drug abuse poses not only to millions of persons but also to whole population groups and even to societies and economies in some countries. To take up the challenge it is necessary to intensify not only measures and programmes directed against the illicit production of and trafficking in drugs but also the activities undertaken to prevent the illicit demand for drugs and to further the treatment and eventual social reintegration of drug addicts."

The current use of psychoactive substances is affecting most countries in the developing world. Governments must work in coordination with each other, fostering the communities' own control of their demand for alcohol and other psychoactive substances; and a heavy responsibility is placed in the hands of industrialised societies to assist those disadvantaged populations which are now being hit the hardest.

At a national level, the conflict between demand reduction and supply control that still pervades most planning decisions, as well as the diverse legal situation of substances, should be discussed to plan coherent health policies on drug related problems.

It is well known that of all the psychoactive substances alcohol and nicotine are the most frequently abused, often in combination with other licit and illicit drugs; and alcohol remains the cause of the greatest number of health and social problems. That is not to diminish the seriousness with which illicit drug problems should be viewed, or indeed the abuse of illicit pharmaceutical products and volatile solvents.

In 1988 WHO sponsored a satellite conference in Australia, following a recommendation of the ICDAIT. In this conference the urgent need for Member States to develop national policies and plans regarding substance abuse was highlighted. It was further advised that national policies should address tobacco, alcohol, and illicit drugs collectively, noting the increasing prevalence of poly-drug use and the commonalities among substances from the public health perspective. It was recognised, however, that national priorities and legal issues may require separate policies for some substances.

For national planners in developing countries, political decision, intersectoral coordination, and outstanding managerial skills will be required to implement and develop national policies to reduce the demand for drugs within a general context of scarcity of resources, competing priorities, and intricate difficulties. The aims of such national plans of action should be:

(i)   the promotion of life free from substance abuse;
(ii) the reduction of the demand for drugs, whether licit or illicit;
(iii) the prevention of new cases of dependence;
(iv) the decrease in the impact of drug use on the health and welfare of individuals and communities;
(v)   the esablishment of accessible services for the effective treatment and rehabilitation of persons affected by drug-related problems.

For a plan to have a meaningful impact on national and international actions, it is essential that clear, measurable objectives be stated, sensitive to the socio-cultural milieu of the country, and consistent with the international context. It will also be necessary to integrate the plans with economic and developmental policies, particularly in the economically disadvantaged nations where drug-related problems have substantial effects on the economy. Demand reduction should be tied to existing structures providing primary health care. There are no simple or easy solutions to the drug problem. Different problems in different societies with specific socioeconomic and cultural contexts do require different approaches. No attempt should therefore be made to reach an internationalisation of homogenous drug policies; activities tailored to regional, national and even local needs are more appropriate. Substance abuse and related problems do not affect only a single sector; multisectoral approaches are required. Although it is entirely appropriate for governments to be 'in front' of the public to lead it forward, policies that are too far in front need to mobilise public concern and involve community participation through information and education.

Last but not least, it would be inaccurate to expect that the public sector could accomplish major social changes alone. Interest groups like providers, industries or political opponents might resist public policies. Alliance with the private sector is then invaluable. Non-governmental organisations (NGOs) that can support the implementation and development of the programmes should be identified for collaboration among businesses, civic associations, religious organisations and community-based groups and initiatives.

The health approach to reduce the demand for drugs

Health complications of substance abuse include lung cancers due to tobacco smoking; violence, accidents and injuries as well as liver diseases and cancers from alcohol drinking; psychiatric diseases and brain damage; suicide and overdoses; foetus damage as well as short- and long-term health care needs of the offspring of pregnant mothers using alcohol and/or cocaine. In more general terms, the disruption of families caused by substance abuse of one or more members creates devastating distress and can result in neglect and personality and emotional disorders.

In developing countries substance-use morbidity and mortality are further exacerbated – particularly among children, adolescents and women – by debilitating factors such as poverty and concomitant malnutrition, infectious and parasitic conditions, illiteracy, lack of sanitation and health services, and cultural barriers which undermine any efforts to assist the affected persons and to educate special risk groups. Other significant contributions to the specific pathology of drug abuse in developing countries are the impurities and poisonous chemicals contained in cheap substances of abuse, like leaded petrol, coca paste, and domestic alcoholic beverages.

Prevention, treatment and rehabilitation of alcohol- and drug-related problems in the countries of the developing world and disadvantaged populations are better dealt with in close collaboration with general practitioners and community health workers rather than specialists in isolated institutions because of the need for a comprehensive approach to complex constellations of health and social problems, usually inextricably linked to both predisposing risk conditions and the actual use of drugs.

Measures to reduce demand should include outreach interventions to protect special risk groups which are not effectively covered by the health system; as well as an increase in training of professionals, community health workers and volunteers. A major emphasis should also be put on action-oriented research to monitor the impact of the programmes and trends of drug use.

The comprehensive approach to alcohol- and drug-related problems has recently been recognised by the *System-wide Plan for Drug Abuse Control* (United Nations, 1990) which includes the following principles:

"Preventive efforts are most likely to succeed when based on sound family structures, broad community participation and supportive services accompanied by the provision of positive alternatives to drug abuse.

A successful treatment programme mitigates the health, social and economic consequences of drug addiction, reduces the illicit demand for drugs and lessens the risk of relapse. It encourages and assists drug dependent persons to return to a drug-free life.

To this end a treatment programme must be linked from the outset to broader rehabilitation and social reintegration measures involving the family, schools, community and the work place, as appropriate, to promote the necessary social support for dependent persons undergoing the treatment process."

Effective responses to the demand for and use of drugs are not only necessary because of medical and humanitarian reasons – as drug dependence is a crippling disease aggravated by a number of miseries – but also to protect the society at large from negative social consequences. The first is that untreated craving and/or dependence constitute the bulk of the inelastic demand for drugs, which stimulates the supply and spreads the use. Second, alcohol and drug users make up the source from which most injuries, accidents and violence, as well as HIV infection come from.

As well as the medical effects of drug use induced by the direct pharmacological or toxic action of the substances on the human body and mind, there are also the social effects of drug use. These are largely dependent on a number of factors which are capable of being both induced and controlled by certain social conditions such as the economic and sociocultural circumstances in which the drugs are taken, or the users' expectations regarding specific drugs, as well as the reasons why some persons take drugs and the reaction of other people.

With regard to the illicit character of the use of specific substances, the rejection and penalisation of drug users and addicts by society may be counterproductive and encourage deviant behaviours and risky lifestyles such as crime and prostitution, and also result in ostracism or increased health risks. Repression towards experimenters or casual users may have the same effect. They should neither be seen as accomplices to drug traffickers, nor as dependent patients. Instead, they should be seen as normal citizens, capable of reasonable control over their own lives provided early identification and simple interventions are available to them. Dramatising and threatening words as well as the hype on drug information, create a paradoxical attraction to drugs, and distort sound prevention and treatment efforts.

The health impact of alcohol abuse

The case of alcohol will be discussed in some detail as a typical example of the negative consequences of licit drug use (Norwegian Ministry of Health and Social Affairs, 1990). The normal use of alcohol does not cause markedly deviant behaviour nor harm the drinker's health, and is socially condoned or even encouraged. Alcohol consumption patterns are strongly influenced by cultural attitudes towards the consumption of, or abstention from, alcoholic beverages. Thus, depending on whether societies are predominantly Hindus, Buddhists or Islamics, distinct attitudes and behaviours regarding alcohol use will prevail. Without idealising the situation, it is reasonable to state that traditional alcohol use in these cultural contexts was well regulated and controlled without major negative consequences.

The contemporary situation, however, is very different. As a consequence of outside political, economic and cultural incursions, rapid urbanisation, increasing global communications and the loosening of traditional social controls result in severe damages to individual, family and community stability as well as to the overall process of development. Aggressive commercial promotion of alcoholic beverages contributes significantly to the above-mentioned negative consequences. All this results in alcohol consumption in many parts of the developing world assuming problematic dimensions. Careful policy and programme initiatives undertaken with due regard to local socio-cultural contexts can go a long way to reversing the current deterioration. It has to be emphasised, though, that in spite of any increases in alcohol consumption, large segments of the population are either abstainers or well-disciplined with respect to alcohol.

The production and consumption of alcoholic beverages are steadily growing in develping countries as a whole. This growth is mostly based on market expansion into countries where alcohol was not previously a commodity. Unlike other products and technologies, alcoholic beverages and alcohol production technology are usually exported from industrialised to industrialising countries without instructions and guidelines on how to use alcohol in a sensible way to cause minimum damage.

Modern industrialised societies have little to be proud of in the way they have handled their alcohol-related problems, although some are now experiencing a decline in alcohol consumption, or at least a slowing down of a long-standing increase for the first time in several decades, suggesting that demand can be limited.

The negative consequences of alcohol abuse exceed the negative consequences of other psychoactive substances, licit or illicit, when measured in terms of years of life lost. This striking fact does not seem to be reflected in national or international preventive programmes and policies. Another disturbing incongruity related to alcohol problems is that they tend to be defined as individual problems with little relation to social processes. Political and public support are given for the treatment and rehabilitation of individuals with alcohol dependence – or alcoholics – but there are no general policies aimed at regulating the availability or the use of alcohol in society at large (Sellaeg, 1990).

The social problems associated with alcohol affect family relationships, the situation of women and children, and are costly to businesses. There are direct costs because money is spent on drink and indirect costs which tend to be underestimated because many elements escape quantification, while others are very difficult or impossible to assess. They include lost productivity, absenteeism, accidents at work, and frequent turnover in personnel. In connection with the workplace, wide-ranging initiatives, including control measures and programmes of prevention and assistance, have been undertaken in highly industrialised societies.

Within the public health framework, primary concern is with the extent to which alcohol causes increased rates of mortality and morbidity. Most alcohol-related deaths before the age of 40 are the outcome of acute intoxication affecting moderate or occasional drinkers (Nakajima, 1991). Drinking has been implicated as an important cause of serious traffic accidents and most other accidents and injuries, including drowning, fatal fires, and leisure and sports accidents. There is also a high rate of alcohol involvement in suicide, homicide, and other forms of violence, particularly domestic violence. In addition to traumatic injury and death, the economic framework adds to the consequences of accidents and criminal violence that result in property destruction, and the legal and administrative costs of arranging insurance payments and litigation.

Alcohol-related damage extends from individuals to their family, immediate community, workplace, other fellow citizens and the broader society as a whole. The impact of this damage is extremely significant in most of the developing world countries, and calls for a systematic review of existing measures for prevention, treatment and rehabilitation, as well as for innovative and cost-effective programmes.

AIDS and substance misuse

Most of the literature concerning the link between AIDS and substance misuse refers to the obvious fact that HIV infection is transmitted to injecting drug users (IDUs) through the sharing of unclean needles and syringes or droppers; in order to reduce the harm of such practices, the free sale or even free distribution of needles, as well as the use of bleach for cleaning the injecting equipment, has already proved to be effective in controlling the spread of HIV infection among particular groups of IDUs in developed countries. It has to be mentioned, however, that drug abuse is also related to the spread of the virus through other ways.

While libido is decreased during excessive drug use, even occasional sexual contact may be sufficient for viral transmission. Furthermore, persons who have been confined for long periods during the course of treatment and rehabilitation or imprisonment, may be unusually prone to have sex with multiple partners.

These are factors to be taken into account when assessing the likely spread of the infection, and it will be necessary to assess the extent to which HIV infection is present in the sexual contacts of drug abusers, including partners and prostitutes, who may become a source of infection among the heterosexual non-drug-user population. These factors should be acknowledged and investigated and sentinel surveillance set up.

There is, however, a distinct possibility that IDUs could be considered as virtually the only source of AIDS within a particular country and that further essentially punitive measures might be taken against them. It is the view of scientists working in this field that no policy of segregation is likely to be effective and that this measure is strongly contraindicated. In fact, the imposition of such measures would be likely to be counterproductive in that IDUs would be driven even further into hiding, thus making the task of combating both problems of drug use and of HIV infection all the more difficult.

Alcohol and sometimes cocaine, which may be used in combination by the same person, are customarily taken to disinhibit sexual behaviour and to facilitate communication with casual partners, particularly among adolescents and prostitutes' clientele. This hedonistic use of drugs happens among people who are neither abusers nor dependents, but are considered as 'normal' or even moderate drinkers. The question arises when the effects of the drug not only trigger sexual boldness, and the feeling of immunity to danger, but interfere with the caution that is required for sexual activities. In developing countries with high illiteracy rates and insufficient information, the increased production and use of alcohol has become a significant catalyst for indulging in unprotected sex, and may counteract the effects of any campaigns to promote safe sex.

Street children and drug abuse

Street children are any minors for whom the street (in the widest sense of the word, including unoccupied dwellings, wasteland) has become their habitual abode, and who are without adequate protection (Report for the Independent Commission on International Humanitarian Issues, 1986).

The phenomenon of street children is not new. They were a common subject of Spanish writers in the early 17th century, and later in Dickens, Twain, Andersen, Gorki, and Hugo. The problem though, and its size have changed both in quantitative and qualitative terms. Street children work, live, sleep, and at times die on the streets in rapidly growing urban centres, mainly in the developing world. Some sell whatever they can, from cigarettes to flowers; some clean and guard cars, shine shoes, carry baggage, beg, and at the end of the day feed themselves from garbage. But there are also some who resort to stealing, selling drugs or are enticed into prostitution.

Deprived of parental love, support and guidance, they are constantly beseiged by hunger and violence. They live in areas with inadequate sanitation, and have no access to education or health and social services. They are extremely vulnerable to abuse, violence, and drug-related problems.

Besides complications due to a lack of pre- and postnatal care, the street child suffers from medical problems such as malnutrition, infectious, parasitic and sexually transmitted diseases including HIV infection, together with accidents and injuries, brain damage and impaired cognitive development.

Specific attention is given to the question of drug use because it represents the most crucial problem facing the world's estimated 100 million street children. For many of them worldwide, drug use represents a form of experimentation and rebellion, or an amusing pastime; it provides them with an escape from the cruel realities of their daily existence: family break-up, parental alcoholism, death of parents, lack of love and care, poverty, hunger and homelessness.

A number of scientific studies have shown that prevalence of drug abuse among street children is higher than in any other groups. Volatile solvents are the substances most frequently used as they are cheap and can be easily procured; other drugs, however, are commonplace, particularly cannabinoids and psychotropic drugs, as well as cocaine (CEBRID, 1990).

Volatile solvent use has deleterious effects on the child's development and may cause irreversible lesions in many organs and the brain. Also, its abuse regularly precedes other forms of illicit drug use (Dinwiddie, 1991). Prevention and treatment of drug abuse must be integrated into community services to enable rehabilitation and social reintegration of the children. Their needs in food, shelter, health assistance, education and job training must be met, and long-term therapy by qualified professionals and volunteers who are familiar with the problems and issues of street life must be made available.

Clinical factors influencing services

If drug abusers remain untreated, their natural history may follow a chronic recurrent course, with gradual exacerbation of individual affliction and social rejection; after years of being exploited by callous traffickers, drug users often become the victims of drug dependence and other harm leading to incapacitating physical and mental deterioration, as well as to premature death. During their long career drug users are gradually ostracised by the community while organising themselves in subcultural groups; in some countries they may eventually become the scapegoats of law enforcement agencies. Such a natural history is typically complicated by problems that also affect the family and the community such as family disintegration, delinquency and crime.

Alcohol and drug users are disabled persons who ought to be assisted if the epidemic of drug-related problems is to be controlled. They may need help to curb their compelling craving. They should be informed about the ways of protecting themselves from HIV infection and other hazards that endanger themselves, their families and indeed the whole society.

It will be necessary to identify the endemic conditions in a particular country to which drug abuse predisposes. For example, malaria, typhoid fever, cysticercosis and tuberculosis may all be associated with drug abuse and will accelerate and aggravate psychotic or confusional disorders associated with the use of alcohol, solvents, and/or cocaine. Pellagra is often a complication of chronic alcohol drinking. Korsakoff amnesic syndrome, as well as polyneuritis, and beriberi cardiac pathology are commonly found among malnourished alcohol and drug abusers. Saturnism has to be investigated in petrol sniffers; and the effects of impurities and chemical precursors should be suspected among users of the by-products of heroin and cocaine preparation and clients of clandestine liquor distilleries. Liver diseases including cirrhosis caused by hepatitis A and schistosomiasis contribute to the impact of alcohol on liver pathology.

Due to the lack of safety in vehicles, roads, and the workplace, serious accidents and injuries are so frequent that repeated bone fractures may be a symptom of alcohol and drug abuse, particularly fractures of the ribs. Head injury may lead to brain damage and epilepsy. In some countries injuries are also a consequence of crime and violence connected to substance use, and the indiscriminate repression injures drug addicts.

Many terminal problems – which in developed societies are only seen among vagrant alcoholics and addicts after more than a decade of heavy abuse – may be present in young users, debilitated by the poverty-ridden conditions of the developing world.

The prudent clinician should always be aware of filtering out these and other prevalent organic conditions, which may be more life-threatening than substance abuse, before deciding how to assist drug dependent persons.

Doctors and health workers in developing countries are seldom aware of the complex links between drug abuse and common physical health problems. There is often a gulf between specialists in addictions and general medicine which has to be overcome through medical education and training of community health workers.

Drug specialists need to be knowledgeable about local epidemiology and public health for clinical practice, and to advocate for good health services for their patients.

General principles of diagnosis and treatment

Substance abuse begins as a kind of psychological crisis, adjustment, or reaction; at this stage, early detection and brief intervention techniques are most cost-effective. Early detection and opportune treatment are components of secondary prevention, which is crucial to prevent actual drug abuse and costly, specialised treatment. All health and social workers, either professionals or volunteers, should be trained to integrate these techniques into their routine work.

When the patient is hooked and dependency established, detoxification (pharmacological treatment of withdrawal symptoms; see section 9.2) is sometimes recommended before making decisions about treatment and rehabilitation. Detoxification is, however, only a short episode in the process of tertiary prevention of drug abuse, which aims at reducing the damage already produced by the drugs, avoiding further deterioration, and extending the remaining years of life in the best possible conditions. Tertiary prevention also includes the alleviation and treatment of medical and social complications, as well as specific techniques for harm reduction, rehabilitation and relapse prevention (see section 9.2). Traditional healers, acupuncturists, and religious leaders in developing countries are frequently skilful therapists and their help may be enough for successful home detoxification if combined with a gradual reduction of the abused drug. Medical support may, however, be necessary for the management of severe intoxication, for the complications of drug abuse, and for the management of rapid withdrawal of drugs like alcohol which cause significant physical dependence.

Detoxification is not a prerequisite for dealing with dependency and other drug-related problems; careful assessment of the complex situation of drug abuse patients should be undertaken to prioritise problems and implement appropriate therapeutic responses.

Even after successful detoxification the patient may be faced with unemployment, stigma, a broken family, and physical and emotional ill health; circumstances like these are usually associated with relapse. To prevent these complications it is best to start organising social and occupational rehabilitation, to ensure social support for the patient, and to link those components of tertiary prevention with medical interventions and aftercare, before raising unrealistic expectations and applying costly interventions which are doomed to failure. The motivation and commitment of drug abuse patients, not only for detoxification but for the whole process of rehabilitation and social reinsertion, must be fostered.

Although specialised services are crucial for the treatment of individuals affected by the most serious drug-related disorders, specialists and hospitals should rather be seen as only elements in a network of alternatives to deal with the varied needs of users in different stages of their natural history. Such a network can also be involved in detecting and assisting special high risk groups, in preventing new cases, as well as in supporting those persons who have undergone treatment, until they are able to live free from the use of drugs.

Drug-related problems should be integrated into the system of primary health care in order to cover the total population and to face all the problems induced by different drugs, with an emphasis on decentralised care and outreach activities, and on giving the family and community participation in the control of their own problems.

Skills to handle drug problems should be essential components of primary health care. Primary health care workers have to be trained in simple but effective techniques, including community mobilisation, the organisation of self-help groups, the ability to encourage healthy life-styles, and the enjoyable use of drug-free leisure time.

To succeed in getting those components into the broad area of primary health care, specialists need to expand their traditional clinical role by carrying out the following new functions:

(i)   Educate and stimulate public awareness and solidarity.
(ii) Act as consultants for cases referred from the community level.
(iii) Decide upon the skills and knowledge to be transferred to the lower levels of the service.
(iv) Visit community health facilities on a regular basis as supervisors, and to encourage preventive interventions and simple research.
(v)   Coordinate and evaluate the whole system, and participate in developing and evaluating national plans and policies.
(vi) Act as advocates to generate public support, and advise government and the mass media on matters related to drugs and alcohol.

To ensure coordination it will be useful for the specialists to create a community action team with representatives from relevant sectors and the community. The members of these teams should be drawn from sectors and groups with a stake in community development, in such a way that they are able to seek answers to questions on the community's perception of drug related problems, and which interventions are best accepted for community report (Grant & Hodgson, 1991).

References

ARGANDOÑA, M. & HAWORTH, A. (1991) *Mission Report: Assessment of Drug Demand Reduction Activities in Afghanistan.* Geneva: WHO.

CEBRID (Centro Brasileiro de Informaçoes Sobre Drogas Psicotrópicas) (1990) *Abuso de Drogas entre Meninos e Meninas de Rua do Brasil.* São Paulo: Departamento de Psicobiología, Escola Paulista de Medicina.

DINWIDDIE, S. H., REICH, T. & CLONINGER, C. (1991) Solvent use as a precursor of intravenous drug abuse. *Comprehensive Psychiatry,* **32,** 133–140.

GRANT, M. & HODGSON, R. (1991) *Responding to Drug and Alcohol Problems in the Community.* Geneva: WHO.

ICDAIT (International Conference on Drug Abuse and Illicit Trafficking) (1988) *Comprehensive Multidsciplinary Outline of Future Activities in Drug Abuse Control.* New York, Vienna: UN.

KITTELSEN, J. & ARGANDOÑA, M. (1992) *Report on the International Workshop on Drug Use and HIV Infection, Chiang-Mai, October 1991.* Geneva: WHO.

NAKAJIMA, H. (1991) *Keynote Address by the Director-General of WHO to the Inter-Regional Meeting on Alcohol-Related Problems.* Tokyo/Geneva: PSA/WHO.

NORWEGIAN MINISTRY OF HEALTH AND SOCIAL AFFAIRS, IN COLLABORATION WITH THE UNO AT VIENNA (1990) *Expert Meeting on the Negative Social Consequences of Alcohol Use, Report of the Meeting.* Oslo, 1990.

OPS (Organización Panamericana de la Salud) (1990) *Abuso de Drogas, Publicación Científica No. 522.* Washington, D.C.

ORFORD, J. (1985) *Excessive Appetites: a Psychological View of Addiction.* Chichester: Wiley.

PORTER, L., *et al* (1986) *The Law and the Treatment of Drug- and Alcohol-Dependent Persons.* Geneva: WHO.

SELLAEG, W. F. (1990) Opening Statement to the Expert Meeting on the Negative Social Consequences of Alcohol Use. Oslo.

UNITED NATIONS (1990) *System-wide Action Plan on Drug Abuse Control.* New York/Vienna: United Nations.

WORLD HEALTH ORGANIZATION (1988) *Health Policies to Combat Drug and Alcohol Problems.* A Satellite Conference to the Healthy Policies Conference, Sydney and Canberra, Australia. Geneva: WHO.

—— (1992a) *Lexicon of Alcohol and Other Drug Terms.* Geneva: WHO.

—— (1992b) *Street Children Project.* Report on Inaugural Meeting of Participants. Geneva: WHO.

9.2 Individual treatment: theoretical and practical approaches

MICHAEL FARRELL and JOHN STRANG

The aim of this section is to provide a brief overview of approaches to individual treatment of alcohol and drug problems. It is worth remembering that many people may make significant changes without using treatment services, and so by definition those who do use treatment services will have failed at attempts at self-change. This section outlines the basic cognitive–behavioural approach to the assessment and the planning of treatment goals for individual patients.

Studies from the United States draw attention to the extent to which a process of 'maturing out' (moving away from illegal drug use with age) may occur, but also draw attention to the conditional nature of this 'maturing out' and identify factors which may slow down the rate of such recovery. In the United Kingdom, Gossop *et al* (1991) have reported on the considerable extent to which heroin addicts in treatment have made previous do-it-yourself attempts at detoxification, employing a variety of strategies with a moderate degree of success in the short term, at least comparable to that achieved in out-patient treatment programmes. The extent to which these approaches may be developed (for example, in the form of self-help manuals) has yet to be evaluated.

Most people who stop smoking do so without any professional assistance. Modification of patterns of alcohol consumption may be strongly mediated by factors such as spouse or family pressure, employer pressure or other lifestyle changes. Environmental supports that promote health changes and healthier lifestyles are important adjuncts to any treatment interventions.

Approaches to treatment

Treatment stages are frequently divided into assessment, treatment and maintenance of abstinence. Treatment can only occur when people are sufficiently motivated to overcome their habitual behaviour. Motivating people to change is, therefore, an important precursor of treatment.

Process of change

The promotion of behaviour change is the key goal of all interventions. Studies of the process demarcate three stages: precontemplation, contemplation, and action. Smokers, drug takers or drinkers who are not concerned about their substance consumption and do not think that the health risks as a result of their pattern of consumption are at the precontemplation stage. The contemplator is the person who has begun to worry that his/her pattern of behaviour may be adversely affecting some dimension of their life. The action stage is reached when the concern becomes more powerful than the reward for continuing substance misuse. It is only then that consumption can be reduced or stopped. This process of change is conceptually simple and is the basis for any treatment intervention.

Motivational interviewing

The motivational interviewer's task is to guide the ambivalent drinker or drug abuser to a position where they develop a robust resolution to modify their behaviour, and then to plan a course of action to achieve this change (Miller, 1983). One of the aims of this approach is to raise health consciousness, and increase the awareness of negative health consequences of substance misuse.

Relapse prevention

Inherent to the management of substance misuse and substance dependence is the reality of relapse. Relapse rapidly leads to the reinstatement of dependence and withdrawal symptoms. One of the major challenges that substance misuse presents is the development of a treatment strategy that will prevent relapse. The treatment course should be easy for the patient to sustain and consolidate and should involve a radical change in his behaviour pattern.

Cognitive–behavioural strategies have been developed that focus specifically on the problem of relapse and have been devised as relapse prevention strategies. Patients are taught to identify the types of situation that put them at risk of relapse and through practised rehearsals are taught to develop alternative coping strategies. For example, efforts should be made into exploring how a patient who has just been detoxified is going to cope with the inevitable intense cravings or urges to use the drug again. Such coping strategies may assist in building up a patient's resistance to the temptation of relapse. High-risk situations may be intrapersonal, interpersonal or environmental.

Approaches to substance-related problems should focus on changing a specific form of behaviour. Underlying psychological and psychiatric issues may also need to be addressed but it should not be expected that their treatment will result in major changes in substance consumption. Rather, it is more likely that a focus on the active change of substance consumption will clarify what issues will subsequently need to be addressed.

Assessing substance problems

A complete assessment of alcohol, drug and smoking behaviour requires a degree of attention and time rarely available to mental health professionals. In most instances, a thorough and detailed history will provide adequate detail to make a comprehensive assessment of the impact of substance use on the overall physical, psychological and social well-being of a patient.

Hospital doctors should always bear in mind that presenting complaints may be alcohol- or drug-induced. Conditions such as pancreatitis and liver cirrhosis should prompt the taking of a more detailed drinking history and where there is evidence of HIV or hepatitis B, a more thorough inquiry into a patient's history of drug injection should be made. It is only by routine enquiry that a clinician can feel comfortable and ensure that her line of questioning is not prompted or indicative of personal prejudice. The self-assessment report provided by the patient is often the only element available on which the clinician is to base her assessment, so that where resources permit, it is useful to confirm a self-report with a urine analysis.

Laboratory investigations

Several studies have confirmed the general reliability of self-report questionnaires in assessing substance use. However, clinical practice and research should not rely on a single measure of drug use; ideally, a wide range of measures should be included in order to validate self-reports. Laboratory investigations are important to provide independent confirmation of self-reports and to objectively monitor drug-free states. In many settings laboratory equipment will be cost-prohibitive and so will take lower priority in the allocation of limited resources. Some health centres may be provided with such facilities through the support of programmes such as the United Nations Demand Reduction Programme.

Laboratory methods include the testing of urine for drugs. Most laboratories use thin layer chromatography (TLC) to detect opiates, amphetamines, cocaine, solvents, barbiturates, benzodiazepines and cannabis (*Lancet*, 1987). However, urine analysis will not detect hallucinogens such as LSD.

Confirmation of a drug within a particular group requires the use of gas liquid chromatography (GLC) or high pressure liquid chromatography (HPLC) which are more expensive. Urine tests provide only a snapshot of drug use which is affected by the half-life of the individual drug. Substances such as cannabis may be present in the urine for up to three weeks after consumption, while others are more rapidly excreted.

Detoxification

Full assessment should provide a detailed picture of the past or current history of drinking and drug abuse. Those individuals who are dependent on alcohol, benzodiazepines, opiates or cocaine may require brief detoxification. Detoxification may be in an in-patient setting, but will most commonly be in an out-patient setting.

Alcohol withdrawal

Alcohol is a cerebral depressant and is the most commonly misused drug in society. Many young people have alcohol-related problems but alcohol dependence is more common among older people. The longer term sequelae are determined by adult drinking patterns. Heavy consumption may be associated with benzodiazepine abuse and the unmanaged combined withdrawal may result in grand mal convulsion.

Alcohol detoxification is usually conducted in the community. It is important that the alcohol-dependent state is fully assessed and withdrawal symptoms identified. Symptoms include restlessness, irritability, disturbed sleep and tremor which may develop into a full alcohol withdrawal state with delirium tremens. This is a potentially life-threatening condition and needs to be appropriately managed.

Benzodiazepines such as diazepam and chlordiazepoxide ($t\frac{1}{2}$ 30–60 hours) are most commonly used in alcohol withdrawal. Chlordiazepoxide is generally administered orally in 20 mg doses four times daily (diazepam 5–10 mg four times daily). Dosages should be adapted according to the severity of the case.

On average, alcohol withdrawal symptoms last approximately 3–6 days. Initial assessment should determine the degree of dependence. The greater the dependence, the more likely will be early morning drinking, early morning nausea, vomiting, or shakings. An anticonvulsant may be given if there is a history of previous withdrawal fits.

Alcohol-dependent patients are prone to depression and often develop suicidal thoughts. A careful mental state assessment should be carried out to identify these conditions.

Withdrawal from opiates

The number of regular opiate users is small compared to the number of alcohol misusers. However, it is this class of drugs that is in highest demand in treatment services in many countries. Heroin is the most commonly used drug in the illicit market but a range of drugs such as codeine, Diconal (dipipanone and cyclizine mixture), dextramoramide (Palfium) and the mixed agonist/antagonist opioid buprenorphine (Temgesic) are also used. No good data are available on how many people have used opiates such as heroin on an 'experimental' basis or what proportion of 'experimenters' go on to develop regular use or dependent use. First use may be associated with nausea and vomiting. Heroin may be smoked or injected or taken intranasally by snorting. Heroin smoking is a common mode of initiation into heroin use which may progress to heroin injecting. Regular use will result in a higher tolerance to opiates. Withdrawal symptoms will give rise to restlessness, irritability, increased bowel activity with diarrhoea and crampy abdominal pain, yawning, sneezing and coryza. Nausea and vomiting may also occur quite frequently. Mild withdrawal symptoms will begin 8–12 hours after the last dose and the peak of symptoms will be reached approximately 36 hours after the last dose. Such withdrawal symptoms will also be associated with intense craving for the drug.

In many countries, the prescription of oral methadone is the commonest approach to the management of opiate withdrawal. In some opiate producing countries other natural opiates have been used as substitute agents but there is limited data available on this practice to date. Methadone dosage is calculated on the basis of a conversion factor of a daily use of one gram of heroin being

TABLE 9.2.1
Withdrawal of opiates using methadone as a substitute

Drug	Dose	Methadone equivalent
Street heroin	Cannot accurately be estimated because street drugs vary in purity. Titrate dose against withdrawal symptoms	
Pharmaceutical heroin	10 mg tablet or ampoule	20 mg
	30 mg ampoule	50 mg
Methadone	10 mg ampoule	10 mg
	Mixture (1 mg/1 ml) 10 ml	10 mg
	Linctus (2 mg/5 ml) 10 ml	4 mg
Morphine	10 mg ampoule	10 mg
Dipipanone (Diconal)	10 mg tablet	4 mg
Dihydrocodeine (DF118)	30 mg tablet	3 mg
Dextromoramide (Palfium)	5 mg tablet	5–10 mg
	10 mg tablet	10–20 mg
Pethidine	50 mg tablet	5 mg
	50 mg ampoule	5 mg
Buprenorphine hydrochloride (Temgesic)	200 microgram tablet	5 mg
	300 microgram ampoule	8 mg
Pentazocine (Fortral)	50 mg capsule	4 mg
	25 mg tablet	2 mg
Codeine linctus 100 ml	300 mg codeine phosphate	10 mg
Codeine phosphate	15 mg tablet	1 mg
	30 mg tablet	2 mg
	60 mg tablet	3 mg
Gee's linctus 100 ml	16 mg anhydrous morphine	10 mg
J. Collis Brown 100 ml	10 mg extract of opium	10 mg

Drug Misuse and Dependence from *Guidelines on Clinical Management* (1991).

equivalent to 80 milligrams of methadone (see Table 9.2.1). In-patient management of withdrawal is a rare facility but where possible the patient should be put on
a 10-day methadone detoxification treatment. Other approaches to withdrawal
include the use of alpha-2 adrenergic agonists such as clonidine or lofexidine as
alternative agents for the management of withdrawal symptoms. Much community-based opiate detoxification takes place on a longer time-scale and efforts
should be made to use this period of treatment to modify other aspects of a
patient's lifestyle.

Maintenance

A 'maintenance' dose of methadone may also be used in longer-term treatment to
facilitate the social rehabilitation of the drug user. This may have the advantage
of reducing heroin injection and HIV transmission. Methadone treatment has
received extensive evaluation in the United States and forms an important part
of the treatment response to opiate dependent misusers (Institute of Medicine, 1990).

Methadone is a long-acting agonist. Recently long-acting oral antagonists
such as naltrexone have been tried as abstinence-based maintenance treatment.
They block any effect from self-administered opiates, but despite their initial
promise, have only found a limited place in the treatment of opiate dependence.

Stimulants

Stimulants like cocaine and amphetamines may be taken intranasally in the form of powder or in solution by injection. Cocaine with the hydrochloride component removed is known as 'crack' and is smokable in this form as it volatises. Stimulants generally produce an elevation of mood and a sense of increased energy with reduction in appetite and a marked reduction in sleep. At higher doses some people may become anxious or irritable, talkative, agitated and some may develop a frank psychosis which may be related to the amount of stimulant consumed. The half-life of cocaine is 50 minutes while the half-life of amphetamines is about 10 hours. Cocaine does not produce dependence but since the rapid growth in the use of cocaine in the United States in the 1980s it has been found that it produces severe psychological dependence which is influenced by the route of administration (Gawin & Ellinwood, 1988). Cocaine smokers may develop dependence more rapidly than snorters. The classic pattern of compulsive consumption is bingeing, lasting from 12 hours to three days which is then followed by a 'crash' with a period of sleepiness, depression and withdrawal and then mounting craving for further cocaine. Cocaine and amphetamines probably exert their reinforcing effect by the release of monoamines. Heavy or prolonged use may result in the depletion of pre-synaptic monoamines which may trigger depression, anxiety or suicidal ideation.

As the number of people using cocaine has increased, so have the reports on the physical complications linked to the toxicity of cocaine (Cregler, 1990). Toxic paranoid psychosis for both amphetamine and cocaine are dose-related and may occur in situations where there is a level of high drug tolerance (Post, 1975). The psychosis may be associated with visual hallucinations, pseudo-hallucination and most classically tactile hallucinations (cocaine bugs). Stereotyped behaviour may occur.

There is limited room for substitute prescribing. The tricyclic antidepressant desipramine has been used in the treatment of stimulant-induced affective disorders and has been reported to reduce cocaine consumption in control studies. Clinical trials of amantidine, bromocriptine and flupenthixol (Gawin & Ellinwood, 1988) have also been undertaken but there is no clear indication of their efficacy. Exposing cocaine users to the cues associated with their drug-taking behaviour can extinguish their cue response behaviour such as craving for the drug. Some treatment trials have reported reduced cocaine use after cue exposure treatment.

Tranquillisers

Barbiturates, benzodiazepines and related compounds

Benzodiazepines are now probably the most common sedative used. Dependence may arise as a result of long-term prescribing as a hypnotic or anxiolytic agent, even when the dose is within the therapeutic range. Benzodiazepines may also be taken in binges or in high doses in excess of up to four times (or multiples thereof) the recommended dose. Although it is not clear whether some benzodiazepines

TABLE 9.2.2
Approximate dosages or common benzodiazepines equivalent to 5 mg diazepam

Drug	Dose
Chlordiazepoxide	15 mg
Diazepam	5 mg
Loprazolam	500 micrograms
Lorazepam	500 micrograms
Oxazepam	15 mg
Temazepam	10 mg
Nitrazepam	5 mg

are more liable to be abused than others, it is postulated that the shorter-acting ones are more so. Management of patients who have developed a dependency on benzodiazepines should be carefully monitored: a plan should be drawn up with a time schedule aimed at shifting away from maintenance prescribing to detoxifying over a three-month period, with regular reduction in dosage. Short-acting benzodiazepines should be replaced by equivalent doses of longer-acting benzodiazepines such as diazepam (see Table 9.2.2) and a gradual reduction begun. Anxiety, stress management and relaxation exercises will help to cope with withdrawal symptoms. Mental state assessment may reveal an underlying psychiatric condition such as depression that has been inappropriately treated. Most individuals can be successfully detoxified in the out-patient setting. However, those with a history of convulsions may require hospital detoxification.

The management of barbiturate dependence is a rare phenomenon in developed countries but some developing countries have experienced an upsurge in barbiturate problems. The problems of overdose and withdrawal fits make the management complicated, and will often require hospitalisation.

Psychedelic drugs (hallucinogens)

MDMA ('Ecstasy')

This is a drug that does not appear to produce dependence or compulsive use and is associated with a rapid development of tolerance. Effects are likely to be that of mild euphoria, a general sense of well-being, increased activity and reduced sleep (Solowil, 1993). At a higher dosage its use may result in a paranoid psychosis (Fahy & Maguire, 1991). To date there are limited studies of the adverse psychological effects but clinical descriptions of affective complications similar to those of stimulants with depression, anxiety and suicidal ideation are now being reported. A small number of cases of chronic paranoid psychosis have been reported. Deaths due to hyperthermia have occurred in previously fit users who are physically active.

LSD (lysergic acid diethylamide)

LSD appears to act particularly on the 5-HT2 receptor. The subjective effect is of visual distortions, disturbance in sense of time and increased sensitivity to colours and sound with a loss of the sense of boundaries between self and the world. Long-term consequences of LSD use are unclear. The most frequently reported adverse effect is that of flashbacks which is a recurrence of the subjective effects long after use of the drug. It may be quite similar to a panic attack but is characterised by distress associated with experiencing the phenomena. Flashbacks may be precipitated by the use of cannabis (marijuana), anxiety, fatigue or movement into a dark environment (Jaffe, 1990). A small number of people may develop long-term psychotic illnesses. It is not clear whether this is a result of LSD use or an indication of pre-morbid or latent psychopathology.

Cannabis (marijuana)

Marijuana is the most commonly used illicit drug in the Western world since the late sixties. The active ingredient is Δ9-tetrahydrocannabinol (Δ9THC) which produces most of the characteristic subjective effects such as relaxation, increased sense of well-being, sleepiness, spontaneous laughter and giggling, distortion in the sense of time and impairment of short-term memory. Higher doses may result in the development of anxiety and paranoid ideas and at sufficiently high doses tetrahydrocannabinol can result in a frank toxic psychosis. The adverse effects of cannabis have been extensively studied. Immediate effect is that of impairment of coordination and psychomotor skills. This may affect driving skills or the capacity to handle machinery. Because of the slow rate of elimination of Δ9THC, residual effects may persist for a number of days after consumption if high doses have been consumed. Long-term cannabis smoking is associated with bronchitis; the smoke is also more carcinogenic than tobacco (Hollister, 1987). Cannabis may induce mild dependence but overall appears to be a weakly reinforcing drug.

Clinical experience indicates that cannabis can be a factor in provoking, aggravating or prolonging psychotic experiences but there is little evidence to support a distinctive clinical syndrome. Cannabis has been linked to the aetiology of schizophrenia (Andreasson *et al*, 1987) in a study of Swedish conscripts.

Cannabis withdrawal does not require a medicated detoxification but a simple cognitive–behavioural strategy aimed at assisting someone in modifying their behaviour and identifying appropriate lifestyle changes.

Volatile substances (glue, solvents)

Volatile substance abuse occurs predominantly in young people and has been particularly noted as a feature of the young homeless in the cities of many developing countries (Chapter 9.1). The popularity may be due to the cheapness and the ready availability of substances, particularly as household products. Gasoline, adhesives, typewriter correcting fluids and paint thinners, butane gas, lighter fuel, fire extinguishers and other aerosols are the most commonly used substances. Vapours may be inhaled from a plastic bag, or aerosols may be directly sprayed onto the back of the larynx resulting in pharyngeal and laryngeal oedema which can result in breathing difficulties. Deaths may result from intoxication, cardiac arrhythmias or from associated accidents and traumatic incidents.

Inhalation initially gives rise to a pleasurable situation but higher dosage use may result in incoordination, confusion and hallucinations. Heavy consumption may result in changes and damage to the kidney, liver, and also to the nervous system with peripheral neuropathies and cerebellar degeneration. Physical complications are reversible on cessation of use but there is still uncertainty about the possibility of long-term neuropsychological deficits (ACMD, 1995).

Rehabilitation

The management of substance abuse requires attention to health and social factors. In many countries considerable emphasis is placed on the role of therapeutic or residential drug- and alcohol-free communities in the rehabilitation of alcohol and drug misusers. There are three main types of programmes: the Concept Based programmes deriving from some of the original American groups, with longer stays and an emphasis on confrontation and need to accept responsibility for one's actions; the 12-step or Minnesota model programme and its slightly modified version, the Hazelden model, based on Alcoholics Anonymous (AA) philosophy, with a shorter-stay approach and a heavy emphasis on the need to engage with anonymous (NA/AA) support groups after discharge from the residential programme (Cook, 1988); and other religious-based programmes such as Christian Therapeutic Communities, where duration of stay ranges from 8 weeks to 18 months.

Rehabilitation may be based in the open community or in specialised residential settings. Rehabilitation programmes focus on the need for psychosocial development and the acquisition of social skills that will sustain independent living.

The self-help movement

Alcoholics Anonymous (AA) originated in the United States but has considerably expanded and adapted. Most countries now have variations of AA tailored to their cultural and social mores. Generally these self-help groups, which also include Narcotics Anonymous and Families Anonymous (support for the other families' members of substance misusers), exist independently of professional organisations and treatment services. Such groups will be an important support for many users and may be particularly valuable in situations where there is very limited availability of treatment. Developing countries need to encourage the maximum development of self-help strategies at an individual and broader social level.

Conclusions

In areas of scare resource there will be limited facilities set aside to respond exclusively to alcohol and drug problems. However, these problems may exact a high social price. A key part of advocacy is the clear identification of the cost burden of substance-related problems. Alcohol and drug use take place in a complex social and economic framework. At international, national and local levels there appear to be ever increasing forces facilitating psychoactive drug use. Policy-makers need to be clearly aware that dependence-inducing substances have particular characteristics and give rise to particular problems. They are more than just commodities in the market place and they have an impact not only on the more visibly disadvantaged drug taker but also on society in general. The line between generating wealth and damaging health needs to be ever more clearly drawn. All governments have the responsibility of promoting the health agenda and to date many have failed badly in this duty. Part of the response should include the provision of treatment for those with substance-related problems.

Further reading

Jaffe (1990) provides detailed information about the clinical pharmacology of drugs of abuse.

References

ANDREASSON, S., ALLBRECK, P., ENGSTROM, A., *et al* (1987) Cannabis and schizophrenia: a longitudinal study of Swedish Conscripts. *Lancet*, **2**, 1483–1486.

COOK, C. C. H. (1988) The Minnesota Model in the Management of Drug and Alcohol Dependency: miracle, method or myth? *British Journal of Addiction*, **83**, 625–634.

CREGLER, L. L. (1989) Adverse consequences of cocaine abuse. *Journal of the National Medical Association*, **81**, 27–38.

DEPARTMENT OF HEALTH (1991) *Drug Misuse and Dependence Guidelines on Clinical Management*. London: HMSO.

GAWIN, F. & ELLINWOOD, E. H. (1988) Cocaine and other stimulants: actions, abuse and treatment. *New England Journal of Medicine*, **318**, 1173–1182.

HOLLISTER, L. (1986) Health aspects of cannabis. *Pharmacological Review*, **38**, 1–20.

GOSSOP, M., BATTERSBY, M. & STRANG, J. (1991) Self-detoxification by opiate addicts. *British Journal of Psychiatry*, **159**, 208–212.

INSTITUTE OF MEDICINE (1990) Broadening the base of treatment for alcohol problems: a report of a study by a committee of the Institute of Medicine, Division of Mental Health and Behavioural Medicine. National Academy of Sciences.

JAFFE, J. (1990) Drug addiction and drug abuse. In (eds L. S. Goodman & L. Gilman) *The Pharmacological Basis of Therapeutics*. New York: Macmillan.

LANCET (1987) Editorial. Screening for drugs of abuse. *Lancet*, **i**, 365–366.

MAGUIRE, P. & FAHY, T. (1991) Chronic psychosis after misuse of MDMA. *British Medical Journal*, **302**, 697.

MILLER, W. (1983) Motivational interviewing with problem drinkers. *Behavioural Psychotherapy*, **11**, 147–172.

POST, R. M. (1975) Cocaine psychoses: a continuum model. *American Journal of Psychiatry*, **132**, 225–231.

10 Depression and bipolar affective disorder

A. VENKOBA RAO

Although the terms 'primary' and 'secondary' depression were first introduced by Woodruff *et al* (1967), a clearer description of these came from Robins *et al* (1972): "a primary affective disorder is one in which the first evidence of diagnosable psychiatric illness is an affective episode; a secondary affective disorder is one in which the affective episode was preceded by another diagnosable psychiatric illness".

Affective disorders resulting from physical illness, medication, infections, neoplasia (Krauthammer & Klerman, 1978) and disabilities are also termed secondary affective disorders. ICD–10 (World Health Organization, 1992) does not accept primary/secondary classification though it is useful in practical clinical application and is one of the best validated.

Mood (affective) disorders in ICD–10 comprise the manic episode (F30.0–30.9), bipolar affective disorder (F31.0–31.9) and depressive episode (F32.0–32.9). There are also separate categories for recurrent depressive disorder (F33.0–33.9), persistent mood (affective) disorders (F34.0–34.9), other mood (affective) disorders (F38.0–38.8) and unspecified mood (affective) disorder (F39).

Depression

Prevalence and distribution

Lifetime prevalence for affective disorders varies between 17–20% (Boyd & Weissman, 1981). Though the men to women ratio for bipolar disorder is almost equal (1:1.2), women are twice as common among monopolar disorders (1:2) (Clayton, 1978). Both monopolar and bipolar depression start earlier in women than in men (average age of first episode 31 and 41 years, respectively (Perris, 1966)). Loranger & Levine (1978) found the age of the first episode of bipolar depression to be 21.1 years in women and 29.1 years for men.

Few studies have addressed the incidence of affective disorders. Boyd & Weissman (1981) report on a one-year incidence of 3% for men and 4–9% for women. The other figures on the occurrence of new cases during a specified period indicate a rate of 4.3 per 1000 person years in men and 7.6 per 1000 person years in women (Rorsman *et al*, 1990), and 2.1 per 1000 person years in men and 2.5 per 1000 person years in women (Murphy *et al*, 1988).

With the formulation of precise diagnostic criteria (predominantly Western world oriented, e.g. DSM, ICD, RDC), with the increasing availability of 'locally' trained psychiatrists and the introduction of general hospital psychiatry (which in countries like India started more than half a century ago), the figures for depression tended to rise. Depression, it came to be realised, occurred at every level of clinical activity.

In primary health care services in India, the estimated prevalence of depression is around 20% (Sen & Williams, 1987), and in general medical practice ranges between 5–20% (Naik & Wig, 1980; Venkoba Rao, 1984). General population surveys measuring the prevalence of depression across India showed varying rates: 30 to 32.9/1000 in South India (Verghese, 1973; Carstairs & Kapur, 1976), 8.9/1000 in Northern India (Sethi *et al*, 1973) and 4.72/1000 in Bengal in Eastern India (Nandi *et al*, 1975). The prevalence of depressive disorder in psychiatric departments of general hospitals in India has ranged from 34.7% (Sethi & Gupta, 1970) to 6% (Venkoba Rao, 1978). For in-patients the figures have varied between 1.85–16.8% (Venkoba Rao, 1986). Recent studies in West Bengal, India, indicate the rising rate of depression *pari passu* with a steep decline of hysteria. Field studies repeated after 10 and 15 years interval respectively in two villages near Calcutta revealed a total mental morbidity unaltered from the base years. However, the prevalence of depressive disorder increased from 61.9% to 77.2% in one village (between 1972 and 1987) and from 27.7% to 53.3% in another village (between 1972 and 1982), confirming that depression is a major mental health problem in India (Nandi *et al*, 1992).

A higher urban frequency of depression noted earlier (Dohrenwend & Dohrenwend, 1974) was not supported by later reports (Coryell *et al*, 1982). Nandi *et al* (1977) observed the disorder to be common among the tribals as well as in the higher castes in an East Indian sample. The symptoms of rural depressive patients not seeking treatment differed little from those seeking clinic treatment (Nandi *et al*, 1976).

German (1987) showed that the prevalence of depression in African countries is comparable to that of the United Kingdom. Cox (1979) compared reports on the psychiatric status of pregnant and puerperal women in Africa and Europe and found that the incidence of depressive neurosis (8%) and depressive psychosis (2%) in Africa is comparable to the rates observed in European countries.

Depression was once considered uncommon in Arab countries, however, Okasha (1977) reported an incidence of 24.5% in out-patients in Egypt. Affective psychosis was the most common reason for admission and depression was most prevalent in middle-aged housewives in Saudi Arabia (Al-Sabaie, 1990).

Pfeiffer (1962) who initially reported a low figure for depression in Indonesia later revised his stand and found that all forms of psychosis seen in Europe and assignable to the World Health Organization (WHO) diagnostic categories occurred in Indonesia (Pfeiffer, 1973). Reports on depression in Korea (Kim & Rhi, 1976), Thailand (Tongyout, 1972) and the Philippines (Lapuz, 1972) indicate that the disorder is similar both in its prevalence and the nature of symptoms to that described in the West. Depression has caused increasing numbers of suicides among Australian Aborigines under custody, hitherto a rare phenomenon (Cawte, 1988).

Among the Latin American countries, depressive illness formed nearly 60% of psychosis surveyed in Peru (Mezzich & Raab, 1980).

Clinical features

A dysphoric mood or a pervasive loss of interest or pleasure is the cardinal feature of depressive disorder. In addition, the presence of at least four of the following symptoms, lasting for a minimum of two weeks and representing a change from previous functioning is required to fulfil the ICD–10 criteria for major depressive disorder: (1) reduced concentration and attention; (2) reduced self-esteem and self-confidence; (3) ideas of guilt and unworthiness; (4) black and pessimistic views of the future; (5) ideas or acts of self-harm or suicide; (6) disturbed sleep; and (7) diminished appetite.

General symptomatology

Many patients appear tired, sick, older than their age and miserable. Some are agitated, while others are slow in movement, slumped in posture and avoidant of gaze.

There are numerous possible symptoms. Weight loss results from loss of appetite. The daily routine demands extra effort (e.g. shaving, bathing, dressing, professional or household work). Absenteeism from work can become a frequent occurrence. The patient feels sad and desperate, but in cases where patients find it difficult to differentiate their current mood from normal sadness, they may not complain of depressed mood unless specifically asked. In Indian patients for instance, the depressed mood is more often an elicited sign than a complained symptom (Venkoba Rao, 1984). There are also cases of 'smiling depression' – the smile serving as a defensive facade.

A progressive decline in interests affects many activities – food, sex, social relations, occupations and ultimately life itself. The loss of interest in one's social environment has been culturally explained in traditional Algerian society as due to 'Tankir' (denial) (Al-Issa, 1989). Letters of resignation from jobs are kept ready to send. Inability to 'feel' for children and spouse is not unusual. The patient suggests to his family not to trust or depend upon him. Unable to enjoy life as others do and sometimes envious of them, the patient feels like an 'island'. The mood may deepen into gloom with feelings of unworthiness, hopelessness and low self-esteem. Life hitherto is seen as a series of mistakes. In serious cases, patients may even plead to be 'done away' with.

Cross-cultural studies have shown that guilt is relatively less common in depressive patients from the Indian sub-continent (Bagadia *et al*, 1977) and Africa (Binitie, 1975) but common in the Japanese (Kimura, 1965). Murphy *et al* (1967) saw guilt as a symptom of depressive illness as a unique feature of Christianity, the degree of guilt being proportionate to the intensity of religious belief. However, a cross-cultural study of 100 Indian depressed patients and two British cohorts showed that the frequency of occurrence of guilt feelings was equivalent in all three groups (Teja *et al*, 1971), although there was a qualitative difference in the content of guilt between the English and Indian groups.

Some regard themselves undeserving of food and help from others. Retardation, mild in earlier stages, may progress to stupor (akinetic mutism). On the other hand restless pacing and frequent changes of position indicate agitation.

Sleep may increase (hypersomnia) or decrease (hyposomnia) both in quality or quantity. Late night ('owl' type) or early morning ('lark' type) insomnia are characteristic of depression, the latter being regarded as a 'biological' feature. Total insomnia is not uncommon. Terminal hypersomnia occurs in some. In the EEG record, the latency between the first onset of sleep (non-rapid eye movement) and the first period of rapid eye movement (REM) sleep is reduced to 15–60 minutes (normal: 70–110 minutes; Kupfer & Thase, 1983). The REM periods are shorter and more frequent than in normal sleep. The themes of dreams reflect low self-esteem, negative events and feelings of death.

In cultures where daily movement of the bowel is a mark of health, constipation brings an exaggerated distress. Fear of diseases such as cancer or of death, panic attacks and obsessions may be distressing. In African patients complaints of forgetfulness and inefficient thinking resulting in confusion and hypochondriasis are noted. The disturbed thinking pattern in African students takes the form of a disorder being imposed from outside – 'Insangana' a result of bewitchment. Another allied disorder is 'Kwetela', 'drowsiness on thinking', noticed in the 'brain fag' syndrome (see below). Though apparently psychotic, in the African context these symptoms are seen as 'spiritual' (related to the supernatural) (Guinness, 1992).

Mood congruent hallucinations and delusions characterise psychotic depression. A voice may accuse or blame the subject of sin or unworthiness. The content of delusions may be bodily health, poverty, guilt or sin. Nihilistic delusions are frequently found in the elderly, who may complain, for example, of 'a rotting brain', 'a bottomless stomach', or 'an absent lung'.

There may be delusions of persecution which are often mood congruent (Vyas, 1992). Some, however, are mood incongruent and unrelated to depressive themes. Such delusions are reported from the French-speaking North African countries Algeria, Tunisia and Morocco. Their themes are of persecution, possession, poisoning and bewitchment but they are responsive to antidepressant therapy rather than to neuroleptics (Al-Issa, 1989). Feelings of being possessed, haunted or spooked which are commensurate with cultural beliefs about bewitchment are also common among other Africans (Guinness, 1992).

In some African depressive people, behaviour disturbances like panic attacks, pseudoseizures, hysterical disassociation and transient psychosis may be present (Guinness, 1992). These may replace the affective and other psychological symptoms of classic depression.

Somatic features and 'somatisation'

It is now accepted that depressive symptomatology may be laden with somatic features and these may be more prominent than the depressed mood itself. Somatisation has been defined as the normative expression of personal and social distress in an idiom of bodily complaints and medical help-seeking (Kleinman, 1986).

These somatic symptoms have been found more commonly in developing countries like India (Teja *et al*, 1971), China (Kleinman, 1986) and Saudi Arabia (Racy, 1980). Puerto Ricans of any age and gender exhibit somatic symptoms more frequently than Mexican Americans and United States non-Hispanic whites. In the case of Los Angeles, Mexican American women older than 40 years display unexplained symptoms, particularly when depressed (Escobar & Canino, 1989). Latin American subjects somatise more than their North American counterparts.

In an Indian study on depression 'somatisation cases' were noted in women in the 25–45 years age group, with a higher education background. The subjects were urbanites and married. Neurotic depression was the commonest diagnosis (62%) and manic depressive psychosis accounted for 10%. The average somatic symptoms per patient was 4.65 and five or more symptoms were reported by 42% of cases (Chaturvedi *et al*, 1987).

Somatic patients are prevalent in primary care and general medical settings. Though somatic presentation of psychological problems is common, the subjects may not be sufficiently depressed for a diagnosis of depressive illness to be made. Goldberg & Bridges (1987) suggest four criteria for defining a patient as being a somatiser: the patient consults for somatic symptoms and the presenting complaints do not include psychological symptoms; the patient attributes his problems to a somatic cause; symptoms of mood disorder are present; a relationship between the mood disorder and presenting complaint is established. Antidepressant treatment is indicated when a definite diagnosis of major depressive episode (ICD–10) is made. It has been found that approximately one-third of somatisers in general medical settings need antidepressants. Chakraborty & Sandel (1984) cautioned that to assume an inverse relationship between the depressed mood and the somatic complaint was an error. On the other hand, they did observe a parallel relationship between the two. In other words, depressive mood is not behind the somatic symptoms but occurs alongside it, and both stem from a common origin. The authors advanced the hypothesis that in India, somatisation is not a substitutive but a normal coping mechanism. They attribute this to the absence in the Indian concept of dichotomy of mind and body. Mind is a sense organ, a component of body, both in Ayurveda and in Indian philosophy.

Nichter (1981) also reported on 'idioms of distress' as alternatives for expression of psychosocial distress in a case study from South India. They relate to indigenous ideas of physiology of routine body cycles: appetite, digestion, sleep and menstruation. Other features include 'hot head' and 'dizziness'.

Depressive psychosis may present as 'chronic pain disorder' as shown in a study by Chatuverdi (1987), where some patients lacked a mood of sadness, but presented with pain at multiple sites. However, the predominant affective symptom was lack of interest in the patient's surroundings, though this was not directly reported. Early morning wakening, loss of appetite and suicidal ideas were noted. The duration of the disorder was less than a year.

In summary, somatisation presents under several forms: it can be a somatic aspect of emotion; an inability to express emotion; a product of 'attention and attribution'; a communication; an idiom of distress; a means of entry into a sick role; or a response to the expectations of the health care system.

Bipolar affective disorder

Prevalence

There are fewer data on the prevalence of mania (ICD–10; F31.0–31.2) than on depression. Recurrent unipolar mania and single episode mania are reported to be more common than bipolar mania or even bipolar depression among the Yorubas of Nigeria (Makanjuola, 1985). Higher numbers of hospital admissions for affective disorder, higher rates of mania and a higher prevalence of affective disorders have been reported among the Afro-Caribbeans in the West Indies, compared to the British in the United Kingdom (Glover, 1989).

The reported rarity of the occurrence of mania in the elderly in Western countries is at variance with reports from developing countries. In a study of affective disorder in old age (Venkoba Rao, 1986), 58 patients had a total of 103 episodes – 67 of depression and 36 mania, yielding a ratio of approximately 2:1. Of 67 depressive attacks, 20 occurred prior to the age of 60 and 47 after 60. Of 36 manic episodes, 28 occurred after the age of 60 while 8 occurred before 60.

Clinical features

ICD–10 criteria for a manic syndrome include a distinct period of abnormally and persistently elevated, expansive or irritable mood. During the period of mood disturbance, several of the following symptoms have persisted and have been present to a significant degree: inflated self-esteem or grandiosity; decreased need for sleep; over-talkativeness; flight of ideas or the subjective experience that thoughts are racing; distraction; increase in directed activities either socially, at work, at school, or in sexual activity, and psychomotor agitation; extensive involvement in pleasurable activities with a high potential for painful consequences; a personal engagement in unrestrained activities: buying sprees, sexual indiscretions or foolish business investments; mood disturbance sufficiently severe to cause marked impairment in occupational or social functioning, or sufficiently severe to require hospitalisation.

Prodromal symptoms of mania and hypomania

Bipolar disorder has a rapid build-up of symptoms, typically within 1–7 days from onset (Post *et al*, 1981). Increased activity is a constant prodromal symptom although elevated mood and decreased need for sleep are also common. There is a striking consistency in the features that precede each of a patient's episodes and many patients can become familiar with their prodromal symptoms and seek early intervention.

General symptomatology of mania and hypomania

The severity of the illness in the developing countries at onset is no less than in the West. In the initial phase, patients appear euphoric (psychological well-being) and eutonic (physical well-being) and believe all their difficulties have been solved, with an exaggerated sense of self-esteem setting in. Gradually, loquaciousness, playfulness, festive mood and an infectious gaiety are noticeable. This mood may change to one of hostile irritability.

A quick sense of humour and wit are noticeable. Indignation and violence may be the response when patients are resisted or may follow the initial euphoric mood. Eroticism colours the talk and jokes. The expansive mood leads to (mood congruent) delusions of grandiosity concerning special abilities, wealth (a wish fulfilment in the poverty-ridden populations) or identity. Religious delusions and feelings of bliss with a spiritual aura are not uncommon.

Delusions and hallucinations of a persecutory nature may also be apparent in mania. The persecutory delusions may be mood-congruent in the sense that the patient believes he is being persecuted because of his superiority and status. Mood incongruent persecutory delusions and hallucinations, and Schneiderian symptoms occur at the height of manic despair (Whybrow *et al*, 1984). Sexual interest may be heightened with consequent marital distress. Periodical sexual excess may be a form of recurrent hypomania or mania. The patients busy themselves with planning for the town or country and get involved in public affairs. Extravagant spending leads to devastating results for the family. There may be gross personal neglect with irregular eating and sleeping. Hallucinations figure in about 10–15% of cases and are visual or auditory. Senses are heightened. 'Possession syndrome' may be a manifestation of mania. Catatonic symptoms like stupor, mutism, negativism and posturing are other occasional psychotic features.

The mean age of onset is around 30 years. The mean duration of the episode of illness in short-term mania is around three months. Though symptomatology appears not dissimilar from that in Western patients, more pronounced distractibility and a persistent embarrassing behaviour are commoner in the Indian setting (Chatterjee & Kulhara, 1989). The resolution of symptoms is quick and recovery noticed in around 90 days with the return to normal function. Only 15% needed to stay as in-patients in hospital at the end of 90 days.

A preponderance of mania in Indian men is reported by Chatterjee & Kulhara (1989) which is at variance with the women's excess in mania observed by Winokur *et al* (1969). This may reflect sociocultural factors in developing countries or differential rates of the illness. Being a male-dominated society, the men being bread-winners receive priority for treatment. There are no current data to favour the differential incidence of illness in the two sexes.

Cycling pattern

The inherent feature of affective disorder is its episodic course. The recurrent episodes are commoner in bipolar disorder. Even within a single depressed episode the diurnal pattern is evident, with symptoms at their worst in the early morning and waning as the day advances. The intervals between episodes of depression may be years, often decades, especially in unipolar illness. In some bipolar patients, a circannual pattern is observable. A few have alternating episodes of depression and mania in cycles as short as 48 hours (Dunner, 1979). Rapid cycling affective disorder (with at least 4 affective episodes of depression, mania, and hypomania per year) form nearly 8% of the cases of major affective illness (Cherian *et al*, 1990).

Dysthymia

The term dysthymia (ICD–10; F34.1) replaces the condition hitherto known as 'neurotic depression'. Considered either as a low grade depression or an expression of a personality disorder, dysthymia currently refers to a mild, chronic depression under the rubric of 'affective disorder'. The lifetime prevalence for dysthymic disorder varies from 3.1% (Eaton & Kessler, 1985) to 4.5% (Weissman & Myers, 1978). Prodromal features of depression, well-defined residual features preceding major depression or depression with partial remission are excluded from dysthymia.

The disorder is characterised by a low grade severity of symptoms of chronic or intermittent course of more than two years' duration. Commencing in childhood and adolescence, the disorder pursues an intermittent or a persistent course.

The clinical features include a depressed mood for the major part of the day, more often expressed than observed. Irritability may replace depressed mood in children and adolescents. Poor appetite or overeating, insomnia or hypersomnia, low energy, fatigue, low self-esteem, poor concentration, indecisiveness and a feeling of hopelessness are other symptoms. There should not have been a symptomless period or evidence of a major depressive episode during the first two years. Manic episodes or hypomanic symptoms are absent. An organic basis or the superimposition of chronic psychotic disorder such as schizophrenia or delusion disorder are not found. Worsening of symptoms towards the later part of the day, with relatively clear mornings differentiates dysthymia from major depression.

Dysthymic disorder may be primary or secondary. In the primary type, the dysphoria is unrelated to a pre-existing chronic non-mood disorder like anorexia nervosa and other psychiatric disorders. Secondary dysthymia is reported to coexist with other psychiatric disorders in 70% of cases over lifetime (Weissman *et al*, 1988). 'Pure' dysthymia, unassociated with other psychiatric disorders forms 10% or less of out-patient populations (Akiskal, 1981).

The course of dysthymia is punctuated by recurrences of depression. The relapses are common and recovery varies. It may take on average up to six years to recover, compared to a lesser period for major depression. Major depression preceded by dysthymia carries a better prognosis than if it is followed by dysthymia. The dysthymic disorder category itself has been said to lack longitudinal stability (Seivewright & Tyrer, 1990). Dysthymic disorder is an ambulatory disorder compatible with stable social functioning.

Postpartum affective disorder

The risk of psychosis in the postpartum period is estimated at 1–2 per 1000 births (Kendell *et al*, 1987). With a history of bipolar affective disorder or postpartum psychosis the risk rises to about 1 in 5. Contrary to earlier reports, recent studies have revealed that affective disorders are commoner than schizophrenia in the postpartum period (Dean & Kendell, 1981; Brockington & Kumar, 1982). The disorders are more common following the first childbirth (Gautam *et al*, 1982). The risk is highest during the first four weeks after delivery with nearly 75% of cases beginning in this period (Inwood, 1989). Fifty per cent of all cases have an onset in the first 7–10 days postpartum. Postpartum psychoses constituted one-third of all female psychiatric admissions in Senegal (Boussat *et al*, 1977), 10–15% in North Africa (Murphy, 1982) while in many parts of the Western world they form 4–5% (Murphy, 1982).

Aetiology

The aetiological search has been directed to biological, psychological, social and interpersonal factors. Thuve (1974) found that children of women treated for psychosis had a significantly higher prevalence of psychiatric disorders. The heavy genetic loading for psychiatric disorders lends support to the theory that puerperal psychoses are closely related to affective illnesses occurring at other times (Kendell *et al*, 1987; Platz & Kendell, 1988). Hormonal theories suggest that rapidly falling postpartum steroid levels trigger psychosis in genetically vulnerable women. Neuroendocrine challenge tests like the dexamethasone suppression test (DST), or thyroid-stimulating hormone (TSH) responses to thyrotropin-releasing hormone (TRH) have not shown any obvious association of abnormalities in the diagnosis of mania, psychotic depression and schizoaffective disorder (Paykell *et al*, 1991). DST non-suppression is notable during 3 to 5 days postpartum in normal women.

There has been a renewed interest in the role of the thyroid in postnatal depression. Postnatal depression is more common in women who are positive for thyroid antibodies than those who are not. An increase in depression was noted irrespective of the status of thyroid function (Harris *et al*, 1992). The predominance of primiparae observed in Western studies (Platz *et al*, 1988) has also been reported in Africa and India. A bimodal distribution has been noted in Morocco with peaks in the first, fourth, and later deliveries (Chkili, 1975). In Indian culture, sons are so desired and prized that postpartum depression has been observed to be more frequent following the birth of baby girls than boys (Guzder & Meenaskshi, 1991).

Cyclothymia (ICD–10; F34.0)

Cyclothymia is a persistent instability of mood, involving numerous episodes of mild depression, and mild elation, none of which have been sufficiently severe or prolonged to fulfil the criteria for bipolar affective disorder or recurrent depressive disorder. It pursues a chronically progressive course with a disturbed interpersonal and marital relationship. There are occasional suicidal ideas, excessive appetite and sexuality, hypersomnia alternating with decreased need for sleep drug and alcohol abuse.

Seasonal affective disorder

The syndrome of seasonal affective disorder (SAD) was described by Rosenthal *et al* (1984). Diagnostic criteria have been suggested as follows:

(a) a regular, temporal relationship between the onset of an episode of bipolar disorder (including bipolar disorder (not otherwise specified, NOS)) or recurrent major depression (including depressive disorder NOS) and a particular 60-day period of the year, e.g. regular appearance of depression between the beginning of October and end of November;

(b) full remission or euthymia or a change from depression or mania, hypomania or hyperthymia also occur within a particular 60-day period of the year (e.g. depression disappearing from mid-February to mid-April);

(c) there have been at least three episodes of mood disturbances in three separate years that demonstrated the temporal seasonal relationship defined in (a) and (b); at least two of the years were consecutive;

(d) seasonal episodes of mood disturbances as described below outnumbered any non-seasonal episodes of such disturbance that may have occurred by more than 3 : 1.

Seasonal depressions have been reported in 15.6% of a large clinic population with recurrent depressive disorders that met the criteria for SAD (Thase, 1989). The 'winter depression' symptoms include decreased activity with a mood of sadness, irritability or anxiety, the 'reversed neuro vegetative symptoms' of increased appetite, carbohydrate craving, increased weight and hypersomnia, daytime drowsiness. The REM latency was not shortened unlike in endogenous depression, and the dexamethasone suppression test (DST) in SAD resembles that found in normal subjects (Rosenthal *et al*, 1984).

The characteristic feature claimed for seasonable depression is its response to light therapy or a change in residence to a lower altitude with longer days and more warmth and light. For example, the occurrence of unipolar winter and summer depression has recently been reported in the Indian sub-continent (Gupta, 1990).

Culture-bound syndromes

Many 'culture-bound syndromes' may be variants of affective disorder.

Dhat syndrome

This is a neurosis common in India, Nepal, Pakistan, Sri Lanka and Bangladesh (Wig, 1984; Bhatia & Malik, 1991). The syndrome is characterised by psycho-sexual complaints like premature ejaculation, impotence, weakness, fatigue, palpitations and sleeplessness. The condition is generally associated with neurotic depression and less often with major depression and anxiety disorder. In many cases a precise diagnostic categorisation is difficult. The response to antidepressant and anti-anxiety drugs is satisfactory. The patients attribute the symptoms to the loss of semen ('dhat' which is prized as a source of robust health) in urine or through masturbation or frequent sexual intercourse. A white discharge in urine is complained of. A depressive mood is a reaction to the draining away of 'dhat'. Assuring the patients on the harmlessness of semen loss amazes them and results in drop-outs. The treatment compliance is better if their ideas are unchallenged.

The counterpart of dhat syndrome in women is leucorrhoea and is a symptom of distress. The symptoms consist of weakness, back pain, 'overheating', poor concentration and feelings of powerlessness to act, 'bones dissolving', and slipping away of vitality and a sense of personal ill-being. There are associated sexual problems. The symptoms are an expression of a disturbed family situation and a state of discord (Nichter, 1981).

Pseudocyesis

Pseudocyesis is the conviction of a non-pregnant woman that she is pregnant and is a phenomenon predominantly found in societies where there is too much cultural pressure on women to have children (Cohen, 1982). It may be considered as a defence against the wish for, or fear of pregnancy or even resolving the conflict between the two (Murray & Abraham, 1978; Zuber & Kelly, 1984). In experimental animals administration of drugs that deplete central catecholamines have induced physiological aspects of pregnancy (Cohen, 1982). Such depletion is noticed in depressive illness and patients with both depression and pseudocyesis have been reported (Starkman *et al*, 1985). Depressive illness occurring after the resolution of pseudocyesis has been reported (Christodoulou, 1978; Silber & Abdalla, 1983). The incidence of pseudocyesis varies. For example 21 cases in four consecutive months in Soweto, South Africa, were reported representing 1 : 2000 new antenatal patients (Brenner, 1976). On the other hand in Boston, USA, less than 10 cases were seen every three years among 20 000 pregnant women (Cohen, 1982).

Bouffée délirante

This is a diagnosis used to refer to certain acute psychotic episodes, and is a term frequently used in francophone Africa (Algeria, Tunisia, Morocco). The clinical picture is marked by an acute onset with hallucinations and delusions. The hallucinations are vivid, and rapid mood swings are accompanied by the clouding of consciousness. The delusional themes are related to religion (prophetic inspiration, divine revelation, end of the world, resurrection, or being a messiah), sexuality, jealousy, poisoning, bewitchment and persecution. The life events that generally precipitate the syndrome are: sudden death in others, migration, forced marriage, sexual abuse and incest. One variety of bouffée délirante, the 'nuptial psychosis' which follows the day of the marriage as a result of stresses of arranged marriages, occurs in women between the age of 20 and 30. Bouffée délirante is most prevalent in Western Africa. For example, in a survey of 2000 patients in Senegal, Collomb (1985) diagnosed bouffée délirante in some 30%.

Vimbusa

This is a manifestation of psychological distress reported from Northern Malawi where it is attributed to bewitchment. The clinical features consist of sleeplessness, palpitation, anorexia, weight loss, irritability, tearfulness and social isolation. Hallucinations and delusions and other psychotic features are significant by their absence. Though they are not considered 'mad', these subjects are 'not their normal selves'. Some patients with vimbusa receive a diagnosis of neurotic depression. The treatment is a complex form of group and family therapy mediated by trance induced by music and with herbs (Rands, 1989). The somatisation is a mode of expression of emotion, since Malawi language seems to offer no terms for such expression.

Koro

This syndrome occurs mostly among South-East Asians. A small sprinkling of cases in an 'incomplete' form has occurred in Western countries along with such disorders as manic depressive illness, fronto-temporal brain tumour, amphetamine intoxication and following a stroke, with the feature of hypochondriacal delusion. The clinical picture is that of an acute anxiety reaction, marked by a desperate fear that the penis is shrinking into the abdomen, resulting in death. Women complain of shrinkage of external genitals. Koro results from cultural, social and psychodynamic influences upon predisposed individuals. Many patients are preoccupied with fears about nocturnal seminal emission, masturbation, sexual fatigue and venery. Isolated cases as well as epidemics of koro have been reported from India (Chowdhury *et al*, 1988). Recent knowledge has suggested that koro is not a unique phenomenon and that while one variety appears to be the culture bound anxiety disorder, another form appears as a delusional disorder.

Emotional distress syndrome (EDS)

Attention has been drawn to a syndrome with an admixture of anxiety and depression resembling the dysthymic disorder (Singh, 1990). An initial stage of emotional numbness, lasting for a few hours to a few days, is followed by a stage of marked anxiety, sadness and hopelessness. In some cases a residual sadness may linger. Clinical recovery with a return to normal functioning invariably occurs within six months. The therapeutic response is good to antidepressants or anti-anxiety drugs. EDS may result from diverse causes and is also considered to be a non-specific reaction to conflict or trauma at the conscious psychic level.

Acute psychotic reaction

The syndrome closely resembles bouffée délirante and the disorder termed brief reactive psychosis. Psychotic reactions of acute onset with precipitant factors, and symptoms reaching a crescendo within 48 hours to a week and then remitting have been reported, particularly in developing countries. Depressive or manic features mark some cases when they are labelled as 'manic depressive psychosis' or schizophrenia. Such brief psychotic reactions have been reported in West Indian immigrants in the United Kingdom (Littlewood & Lipsedge, 1977), in Nigeria (Lambo, 1965), India (Singh & Sachdeva, 1980) and other developing countries (Littlewood & Lipsedge, 1977). In one study, 25% of the cases of acute psychotic reactions received a diagnosis of manic depressive psychosis both at index and a year later (Indian Council of Medical Research, 1986). Such acute presentations of depressive or manic pictures are to be differentiated from other acute psychotic manifestations with schizophrenic symptomatology and psychoses 'not otherwise specified'. Acute psychoses *with* precipitant factors and considered as reactive psychoses were found to resemble affective psychoses, while acute psychoses *without* precipitating stress simulated schizophrenia (Kapur & Pandurangi, 1979).

Brain fag syndrome

Prince (1962) described a syndrome with five symptoms: head symptoms (aching, burning, crawling sensations), eye symptoms (blurring, watering, aching), difficulty in grasping the meaning of spoken or printed words, poor retentiveness, and sleepiness on studying. Nigerian students named it 'brain fag'. It is now found to be a form of somatised anxiety associated with the education process and a type of 'transitional syndrome' occurring in those at the interface of Western and traditional cultures. Diverse theories of social aetiology have been advanced: for example, disruptive effects or urbanisation and destruction of cultural patterns in Nigeria (Anumonye, 1980); over-expectations of education (Thebaud & Rigamer, 1972); and disparity between students' origins and ambitions (Minde, 1974). The financial sacrifice undergone by the family to procure education may induce brain fag anxiety in the student. Currently, the syndrome is being related to the complex social changes and rapid social transition in which education plays a major role. Symptoms of depression occur in brain fag syndrome, which leads to the suggestion that it is a form of 'masked depression' – 'masked' because the depressive features are not verbalised in Western fashion (Rwegellera, 1981).

Differential diagnosis

Depression and mania are to be differentiated from other psychiatric syndromes and (organic) physical disorders whose symptomatology may carry affective components.

Given a picture of progressive loss of appetite and weight, and persistent constipation, an appreciable number of cases are diagnosed as cancer of the large bowel or stomach, especially in the elderly. These patients reach the psychiatrist after a period of fruitless investigations by surgeons, physicians and gastroenterologists. A similar situation is likely to occur when pain is the leading symptom and patients pass between cardiologists, neurologists, neurosurgeons, orthopaedists, gynaecologists and pain clinics. A few patients with abdominal pain go through exploratory laparotomy too.

Among the organic syndromes that manifest with affective symptoms are a host of clinical situations: (1) malignancy, both occult (where affective prodromes are common) and manifest of brain, lung and pancreas; (2) infections like syphilis, AIDS, infectious hepatitis, mononucleosis, postinfluenza, post (TB) meningitis; (3) metabolic disorders such as Cushing's syndrome and hypothyroidism; (4) medication with corticosteroids, reserpine, alpha methyldopa, levodopa, indomethacin, cimetidine, ranitidine (H_2 receptor antagonists), propranolol, amphetamine withdrawal and oral contraceptives.

Among the psychiatric syndromes to be excluded are schizophrenic disorders, schizoaffective disorders, generalised anxiety disorder, obsessive–compulsive neurosis, dementia, alcoholism, drug abuse and borderline personality disorder.

The differentiation of depressive pseudodementia from primary dementia (especially in the elderly) may be a simple affair or a difficult clinical exercise. The fluctuations of mood, the exaggerated form of complaining of the symptoms, absence of neurological features, clearing of depressed mood and cognitive disturbance with antidepressant therapy – all these favour a diagnosis of depression. Agnosia (unawareness) of memory impairment characterises primary dementia, while in pseudodemented depression the patient retains his awareness of amnesic difficulties.

Acute manic excitement is to be differentiated from excitement of catatonic schizophrenia. However, perseveratory speech with neologisms, repetitive activities and flat affect point to schizophrenia. A variety in the theme of talk, distractibility, pliability of mood, its infectious nature mark mania. Family history, premorbid personality and earlier affective episodes are to be taken into account.

Depressive symptomatology in epilepsy has been recorded in developing countries. Manic episodes were reported by Bagadia *et al* (1973) in 4.7% of 536 patients with epilepsy. Six per cent of 150 cases of epileptic psychosis were found to be manic (Satyanarayana Swamy *et al*, 1986). A significant sub-population of 60 cases of epileptic psychosis had pathological elevation of mood (Fernandez *et al*, 1988) with grandiose delusions as the second most common type of delusion. Some Indian studies do not indicate a higher incidence of depression or suicide in epileptics (Bagadia *et al*, 1973; Venkoba Rao *et al*, 1974).

It is not only the current organic factors that are of diagnostic relevance. Cerebral insults from past infections, toxic agents, marginal nutritional status operating at critical developmental periods may have affected the neural substrate of psyche and predispose to psychotic breakdown under later stresses (German, 1992). There is a greater component of organic factors in psychiatry of the developing world compared to the Western world.

Depressive disorder and suicidal behaviour

Individuals with suicidal behaviour are trichotomised into those contemplating suicide (ideators), those who have survived suicidal attempt(s) (attempters) and those whose attempts are fatal (completers) (Beck *et al*, 1973). Patients with a depressive disorder can fall into all three categories. Diagnoses associated with suicide include depression, alcoholism, schizophrenia, personality disorder and drug addiction.

The lifetime prevalence of suicide attempts was assessed in a study in the Epidemiologic Catchment Area Program in the US among those with a life history of various mental disorders. The rate of suicide attempts was 1% among those with lifetime history of depressive disorder, 24% for those with bipolar disorder, 18% for those with major depression and 17% for those with dysthymia (Regier & Moscicki, 1987).

Follow-up studies of depression (endogenous) over a period of 15 years revealed that one in six deaths (about 15%) was from suicide, a figure 15 times higher than expected (Sainsbury, 1980). More important data were uncovered through 'psychological autopsy'. Robins *et al* (1959) were the first to initiate such studies and attributed 45% of the completed suicides (out of 134) to manic depressive illness. Dorpat & Ripley (1960) diagnosed 30% of suicides in Seattle as arising from depression. Barraclough *et al* (1974), studying the detailed records of 100 consecutive suicides and 150 controls in two county areas in England found 64% to be uncomplicated cases of primary depression.

There are nevertheless cultures in which suicides among depressive patients do not match Western figures. A 3–13 years follow-up of 122 cases of depression by Venkoba Rao & Nammalvar (1977) in India revealed one suicide, and similar findings have been reported from Nigeria (Binitie, 1975) and Egypt (Okasha, 1980).

Many factors influence the progression from suicidal ideas and attempts to completed suicide. Important in such cultural contexts are the so-called 'suicide counters' reported by Venkoba Rao (1978). They are of religious, ethical, economic or familial nature. It is not uncommon to hear suicide-prone subjects say: "But for my family and children, I would have committed suicide"; "If I commit suicide, who will marry my daughter thus stigmatised?"; "If I die by suicide, my soul may be denied salvation". The counters may offset the strength of suicide impulses, though this is less likely in severe depression and anguish.

The rate of suicide among the Indians who migrated to Singapore before the war is quite high: 20.4/100 000 as against 12.4/100 000 mean annual suicide rate for the general population of Singapore (Kua & Ko, 1992). Such findings also apply to Indians in Malaysia and Fiji (Haynes, 1984). Suicide is attributed to being less successful and a reluctance to return to homeland to avoid a loss of face. Suicide among elderly Indians (over 65 years) was higher, 30.5/100 000 – more than double the figure for the youngsters. The elderly who were unmarried and those without pension and dependent on their children were at maximum risk. The highest suicide rates in Sri Lanka are in the predominantly Tamil areas (43.5/100 000 as against the general population rate of 22.1/100 000) with migrants from South India. Those high rates are attributed to unemployment, internal migration and psychological stresses arising from disruption of the customary bonds of family and community (Kearney & Miller, 1985). Depressive disorder, physical illness, and poor social support among the elderly Chinese women in Singapore have been correlated with suicide.

Suicide rates in the Islamic countries and also the Malay community (with Islamic faith) of Malaysia and Singapore are considerably lower, possibly due to strong Islamic beliefs which reject the taking of one's life (Kua & Ko, 1992). However, in the urban areas of Muslim countries suicide among youngsters and the unemployed has been increasing, while in the traditional rural sector the rate is still low. The lowest rate is observed during the Muslim fasting month of Ramadan (Al-Issa, 1989).

Aetiological theories

Genetic predisposition

Depression runs in families and there is good evidence for familial clustering due to genetic influences. The first degree relatives (FDRs) of the subjects run a risk of illness of between 7.8 and 32.9% as against 2–4% in the general population. The concordance rate in bipolar monozygotic twins is around 79% and for unipolar monozygotic twins 54%. The figure for dizygotic twins varies from 19–29% irrespective of polarity. The risk of primary affective disorder in bipolar FDRs is 20% and more while among the monopolar FDRs the risk is less than 11–13%. An eightfold increase of depression and a 15-fold increase of suicide is reported in the biological relatives of depressive adoptees compared to the non-adoptive relatives.

A reported transmission by an X-linked gene is now believed to affect only a minority of inherited forms of affective disorders. Chromosome-11 has been implicated in that there is a linkage between the locus on this chromosome and the gene for bipolar disorder among the Amish of Pennsylvania (Egeland *et al*, 1987). However, this could not be confirmed in other North American, Icelandic and Irish pedigrees. Genetic linkage has been observed between affective disorder and Down's syndrome and thalassaemia minor (Joffe *et al*, 1986).

What one inherits is the predisposition rather than the disorder itself. A multifactorial liability-threshold model has been hypothesised in which the variable 'liability to develop the disorder' is found to be normally distributed in the population.

Biochemical hypothesis

The clinical efficacy of antidepressant drugs in affective disorders and their neurochemical effects in animals led to the monoamine hypothesis (MA) of affective disorders. The classical monoamine hypothesis states that depression is associated with a functional deficit of one or more neurotransmitters, especially catecholamines like noradrenaline, and dopamine and indoleamines like serotonin at the critical synapses of the central nervous system. Conversely mania is associated with their functional excess. This hypothesis, with its 'too much or too little' amine concept is now seen as too simplistic, and the amine hypothesis has been extended to include the cholinergic system, endorphins and encephalins (Janowski *et al*, 1972; Watson *et al*, 1980).

There are two views of MA transmitter theories: the more common one relates emotions to the balance of the available transmitters at the receptors, for example, acetylcholine and noradrenaline or dopamine and noradrenaline. The second theory relates the mood to the deficit in central serotonergic transmission which 'permits' affective disorder but is an insufficient cause in itself. Given this deficit the affective disorder is precipitated by changes in central catecholamine function – low norepinephrine causing depression and high norepinephrine causing mania. This 'permissive hypothesis' was formulated by Prante *et al* (1974). The 'pharmacological bridge' between the MA hypothesis and affective disorder has its robust support from the action of antidepressant drugs, especially first generation tricyclics that tend to elevate the levels of catecholamines. Certain antimanic drugs, chlorpromazine, haloperidol and pimozide tend to lower their levels.

The concept, however, weakens when one takes into consideration the effects of the newer antidepressant drugs. Iprindole, trazodone and mianserin are clinically effective against depression, with little effect on serotonin or noradrenaline reuptake. Paradoxically Tianeptine, a new tricyclic antidepressant, increases serotonin reuptake. Further difficulty with the amine hypothesis is that inhibition of reuptake, though evident from the first dose, does not parallel clinical improvement which should be observed by the second or the third week. Knowledge of chronic administration effects is needed to explain antidepressant properties. Low serotonin levels (5-HIAA in cerebrospinal fluid) persist in some clinically recovered patients following antidepressant therapy. The normal slow wave sleep disturbance in stage 4 (dependent upon serotonin) also persists. A low level of urinary methoxyhydroxyphenylglycol, a major metabolite of norepinephrine persists in depressive patients on recovery. It has been reported that mood variations precede the biochemical shift by several days and mania and depression are not necessarily bipolar (Court, 1972). Computerised tomography scan studies have revealed enlargement of the cerebral ventricular system, especially in aged depressed individuals. This favours structural rather than biochemical predisposition to depression. There is yet no convincing proof for an amine hypothesis.

The receptor hypothesis states that super-sensitivity of beta-adrenergic receptors and low post-synaptic alpha-2-adrenergic receptors are related to depression. Recently, neurobiological research has extended to the 'second messenger' adenylate cyclase system linked to the post-synaptic beta-receptor and inositol 1,4,5-triphosphate (IP3).

Dexamethasone suppression test

The dexamethasone suppression test (DST) has been used to distinguish adult patients with 'endogenous' depression from those with 'neurotic' depressive conditions (Carroll *et al*, 1981; Dam *et al*, 1985). Dexamethasone is a synthetic corticosteroid which suppresses the adrenocorticotropic hormone (ACTH) and cortisol secretion in normal subjects. DST non-suppression has been reported in 68% of cases of 'endogenous' depression by Carroll *et al* (1981). The remainder form another subgroup with no abnormal DST. Among patients with endogenous depression and melancholic features, a sample population has shown raised values of plasma cortisol following administration of dexamethasone 17–24 hours earlier (Arana *et al*, 1985). The DST positives are likely to respond better to noradrenaline potentiating antidepressants and to electroconvulsive therapy (ECT), and in general carry a more favourable prognosis. They are thought to be less likely to respond to cognitive and other non-pharmacological treatments for depression, though this is still in debate (Rush, 1984; Brown *et al*,

1987). Conversely, the normal DST-depressed patients respond to 5-HT potentiating antidepressants (Brown *et al*, 1981). There is a correlation between a normal DST and a low CSF 5-HIAA (Carroll, 1980).

Psychoanalytic theory

In early analytical theory, 'primary parathymia' is the infantile depression consequent to a succession of frustrations and is the forerunner of the later clinical depression. This concept has been elaborated by the addition of the concepts of object loss, introspection over the lost object, vilification of the internalised effigy of the lost object, and aggression towards the ambivalently loved and hated introjected object. The turning of hostility and aggression (reversal of aggression) inwards has been a fundamental concept in classical psychoanalytical theory. This explains the self-reproach, guilt, poor esteem and suicide attempts in depression.

Freud drew attention to the similarities and differences between mourning and melancholia. Bowlby states that early relationships serve as a root type for all subsequent bonds with other people and with the world at large. The adult's predisposition to depression is held to be directly related to whether early separation from important loved ones was successfully coped with.

Cognitive theories

Cognitive theories assign a central role to negative patterns of thinking in the genesis of depression. Basic to the mood of depression are the distorted cognitions of the individual towards the environment, to himself and to the future. Such a negative 'cognitive triad' is a reaction to the experiences of the individual in early life. Depressive 'schemas' (established patterns of thinking) become a stable cognitive background, against which incoming stimuli are interpreted.

The schemas lie dormant until they are activated by a stressful event. The resulting cognitive errors comprise: arbitrary inferences (drawing a negative conclusion from neutral evidence); selective abstraction (focusing on a single negative aspect of a larger situation); over-generalisation (drawing broad conclusion from a single bit of information); and magnification (exaggerating the negative aspects of something). The lowering of mood that follows these thoughts also enhances them.

Life events and their relationship to aetiological theories

Compared with the general population, depressed patients experience three times as many life events in the six months preceding investigation. The stressful life events that relate to severe depression fall into three general categories: death of a loved one, failure in an important interpersonal relationship (usually with one's spouse) and a severe set-back in work or other goals to which the individual has been devoted.

Many have documented the pathogenicity of a single event like bereavement in the occurrence of depression. A prospective epidemiological study revealed that 35% of the widows and widowers participating suffered depression 18 months after being widowed (Clayton *et al*, 1968).

Paradoxically 'post' bereavement acute mania has also been reported. The notion of 'manic defence' was postulated by Melanie Klein (1940). She suggested that when loss or sadness is too sudden and severe the ego is unable to cope with disaster. This explanation has also been offered for mania occurring in cases of terminal illness.

Apart from initiating the first onset of depression, life events have also preceded relapses (Paykel, 1979; Paykel & Tanner, 1976). The clustering of events as against isolated ones during the two-year period prior to depression has been observed (Venkoba Rao & Nammalvar, 1976). Loss of mother in early childhood increases vulnerability to depression in later life in response to later life events (Brown & Harris, 1978). Reports from India on the association between early parental deprivation and late depression are conflicting (Wig *et al*, 1969; Venkoba Rao, 1979), however, Indian studies note that two events within a year are generally 'tolerable' (Singh *et al*, 1981) and that the 'clustering' of events is the rule in the pre-depressive state (Venkoba Rao & Nammalvar, 1976; Chatterjee *et al*, 1981).

Life events by themselves may not matter. Much depends on the psychosocial milieu, genetic factors and personality. Paykel's (1974) observation that only around 10% of those who have experienced 'exit' events suffer depression testifies to this point. Recently, the tendency to encounter or to report threatening life events has itself been found to be familial. Thus life events associated with depression may occur in individuals who are vulnerable in part because of personality factors or familial cognitive style.

The association between life events and affective disorder has been hitherto more with minor and monopolar depressions and less with bipolar depressions. However, recent studies have revealed the occurrence of depressive symptoms in the relatives of probands with both endogenous (non-reactive) and reactive depression (stress-related). Thus, life events' research fails to support the dichotomy of 'neurotic–reactive' and 'endogenous' depression (Farmer & McGuffin, 1989).

Recent neuroendocrine research has suggested that any one of the steps in the hypothalamo-pituitary-adrenal axis may be the target for stressful life events. The noradrenergic projections from the brainstem to the hypothalamus, the secretions of corticotropin-releasing factor, ACTH and corticosteroids and the action of corticosteroids on type II corticosteroid receptors in the brain are the suggested foci of activation (Checkley, 1992).

Treatment of affective disorder

The comprehensive treatment of affective disorder comprises three phases: treatment of the acute episode, maintenance following control of the symptoms and prevention of recurrences. In addition, measures to minimise the onset of chronicity and its management are included. Functional and social impairment that accompany chronicity must also be targeted. Pharmacological agents include antidepressants, antimanic agents, tranquillisers, lithium, carbamazepine, and sodium valproate. Other measures include advice to the family and social support. Wherever organic causes are found to be contributory or comorbid with affective disorder they should be treated appropriately (for individual drugs, see chapter on treatments).

Acute depression

Drug treatments

Acute depression can be a psychiatric emergency. In the most acute stage, refusal of food or drink, non-compliance for drug taking and threats of suicide may necessitate hospitalisation. Important methods of intervention are the use of antidepressant drugs, and ECT. Tricyclic antidepressants (e.g. imipramine, amitriptyline, doxepine, clomipramine) continue to be widely used for acute episodes. Controlled clinical trials have established their effectiveness in acute states, although a review of literature shows that these are no more effective than the newer drugs. Other antidepressants are tetracyclics (mianserin) and serotonin reuptake inhibitors (e.g. fluoxetine and fluoxamine). Recently there has been a revival of interest in monoamine oxidase inhibitors (MAOI) such as moclobemide which inhibits the 'A' form of MAOI and is characterised by a reversible binding with monoamine oxidase, unlike earlier MAOI drugs whose binding was irreversible and hence was the cause of the 'cheese' reaction.

For the earlier claims that the dosage of antidepressants varies between cultures, there is no unequivocal evidence from control studies. Adequate dosage ensures good response with a time lag of 2–4 weeks. Notwithstanding this, sleep inducing and anxiolytic properties of tricyclics come on rapidly, encouraging compliance. The use of more than one antidepressant does not ensure any improved effectiveness. Nor is the time-lag shortened by parenteral administration of the drug. Nearly 60–70% of all depressed patients respond to the first antidepressant drug used, while a further 10–15% respond to an alternative antidepressant (or ECT) (Keilholz *et al*, 1982). The dosage of 125–150 mg per day of imipramine is the recommended standard and medication is to be continued for at least six months following recovery from acute symptoms in order to minimise the risk of early relapse. Although all the antidepressants in use are known to be effective and superior to placebo, their side-effects profile determines the choice.

Anticholinergic side-effects occur with all tricyclic antidepressants: most common are dryness of the mouth, blurring of vision, difficulty in micturition, constipation, partial impotence and anorgasmia. Compliance improves if the possible side-effects are explained beforehand to patients. Adverse effects on cardiac conduction and myocardial contractility with an increased risk of dysrhythmias can occur with tricyclics, especially when there is pre-existing cardiac disease. They are less likely with the tetracyclics and the newer antidepressants. Monitoring serum levels of the drugs continues to be a research procedure not generally practised in developing countries. In 30% of patients response to tricyclics is inadequate. MAOIs or lithium supplementation are then most likely to be effective. For the control of delusions and hallucinations, antidepressants alone are not sufficient, and need to be supplemented with neuroleptics (Spiker *et al*, 1985). However, that delusional forms of depression respond well to antidepressants alone has been reported in North Africa.

Electroconvulsive therapy

ECT is most useful for severe depression. In developing countries, ECT offers an advantage in treating large numbers of patients crowding the state-run and private hospitals, and in overcoming poor compliance, the irregular supply of drugs, and the inability of patients to pay for their drugs. ECT exerts a remarkable effect, particularly in acute depression where psychomotor retardation or agitation, loss of weight, psychotic features like delusions and hallucinations and suicide risk are present. Control studies of ECT have shown that the presence of delusions is the most reliable indicator of good response (Quitkin *et al*, 1978). It is also useful in cases of poor response to antidepressants or when these are contraindicated in the presence of cardiac disease, pregnancy and in elderly patients with low tolerance levels to medication. The policy of three treatments (maybe 7 or 8 in some cases) administered unilaterally and under anaesthesia is recommended and achieves a satisfactory clinical response. The unilateral technique minimises memory impairment and confusion associated with bilateral technique (see also Chapter 6).

Acute mania

Acute mania is a psychiatric emergency; patients need intensive measures which are best provided either in state or private hospitals. Admission is necessary to prevent exhaustion and overactivity, and to overcome social disturbances. Among the drugs that are in common use for treatment are neuroleptics, lithium, carbamazepine and sodium valproate. Chlorpromazine administered either orally or parenterally is the preferred drug. Haloperidol is useful to control aggressive behaviour and for abatement of increased psychomotor activities. Diazepam may be necessary either parenterally or orally as an adjuvant. Lithium and carbamazepine are also used in acute manic episodes, but are slower than neuroleptics. Sodium valproate has been used in acute episodes (Emrich *et al*, 1985). ECT is also useful as an antimanic administered in conjunction with the drugs. Although lithium could be started along with haloperidol, it is safer to avoid the combination. Lithium may be introduced after the initial management with neuroleptics.

In patients who are violent and assaultive, not uncommon in developing countries, parenteral diazepam is preferred for immediate control. Minimal physical restraint may then be sufficient. Other supportive measures are control over nutrition and fluids, and prevention of injury through overactivity.

Prophylaxis of affective disorder

According to a 1989 consensus statement of a group of WHO Mental Health Collaborating Centres, if a patient has had more than one severe episode of depressive illness (especially in the last five years), long-term prophylactic therapy is to be considered. This may be with a tricyclic antidepressant, lithium or carbamazepine and sodium valproate. There is no significant difference between tricyclics and lithium in monopolar depression but lithium is more effective in preventing relapses of both manic and depressive episodes in bipolar disorder. Carbamazepine is used as an alternative prophylactic in both monopolar and bipolar disorder. Sodium valproate or carbamazepine alone or in combination with lithium have been found in rapid cycling bipolar disorder (Calabrese, 1993).

The use of lithium has been shown to reduce the number of relapses and to prolong the period of remission between the relapses. Owing to its teratogenic effect, the drug is withheld during pregnancy, especially in the first trimester, but it may be used as a prophylactic against postnatal affective disorder. There is a risk of lithium toxicity to the newborn child when the drug is administered before childbirth, or during breastfeeding. Monitoring frequency of lithium levels varies from once within 1–3 months to once or twice a year (King *et al*, 1991).

The common tendency to prescribe suboptimal dosage of antidepressants in general practice has come in for criticism (Catalan *et al*, 1988). However, recent studies have reconfirmed the use of lower doses and also for a lesser period of maintenance therapy. It has been observed that the prophylactic effect of antidepressants is the same as lithium over a 3-year period in monopolar depression. Beyond this, no clear knowledge is available on the benefits of longer term (over 3–5 years) maintenance treatment (Kerr, 1991). Evidence at present seems to indicate that there may not be a need for drugs for more than three years.

Life events are known to play an important part in precipitating recurrences and also in perpetuating the illness. Advice is given to enable the patient to cope with stressful life events. Marital support for depressed women can facilitate and maintain recovery while lack of support from spouses can lead to a poor outcome.

The most important advice is regarding drug compliance. In addition, approximately 1% of all depressed patients die by consuming their prescribed drugs in overdose (Henry, 1992). The risk of using antidepressants for suicidal purposes is currently uncommon in developing countries, probably because other methods are available and antidepressants are not as popular as 'sleeping pills'.

Psychotherapy (see chapter 9.2)

The question has been raised whether psychotherapy is necessary or possible in the developing world (MbWambo *et al*, 1992), and if used, what forms it should take and what skills are expected of the therapist. The twin constraints are the cost which may be beyond the economic reach of the average patient and the small number of therapists available. The most important role for the psychiatrists in such situations will be to train the primary care physicians in basic psychotherapeutic techniques targeted at recognition of distress, sensitivity to patients' feelings and 'problem solving'. This approach enables a better rapport and improves compliance in drug treatment.

References to psychotherapy for depression in developing countries are scanty. Varma & Ghosh (1976) in their study of 132 patients showed that 28% of the patients were receiving psychotherapy as the sole treatment and 64.4% were administered drugs in combination with psychotherapy; manic depressive psychosis contributed to three cases. Though neurosis accounted for 55.2% of all the diagnostic categories, the respondents did not state the number of neurotic depressive patients included for psychotherapy. Though some responders pointed out that the Western model did not suit their patients, no specific model for use was suggested. There have been reports on cognitive–behavioural therapy for neurotic and endogenous depression (Kuruvilla, 1989), psychotherapy for endogenous depression (Agarwal, 1980), behaviour therapy in depression (Sen, 1974, 1975) supportive psychotherapy for depression in general practice (Jayaram, 1980). Psychoanalytical psychotherapy is also used in rural and urban depressive patients, utilising classical psychoanalytical principles (Nandi, 1978), yoga in neurotic depression (Vahia *et al*, 1975), and a liberal and holistic approach with brief group and comprehensive strategies in depression (Sethi, 1979).

Interpersonal therapy

Interpersonal therapy is based on the theory that the depressed person's interaction with his social environment is crucial for the occurrence as well as resolution of depression. McLean (1976) holds that depression results when the individual loses the ability to control the interpersonal environment due to ineffective coping techniques. Interpersonal therapy incorporates the techniques of behaviour and cognitive therapies. The specific components of therapy are communication training, behavioural productivity, social interaction, assertiveness, decision-making and problem solving, and cognitive control.

Weissman *et al* (1979) reported on an evaluation of interpersonal psychotherapy in four groups: one receiving amitriptyline, another receiving interpersonal therapy, the third receiving both the drug and interpersonal psychotherapy, and the fourth group who were offered supportive psychotherapy on demand. Their findings were that amitriptyline and psychotherapy were equally effective in symptom reduction. However, the drug used in combination with psychotherapy conferred an improved symptom reduction. The antidepressant controlled such symptoms as sleep and appetite, while psychotherapy influenced mood, suicidal ideation, work and interest. The group on supportive therapy fared worst. Interpersonal psychotherapy or tricyclics medication alone were useful in reactive depression. Endogenous depression failed to react to interpersonal psychotherapy alone but with added antidepressants the response was good. Besides, the group receiving psychotherapy functioned better socially and in interpersonal relationships. In a related study it was found that the use of antidepressants and not psychotherapy prevented the relapse of symptoms.

Behavioural therapy

This is based on the concept that depression results from behaviours not followed by positive reinforcement. The therapy aims to alter the quality and quantity of the patient's interactions with other people and the environment by increasing those that have positive outcomes and decreasing those that are negative. A course is limited to 12 structured sessions. The initial diagnostic phase of the therapy consists in identifying the specific interactions that lead to depressive symptoms. The ultimate objective of the treatment is to make the depressed person learn new skills that can be used to change the established pattern of behaviour. At present this treatment is useful for less severely depressed patients.

Cognitive therapy

This therapy is directed at the involuntary and automatic negative cognitions that contribute to depression (see above) (Rush & Beck, 1978). The therapy aims to rectify the negative patterns of thought and so ameliorate depressive symptoms. The therapy itself is short-term with a maximum of 20 sessions over 10 to 12 weeks.

There is substantial evidence that cognitive therapy produces lasting results in depressed persons with prior poor response to antidepressant agents. Rush *et al* (1977) reported that cognitive therapy was more effective than tricyclics in 41 moderately to severely depressed patients. It has produced improvements in chronic depression with suicidal tendency.

Kuruvilla (1980) reported on cognitive–behavioural therapy as the only method of treatment in 20 neurotic depressive patients and in 14 endogenous depressive patients with added antidepressant medication. He reported encouraging results at the time of termination of treatment and on follow-up.

However, there is a group of depressive subjects with a high genetic loading with mostly endogenous symptoms who are less likely to respond to cognitive therapy (Rush, 1984).

Combined psychotherapy and antidepressant drugs

There has been growing evidence of successful outcome with the combined use of psychotherapies and antidepressants (Weissman, 1979). The combination has produced additive effects on different symptoms of the illness. Lesse (1962) reported favourable results with a combination of psychoanalytical psychotherapy and antidepressants. He found the combination much better than drugs or ECT alone.

In four controlled studies using combined drugs and psychotherapy, three for maintenance and one for the acute illness (Klerman *et al*, 1974; Covi *et al*, 1974; Friedman, 1975), all demonstrated benefit from psychotherapy, especially in areas related to problems of living, social functioning, interpersonal relationship and family participation. The therapy did not affect symptoms appreciably. Early control of symptoms like sleeplessness or anorexia by drugs rendered the patients more amenable to psychotherapy. Psychotherapy improved suicidal ideation and depressed mood at 4 to 8 weeks. Drugs prevented relapse of symptoms but exercised poor effect on problems of living.

'Therapy resistant' depression

Although it is recognised that some patients may become resistant to all available antidepressant measures, the entity 'therapy resistance' awaits a clear definition. Those who fail to respond to multiple drug combination followed by ECT for a minimum period of two years may be described as treatment resistant. Among the factors that are responsible are inappropriate drugs or their dosage, and duration of treatment, low therapeutic tissue levels of the drugs used and the use of drugs that interfere with the transport or metabolism of the antidepressant used. Rapid cycling affective disorder and comorbidity of physical disorders such as thyroid dysfunction are other causes of resistance. The use of lithium in combination with tricyclic antidepressants, use of standard or the new reversible MAOIs, administration of thyroid hormone, use of sleep deprivation, use of specific serotonin reuptake inhibitors, and ECT have been recommended. Before refractoriness to tricyclics is pronounced the patient should have received imipramine 300 mg or equivalent or phenelzine 70 mg or equivalent. The relationship between lithium and the newer non-tricyclic antidepressants is not yet clear. Non-pharmacological factors to be explored relate to alcoholism or substance abuse in the patient, unresolved marital or family conflicts, personality and other psychiatric disorders such as schizophrenia.

Course and outcome of affective disorder

The course and outcome of affective disorder, besides including lasting remission, recurrence, chronicity and social impairment is punctuated by suicide behaviour.

Recurrences

Recurrences characterise affective disorder. Few studies are available from the developing world focusing on the long-term outcome of affective disorder. Follow-up periods varying from 3–13 years and 5–15 years have indicated freedom from recurrences following the first episode in 28% (Venkoba Rao & Nammalvar, 1977) and 36.6% (Gada, 1989) of patients respectively. Recurrences of either depression alone or together with mania have been reported in 62% of cases (Venkoba Rao & Nammalvar, 1977). Manic recurrences were twice as common as depression in bipolar disorder. The occurrence of the first episode of mania following the single or more episodes of depression occurred within the first three years after the initial episode, although such a shift could be observed in a few individuals 3–13 years after the first episode of depression (Venkoba Rao & Nammalvar, 1977). The number of episodes in monopolar depression is on average 3.5, fewer than in the bipolar variety. Recurrences are more common if the illness starts in the second or the third decade of life (Venkoba Rao & Nammalvar, 1977).

Chronicity

Several studies point out that appreciably one-fifth of patients develop chronic disorder after the first episode. Carlson *et al* (1974) described one-third of their series of 47 bipolar patients as becoming chronic. Chronicity (defined as persistence of affective symptoms at 3–13 years follow-up) was observed in 10% of subjects by Venkoba Rao & Nammalvar (1977).

A poor prognosis following an episode of major depression has been reported in both medium (2 years) and long-term (over 15 years) outcome studies and is observed in both community and hospitalised depressive patients (Keller *et al*, 1984; Kiloh *et al*, 1988; Lee & Murray, 1988).

The chronic course is reported to evolve in 12–15% of cases if one takes into account those studies in which chronicity has been defined as the persistence of symptoms on follow-up of two or more years until death (Scott, 1988). The chronicity rate has been constant for several decades, uninfluenced by the advent of ECT, antidepressants and other forms of therapy. In the study of Venkoba Rao & Nammalvar (1977), later onset (after 40 years) predisposed to chronicity, while earlier onset was related to recurrence. Social impairment, however, is known to occur as a consequence of persistent and even trivial depressive symptoms (Bebbington, 1982). These could pose a problem even after recovery from the illness (Weissman & Paykel, 1974). A depressive defect state has been described as a result of personality changes (Helmchen, 1974).

Chronicity is known to be related to positive history of affective disorders in the first degree relatives and being a woman. Monopolar depression figures more prominently than bipolar disorder among chronic depressive patients. Life events contribute to the maintenance of depressive episodes (Paykel, 1979), particularly in chronic depressive women. Examples are the loss of a first degree relative, and a serious illness in an immediate member of the family (Cassano *et al*, 1983). The occurrence of thyroid dysfunction among chronic depressive women is an important observation. This has been shown not to be a consequence of lithium therapy or other medication (Johnstone *et al*, 1986; Barker, 1988).

The duration of an illness episode seems to be the most significant predictor of chronicity. The greater the length of the episode prior to treatment, the more likely the illness is to become chronic (Keller *et al*, 1986). An incomplete recovery at the time of discharge is yet another predictor of symptomatic chronicity (Toone & Ron, 1977).

The other suspected causes of chronicity are inadequate and inappropriate treatment. The pace of recovery is known to slow down with time: 64% recover within six months: 74% within 12 months, but only 79% recover within two years (Keller *et al*, 1984).

Mania is reported to run a chronic non-cyclic course among the Bantus of South Africa (nearly 81% of bipolar disorder), whereas the whites in the same country showed a lower rate of chronic manic illness (26%). The lack of cycling of mania among the Nigerian Yorubas has also been reported by Makanjuola (1985). Though the significance of non-cycling chronic course of mania in the Africans is not known, it has been suggested that the proportion of manic reactions may decline with increasing education (Murphy, 1982).

Chronicity in the elderly is an important area of clinical concern. The clinical stereotype of depression after 65 years with a predominance of somatic symptoms, hypochondriasis, paranoid tendency, marked agitation and a greater tendency for chronicity has been re-examined in recent studies. These indicate that those patients above 65 years of age experience more 'single' episodes of depression precipitated by psychosocial circumstances (Musetti *et al*, 1989). Uncomplicated depression in old age tends to have a good prognosis. Conversely, when physical illness and adverse psychosocial circumstances exist, the prognosis is poor. Indeed Murphy *et al* (1988) have shown that physical illness at referral in a group of elderly depressed patients resulted in an increased mortality in a four-year period as against age and gender matched controls. The chief contributory factors towards higher mortality in late life depression are cardiovascular and cerebrovascular disease, and occult or frank malignancy.

Features of cultural interest

These are related not only to the beliefs, superstitions, attitudes, cultural practices, illiteracy and economic poverty but also to the philosophies and medical systems of the countries.

Moderately depressed patients, unlike the severely depressed or physically ill are misunderstood, since their distress is seldom comprehensible to family relations, friends or even to the medical practitioners. An assurance by the medical practitioner that there is nothing physically wrong with them is demoralising. Many are blamed as idlers, and young housewives are often faulted as avoiding work and are threatened with divorce or being returned to their parental home. The biological basis of the disorder is not recognised and the patients are advised to 'change their mind'.

Cultural concepts of mental illness in the developing countries are related to such factors as possession, evil spirits, bewitchment, evil eye, sorcery, and witchcraft (Campoling, 1989). These 'spiritual' (supernatural) causes of mental illness lie external to the individual. Each culture has its own lexicon for the 'spirits' and insanity. For example, 'Jinn' indicates spirits and 'Jinnon' madness in Arabic countries. The evil eye is motivated by envy, jealousy or even admiration of an enemy or friend. The state of social withdrawal called 'tankir' is believed to be induced by a witch in the francophone North African Arabs (Al-Issa, 1989). Becoming possessed by the ghosts of ancestors or someone else is part of a belief system in many cultures and such behaviours have social sanctions. To hear the voice of an ancestor does not mean that one is mad. Similarly, to struggle at night with ghosts and finally to become 'possessed' is not pathological but part of a belief system in Zimbabwe.

Cultural factors come into prominence during the maintenance of prophylactic therapy. It is a common notion that medicines are needed only for illness. In a disease-free state, drugs are not required, thus compliance becomes difficult. Among Muslim patients compliance may be affected by fasting during the Ramadan month. Prophylaxis with lithium, carbamazepine or antidepressants meets with difficulty even when the subject is informed about the potential for recurrence. When relapse occurs, ineffective treatment of the earlier episode is blamed and a different psychiatrist is consulted. Alternatively, patients may switch over to other systems of treatment, for example ayurveda, yoga, homeopathy, acupuncture or traditional healing. Recently, there has been a tendency to revert to traditional therapies and indigenous remedies in African countries like Algeria and other Arab societies.

References

AGARWAL, A. K. (1980) Psychotherapy in endogenous depression. In *Depressive Illness* (eds A. Venkoba Rao & S. Parvathi Devi). Madurai: Vaigai Achagam.

AKISKAL, H. S. (1981) Subaffective disorders, dysthymic cyclothymic and bipolar II disorders in the 'borderline' realm. *Psychiatric Clinics of North America,* **4,** 25–46.

AL-ISSA, I. (1989) Psychiatry in Algeria. *Psychiatric Bulletin,* **13,** 240–245.

AL-SABAIE, A. (1990) Psychiatry in Saudi Arabia: an overview. *Psychiatric Bulletin,* **14,** 298–300.

ANUMONYE, A. (1980) *Brain Fag Syndrome.* CIPAT Lausanne: ICAA.

ARANA, G. W., BALDESSARINI, R. J. & ORNSTEEN, M. (1985) The dexamethasone suppression test for diagnosis and prognosis in psychiatry. *Archives of General Psychiatry*, **42**, 1193–1204.

BAGADIA, V. N., JESTE, D. V., CHAREGAONKAR, A. S., *et al* (1973) Psychological study of 180 cases of epilepsy. *Indian Journal of Psychiatry*, **15**, 391.

———, ———, DAVE, K. P., *et al* (1977) A prospective epidemiological study of 233 cases of depression. *Indian Journal of Psychiatry*, **12**, 44–46.

BARKER, W. A. & ECCLESTON, D. (1988) The Newcastle chronic depression study. Patient characteristics and factors associated with chronicity. *British Journal of Psychiatry*, **152**, 28–33.

BARRACLOUGH, B., BUNCH, J., NELSON, B., *et al* (1974) A hundred cases of suicide: clinical aspects. *British Journal of Psychiatry*, **125**, 355–373.

BEBBINGTON, P. E. (1982) The course and prognosis of affective disorders. In *Cambridge Handbook of Psychiatry: 3. Psychoses of Uncertain Aetiology* (ed. J. K. Wing). Cambridge: Cambridge University Press.

BECK, A. T., DAVIS, J. H., FREDERICK, C. J., *et al* (1973) Classification and nomenclature. In *Suicide Prevention in the Seventies* (eds H. L. P. Resnik & B. C. Hathorne). Rockville, MD: National Institute of Mental Health Center for Studies on Suicide Prevention.

BHATIA, M. S. & MALIK, S. C. (1991) Dhat syndrome – A useful diagnostic entity in Indian culture. *British Journal of Psychiatry*, **159**, 691–695.

BINITIE, A. (1975) A factor-analytical study of depression across cultures (African and European). *British Journal of Psychiatry*, **127**, 559–563.

BOUSSAT, M., GUEYE, M., HANCK, C., *et al* (1977) *Comparative Psychiatry*. New York: Springer-Verlag.

BOYD, J. H. & WEISSMAN, M. M. (1981) Epidemiology of affective disorder: a re-examination and future direction. *Archives of General Psychiatry*, **38**, 1039–1046.

BRENNER, B. M. (1976) Pseudocyesis in blacks. *South African Medical Journal*, **50**, 1757.

BROCKINGTON, I. F. & KUMAR, R. (1982) *Motherhood and Mental Illness*. New York: Grune & Stratton.

BROWN, G. W. & HARRIS, T. O. (1978) *Social Origins of Depression*. London: Free Press.

BROWN, W. A. & QUALLS, C. B. (1981) Pituitary adrenal disinhibition on depression: marker of a subtype with characteristic clinical feature and response to treatment. *Psychiatric Research*, **4**, 115.

———, SHRIVASTAVA, R. & ARATO, M. (1987) Pretreatment pituitary-adrenocortical status and placebo response in depression. *Psychopharmacology Bulletin*, **23**, 155–159.

CALABRESE, J. E., RAPPORT, D. T., KIMMEL, S. E., *et al* (1993) Rapid cycling bipolar disorder and its treatment with valproate. *Canadian Journal of Psychiatry*, **38** (Suppl. 2), S57–61.

CAMPLING, P. (1989) Race, culture and psychotherapy. *Psychiatric Bulletin*, **13**, 550–551.

CARLSON, G. A., KOTIN, J., DAVENPORT, Y. B., *et al* (1974) Follow-up of 53 bipolar manic depressive patients. *British Journal of Psychiatry*, **124**, 134.

CARROLL, B. J. (1980) Disinhibition of cortisol secretion in depression. Paper read at the 12th Congress of Collegium International Neuropsychopharmacology, Gotebery, 22 June 1980.

———, FEINBERG, M., GREDEN, J. F., *et al* (1981) A specific laboratory test for the diagnosis of melancholia: standardisation, validation and clinical utility. *Archives of General Psychiatry*, **38**, 15–22.

CARSTAIRS, G. M. & KAPUR, R. L. (1976) *The Great Universe of Kota: Stress Changes and Mental Disorder in an Indian Village*. London: The Hogarth Press.

CASSANO, G. B., MAGGINI, C. & AKISKAL, H. (1983) Short-term subchronic sequelae of affective disorders. *Psychiatric Clinics of North America*, **6**, 55–68.

CATALAN, J., GATH, D. H. & BOND, A., *et al* (1988) General practice patients on long-term psychotropic drugs. A controlled investigation. *British Journal of Psychiatry*, **152**, 399–406.

CAWTE, J. (1988) Aboriginal death in custody: the views of aboriginal health workers. *Australian Journal of Forensic Sciences*, **20**, 244–253.

CHAKRABORTY, A. & SANDEL, B. (1984) Somatic complaints syndrome in India. *Transcultural Psychiatric Research Review*, **21**, 212.

CHATTERJEE, R. N., MUKHERJEE, S. P. & NANDI, D. N. (1981) Life events and depression. *Indian Journal of Psychiatry*, **23**, 333.

——— & KULHARA, P. (1989) Symptomatology symptom resolution and short term course in mania. *Indian Journal of Psychiatry*, **31**, 213–218.

CHATURVEDI, S. K. (1987) Depressive psychosis presenting as chronic pain disorder. *Indian Journal of Psychiatry*, **29**, 235–238.

CHECKLEY, S. (1992) Neuroendocrine mechanisms and the precipitation of depression by life events. *British Journal of Psychiatry*, **160** (Suppl. 15), 7–17.

CHERIAN, A., KURUVILLA, K. & PRABHAKAR, S. (1990) Rapid cycling and affective disorder associated with EEG abnormality. *Indian Journal of Psychiatry*, **32**, 89–92.

CHKILI, T. & EL KHAMLICHI, A. (1975) Les psychoses puerpérales en milieu Marocain. *La Tunisie Médicale*, **53**, 375–392.

CHOWDHURY, A. N., CHATTERJEE, A., PAL, P., *et al* (1988) Analysis of North Bengal koro epidemic with three years follow-up. *Indian Journal of Psychiatry*, **30**, 69–72.

CHRISTODOULOU, G. N. (1978) Pseudocyesis. *Acta Psychiatrica Belgia*, **78**, 224–234.

CLAYTON, P. J., DESMARAIS, L. & WINOKUR, G. (1968) A study of normal bereavement. *American Journal of Psychiatry*, **125**, 168.

———— (1978) Bipolar Affective disorder: techniques and result of treatment. *American Journal of Psychiatry*, **32**, 81–92.

COHEN, L. M. (1982) A current perspective of pseudocyesis. *American Journal of Psychiatry*, **139**, 1140–1144.

COLLOMB, H. (1965) Bouffées délirantes en psychiatrie Africaine (Abstract). *Transcultural Psychiatric Research Review*, **3**, 29–34.

CORYELL, W., SCHLESSER, M. (1981) Suicide and DST in unipolar depression. *American Journal of Psychiatry*, **138**, 1120–1121.

————, WINOKUR, G. & ANDERSON, N. (1982) Effect of case of definition on affective disorder rate. Epidemiology of affective disorder. *Archives of General Psychiatry*, **39**, 35–46.

COURT, J. H. (1972) The continuum model as a resolution of paradoxes in manic depressive psychosis. *British Journal of Psychiatry*, **129**, 342.

COVI, L., LIPMAN, R., DEROGATIS, L., *et al* (1974) Drugs and group psychotherapy in neurotic depression. *American Journal of Psychiatry*, **131**, 191.

COX, J. L. (1979) Psychiatric morbidity and pregnancy: a controlled study of 263 semi-rural Ugandan women. *Psychiatry*, **134**, 401–405.

DAM, H., MELLERUP, E. T. & RAFAELSEN, O. J. (1985) The dexamethasone suppression test in depression. *Journal of Affective Disorders*, **8**, 95–103.

DEAN, C. & KENDELL, R. E. (1981) The symptomatology of puerperal illness. *British Journal of Psychiatry*, **139**, 128–133.

DOHRENWEND, B. P. & DOHRENWEND, P. S. (1974) Psychiatric disorders in urban settings. In *American Handbook of Psychiatry*, Vol. 2 (ed. G. Caplan). New York: Basic Books.

DORPAT, R. & RIPLEY, H. S. (1960) A study of suicide in the Seattle area. *Comprehensive Psychiatry*, **1**, 349.

DUNNER, D. L. (1979) Rapid cycling bipolar manic depressive illness. *Psychiatric Clinics of North America*, **2**, 461–467.

EATON, W. W. & KESSLER, L. G. (1985) *Epidemiological Field Methods in Psychiatry. The Epidemiological Catchment Area Programme*. New York: Academic Press.

EGELAND, J. A., GERHARD, D. S., PAULS, D. L., *et al* (1987) Bipolar affective disorder linked to DNS markers on chromosome 11. *Nature*, **325**, 783–787.

EMRICH, H. M., DOSE, M. & VON ZERSSEN, D. (1985) The use of sodium valproate, carbamazepine and oxcabazine in patients with affective disorders. *Journal of Affective Disorders*, **8**, 243–250.

ESCOBAR, J. I. & CANINO, G. (1989) Unexplained physical complaints: psychopathology and epidemiological correlates. *British Journal of Psychiatry*, **154** (Suppl. 4), 24–27.

FARMER, A. E. & McGUFFIN, P. (1989) Classification of depression: Contemporary confusion revisited. *British Journal of Psychiatry*, **155**, 437–443.

FERNANDEZ, A., KHANNA, S. & CHANNABASAVANNA, S. M. (1988) Epileptic psychosis. A retrospective study. *Indian Journal of Psychiatry*, **30**, 95–101.

FRIEDMAN, A. S. (1975) Interaction of drug therapy with marital therapy in depressed patients. *Archives of General Psychiatry*, **32**, 619.

GADA, M. (1989) The course of depressive illness. A follow-up investigation of 92 cases. *Indian Journal of Psychiatry*, **31**, 196–200.

GAUTAM, S., NIJHAWAN, M. & GEHLOT, P. S. (1982) Postpartum psychiatric syndromes: an analysis of 100 consecutive cases. *Indian Journal of Psychiatry*, **24**, 383–386.

GERMAN G. A. (1982) *The Schizophrenia Enigma*. Academic Address of the Australian Society for Psychiatric Research.

———— (1987) Mental health in Africa: I. The extent of mental health problems in Africa today. An update of epidemiological knowledge. *British Journal of Psychiatry*, **151**, 435–439.

GLOVER, G. R. (1989) The pattern of psychiatric admissions of Caribbean-born immigrants in London. *Social Psychiatry and Psychiatric Epidemiology*, **24**, 49–56.

GOLDBERG, D. & BRIDGES, K. (1987) Screening for psychiatric illness in general practice: the general practitioner versus the screening questionnaire. *Journal of the Royal College of General Practitioners*, **37**, 15–18.

GUINNESS, E. A. (1992) Patterns of mental illness in the early stages of urbanisation. *British Journal of Psychiatry*, **160** (Suppl. 16), 4–72.

GUPTA, R. (1990) Unipolar summer and winter depression a report from North India. *Indian Journal of Psychiatry*, **32**, 201–203.

GUZDER, J. & MEENAKSHI, K. (1991) Sita-Shakti: cultural paradigms for Indian women. *Transcultural Psychiatric Research Review*, **4**, 257–302.

HARRIS, B., OTHMAN, G., DAVIES, J. A., *et al* (1992) Association between postpartum thyroid dysfunction and thyroid antibodies and depression. *British Medical Journal*, **305**, 152–156.

HAYNES, R. H. (1984) Suicide in Fiji: a preliminary study. *British Journal of Psychiatry*, **145**, 433–438.

HELMCHEN, H. (1974) Symptomatology of therapy-resistant depression. *Pharmacopsychiatria*, **7**, 145–155.

HENRY, A. (1992) The safety of antidepressants. *British Journal of Psychiatry*, **160**, 439–441.

INDIAN COUNCIL OF MEDICAL RESEARCH (1986) The phenomenology and natural history of acute psychosis. Final report of the project. New Delhi.

INWOOD, D. G. (1989) Postpartum psychotic disorders. In *Comprehensive Textbook of Psychiatry* (5th edn) (eds H. I. Kaplan & B. J. Sadock), pp. 852–858. Baltimore: Williams & Wilkins.

JANOWSKI, D. S., EL YOUSEF, M. K., DAVIS, J. M., *et al* (1972) A cholinergic adrenergic hypothesis of mania and depression. *Lancet*, **ii**, 632.

JAYARAM, S. S. (1980) General practitioner and psychological treatment in depressive illness. In *Depressive Illness* (eds A. Venkoba Rao & S. Parvathi Devi). Madurai: Vaigai Achagam.

JOFFE, R. T., HORVATH, Z. & TARVYDAS, I. (1986) Bipolar affective disorder and thalassaemia minor. *American Journal of Psychiatry*, **143**, 933.

JOHNSTONE, E. C., OWENS, D. G. C., CROW, T. J., *et al* (1986) Hypothyroidism as a correlate of lateral ventricular enlargement in manic depressive and neurotic illness. *British Journal of Psychiatry*, **148**, 317–321.

KADRMAS, A., WINOKUR, G. & CROW, R. (1979) Postpartum mania. *British Journal of Psychiatry*, **135**, 551–554.

KAPUR, R. L. & PANDURANGI, A. K. (1979) A comparative study of reactive psychosis and acute psychosis without precipitating stress. *British Journal of Psychiatry*, **133**, 544–560.

KEARNEY, R. N. & MILLER, V. D. (1985) The spiral of suicide and social changes in Sri Lanka. *Journal of Asian Studies*, **45**, 81–101.

KEILHOLZ, P., TERZANI, S., GASPAR, M., *et al* (1982) Zur Behandlung therapie resistenter Depressionen: Ergebnisse einer Kombinserten Infusion-therapie. *Schwiezerische Medizinische Wochenschrift*, **112**, 1090–1095.

KELLER, M. B., KLERMAN, G. L., LAVORI, P. W., *et al* (1984) Long term outcome of episode of major depression. *Journal of the American Medical Association*, **252**, 788–792.

———, LAVORI, P. W., RICE, J., *et al* (1986) The persistent risk of chronicity in recurrent episodes of non bipolar major depressive disorder. A prospective follow-up. *American Journal of Psychiatry*, **143**, 24–28.

KENDELL, R. E. (1985) Emotional and physical factors in the genesis of puerperal mental disorders. *Journal of Psychosomatic Research*, **29**, 3–11.

———, CHALMERS, J. C. & PLATZ, C. (1987) Epidemiology of puerperal psychosis. *British Journal of Psychiatry*, **150**, 662–673.

KERR, P. (1991) Antidepressant prescribing in general practice – how long can this go on? *Psychiatric Bulletin*, **15**, 281–283.

KILOH, L. G., ANDREWS, G. & NEILSON, M. (1988) The long-term outcome of depressive illness. *British Journal of Psychiatry*, **153**, 752–757.

KIM, K. I. & RHI, B. Y. (1976) A review of Korean culture psychiatry. *Transcultural Psychiatric Research Review*, **13**, 101.

KIMURA, B. (1965) Comparative investigations of depression in Japan and Germany. *Fortschritte für Neurologie-Psychiatrie*, **33**, 202–215.

KING, J. R., PHILLIPS, J. D., JUDGE, R., *et al* (1991) Instant lithium monitoring. *Psychiatric Bulletin*, **15**, 138–139.

KLEINMAN, A. (1986) *Social Origins of Distress and Disease: Depression, Neurasthenia, and Pain in Modern China*. New Haven: Yale University Press.

KLERMAN, G. L., DIMASCIO, A., WEISSMAN, M. M., *et al* (1974) Treatment of depression by drugs and psychotherapy. *American Journal of Psychiatry*, **131**, 186.

KRAUTHAMMER, C. & KLERMAN, G. (1978) Secondary mania. Manic syndromes associated with antecedent physical illness of drugs. *Archives of General Psychiatry*, **35**, 1333–1339.

KUA, E. H. & KO, S. M. (1992) A cross cultural study of suicide among the elderly in Singapore. *British Journal of Psychiatry*, **160**, 558–559.

KUPFER, D. J. & THASE, M. E. (1983) The use of sleep laboratory in the diagnosis of affective disorders. *Psychiatric Clinics of North America*, **36**, 635–643.

KURUVILLA, K. (1980) Cognitive behaviour therapy in the treatment of depression. In *Depressive Illness* 223 (eds A. Venkoba Rao & S. Parvathi Devi). Madurai: Vaigai Achagam.

LAMBO, T. A. (1965) Schizophrenia and borderline states. In *Transcultural Psychiatry* (eds A. V. S. de Reuck & R. Porter). (Ciba Foundation Symposium). London: Churchill.

LAPUZ, L. (1972) A study of psychopathology in a group of Fillipino patients. In *Transcultural Research in Mental Health* (Vol. 11) (ed. W. P. Lebra), pp. 172. Honolulu: University of Hawaii Press.

LEE, A. S. & MURRAY, R. M. (1988) The long term outcome of Maudsley depressives. *British Journal of Psychiatry*, **153**, 741–751.

LESSE, S. (1962) Psychotherapy in combination with antidepressant drugs. *American Journal of Psychotherapy*, **16**, 407.

LITTLEWOOD, R. & LIPSEDGE, M. (1985) Culture-bound syndromes. In *Recent Advances in Clinical Psychiatry*, No. 5 (ed. K. Granville-Grossman), pp. 105–142. Edinburgh: Churchill Livingstone.

LORANGER, A. W. & LEVINE, P. M. (1978) Age at onset of bipolar affective illness. *Archives of General Psychiatry*, **35**, 1345–1348.

MAKANJUOLA, R. O. A. (1985) Recurrent unipolar manic disorder in the Yoruba Nigerian: further evidence. *British Journal of Psychiatry*, **147**, 434–437.

MBWAMBO, J., APPLEBY, L., GATER, R. (1992) Training matters: the training of psychiatrists for the developing world. *Psychiatric Bulletin*, **16**, 352–354.

MCLEAN, P. (1976) Therapeutic decision making in the behavioural treatment of depression. In *The Behavioural Management of Anxiety, Depression and Pain* (ed. P. O. Davidson). New York: Brunner-Mazel.

MEZZICH, J. E. & RAAB, E. S. (1980) Depressive symptomatology across the Americas. *Archives of General Psychiatry*, **37**, 818.

MINDE, K. (1974) Study problems in Ugandan secondary school students. *British Journal of Psychiatry*, **125**, 131–137.

MURPHY, H. B. M., WITTKOWER, E. D. & CHANCE, N. A. (1967) Cross cultural enquiry into symptomatology of depression: a preliminary report. *International Journal of Psychiatry*, **3**, 6–15.

—— (1982) *Comparative Psychiatry*. New York: Springer Verlag.

MURPHY, J. M., OLIVER, D. C., MONSON, R. R., *et al* (1988) Incidence of depression and anxiety: the Stirling country study. *American Journal of Public Health*, **5**, 534–540.

MURRAY, J. L. & ABRAHAM, G. E. (1978) Pseudocyesis – a review. *Obstetrics and Gynecology*, **51**, 627–631.

MUSETTI, L., PERUGI, G., SORIANI, A., *et al* (1989) Depression before and after 65. A re-examination. *British Journal of Psychiatry*, **155**, 330.

NAIK, U. & WIG, N. N. (1980) A study of depressive disorders in a general hospital out-patient service. In *Depressive Illness* (eds A. Venkoba Rao & S. Parvathi Devi). Madurai, India: Vaigai Achagam.

NANDI, D. N., AJMANY, S., GANGULI, H., *et al* (1975) Psychiatric disorders in a rural community in West Bengal – An epidemiological study. *Indian Journal of Psychiatry*, **17**, 87.

——, ——, ——, *et al* (1976) A clinical evaluation of depressives found in a rural survey in India. *British Journal of Psychiatry*, **128**, 523.

——, KUKHERJEE, S. P., BORAL, G. C., *et al* (1977) Prevalence of psychiatric morbidity in two tribal communities in certain villages of West Bengal – A cross-cultural study. *Indian Journal of Psychiatry*, **19**, 32.

—— (1978) Psychoanalysis in India. In *Psychotherapeutic Processes*, (Vol. 21) (eds M. Kapu, V. N. Murthy, K. Sathyavathi, *et al*). Bangalore: National Institute of Mental Health and Neurosciences.

——, BANERJEE, G., NANDI, S., *et al* (1992) Is hysteria on the wane? A community survey in West Bengal, India. *British Journal of Psychiatry*, **160**, 87–91.

NICHTER, M. (1981) Idioms of distress: alternatives in the expression of psychosocial distress: a case study from South India. *Culture, Medicine and Psychiatry*, **3**, 379–408.

OBEYESKERE, M. (1976) The impact of Ayurvedic ideas on the culture and the individual in Sri Lanka. In *Asian Medical Systems: a Comparative Study* (ed. C. Leslie). Berkeley: University of California Press.

OKASHA, A. (1977) Psychiatric symptomatology in Egypt. In *Mental Health and Society*. Basel: Karger. 4, 121–125.

—— (1980) Differential aspects of the psychopathology of Egyptian depressives. In *Psychopathology of Depression* (eds K. Achte, V. Ashberg & J. Lonngrist), pp. 135. Psychiatrie Fennica Supplement. Helsinki.

PAYKEL, E. S. (1974) Recent life events and clinical depression. In *Life Stress and Illness* (eds E. K. Gunderson & R. H. Rahe), p. 134. Springfield, Illinois: Charles Thomas.

—— & TANNER, J. (1976) Life events, depressive relapse and maintenance treatment. *Psychological Medicine*, **6**, 481–485.

—— (1979) Recent life events in the development of depressive disorders. In *The Psychobiology of the Depressive Disorders – Implications for the Effects of Stress* (ed. R. A. Depue). New York: Academic Press.

PERRIS, C. (1966) A study of bipolar and unipolar recurrent depressive illness. *Acta Psychiatrica Scandinavica*, **42** (Suppl. 194).

PFEIFFER, W. M. (1973) Mental disorders in a traditional culture, Nias, Indonesia. *Transcultural Psychiatric Research Review*, **13**, 101.

PLATZ, C. & KENDELL, R. E. (1988) A matched-control follow-up and family study of 'puerperal psychosis'. *British Journal of Psychiatry*, **153**, 90–94.

POST, R. M., BALLENGER, J. C., REY, A. C., *et al* (1981) Slow and rapid onset of manic episodes. *Psychiatry Research*, **4**, 229–237.

PRANGE, A. J., WILSON, I. C., LYNN, C. W., *et al* (1974) L-tryptophan in mania: contribution to the permissive hypothesis of affective disorders. *Archives of General Psychiatry*, **30**, 56–62.

PRINCE, R. H. (1968) The changing picture of depressive syndromes in Africa. Is it fact or diagnostic fashion? *Canadian Journal of African Studies*, **1**, 177–192.

QUITKIN, F., RIFKIN, A. & KLEIN, D. F. (1978) Imipramine response in deluded depressive patients. *American Journal of Psychiatry*, **135**, 806–811.

RACY, J. (1980) Somatisation in Saudi women: a therapeutic challenge. *British Journal of Psychiatry*, **137**, 212–216.

RANDS, G. (1989) Psychiatry, traditional healers, and the vimbusa in northern Malawi. *Psychiatric Bulletin*, **13**, 622–625.

REGIER, D. A. & MOSCICKI, E. D. (1987) *Reduction of the Suicide Rate in Young People*. Progress Review. Washington DC: US Department of Health and Human Services, Office of the Assistant Secretary of Health.

ROBINS, E., MURPHY, G. E., WILKINSON, R. H., *et al* (1959) Some clinical considerations in the prevention of suicide based on a study of 134 successful suicides. *American Journal of Public Health*, **49**, 888–889.

—— & CUZE, S. B. (1972) Classification of affective disorders: the primary-secondary, the endogenous and the neurotic-psychotic concepts. In *Recent Advances in the Psychology of Depressive Illness* (eds T. A. Williams, M. M. Katz & J. A. Shield). Washington, DC: Department of Health, Education and Welfare.

——, MUNOZ, R. A., MARTIN, S., *et al* (1972) Primary and secondary affective disorders. In *Disorders of Mood* (eds J. Zubin & F. A. Freyhan), pp. 33–45. Baltimore MD: Johns Hopkins Press.

RORSMAN, B., GRASBECK, A., HAGNELL, O., *et al* (1990) A prospective study of first incidence depression. The Lundby study, 1957–1972. *British Journal of Psychiatry*, **156**, 336–342.

ROSENTHAL, N. E., SAC, D. A., GILLIN, J. C., *et al* (1984) Seasonal affective disorder. A description of the syndrome and preliminary findings with light therapy. *Archives of General Psychiatry*, **4**, 72–80.

RUSH, A. J., BECK, A. T., KOVACS, M., *et al* (1977) Comparative efficacy of cognitive therapy and pharmacotherapy in the treatment of depressed outpatients. *Cognitive Therapy Research*, **1**, 17.

—— & —— (1978) Cognitive therapy of depression and suicide. *American Journal of Psychotherapy*, **32**, 201.

—— (1984) A phase II study of cognitive therapy of depression. In *Psychotherapy Research* (eds J. B. W. Williams & R. L. Spitzer). New York: Guilford Press.

RWEGELLERA, G. G. C. (1981) Cultural aspects of depressive illness, clinical aspects and psychopathology. *Psychopathologie Africaine*, **17**, 41–63.

SAINSBURY, P. (1980) Suicide and depression. In *Psychopathology of Depression* (eds K. Achte, V. Ashberg & J. Lonngrist), pp. 259. Psychiatrica Fennica Supplment. Helsinki.

SATYANARAYANA SWAMY, H., MALLIKARJUNAIAH, M., BETTI, H. S., *et al* (1986) A study of epileptic psychoses – 150 cases. *Indian Journal of Psychiatry*, **28**, 486–493.

SCOTT, J. (1988) Chronic depression. *British Journal of Psychiatry*, **153**, 287–297.

SEIVEWRIGHT, N. & TYRER, P. (1990) Relationship of dysthymia to anxiety and other neurotic disorders. In *Dysthymic Disorder* (eds S. W. Burton & H. S. Akiskal), pp. 24–36. London: Gaskell.

SEN, B. & WILLIAMS, P. (1987) The extent and nature of depressive phenomena in primary health care. A study in Calcutta, India. *British Journal of Psychiatry*, **151**, 486–493.

SEN, N. N. (1974) Behaviour therapy in depression. I – Experimental analysis. *Indian Journal of Clinical Psychology*, **1**, 53.

—— (1975) Behaviour therapy in depressions. II – Plan and procedure of case analysis and treatment. *Indian Journal of Clinical Psychology,* **2**, 77.

SETHI, B. B. & GUPTA, S. C. (1970) An epidemiological and cultural study of depression. *Indian Journal of Psychiatry,* **12**, 14.

——, NATHAWAT, S. S. & GUPTA, S. C. (1973) Depression in India. *Journal of Social Psychology,* **91**, 3.

—— (1979) Psychotherapy of depressive conditions. In *Prevention and Treatment of Depression,* (eds T. A. Ban, R. Gonzales, A. S. Jablensky, *et al*). Baltimore: University Park Press.

SILBER, T. J. & ABDALLA, W. (1983) Pseudocyesis in adolescent females. *Journal of Adolescent Health Care,* **4**, 109–112.

SINGH, G. & SACHDEVA, J. S. (1980) A clinical and follow-up study of atypical psychosis. *Indian Journal of Psychiatry,* **22**, 167–172.

——, KAUR, D. & KAUR, H. (1981) Presumptive stressful events scale (PSE Scale). *Indian Journal of Clinical Psychology,* **8**, 173.

SPIKER, D. G., WEISS, J. C., DEALY, R. S., *et al* (1985) The pharmacological treatment of delusional depression. *American Journal of Psychiatry,* **142**, 430–436.

STARKMAN, M. N., MARSHALL, J. C., LA FERLA, J., *et al* (1985) Pseudocyesis; psychologic and neuroendocrine inter-relationships. *Psychosomatic Medicine,* **47**, 46–57.

TEJA, J. S., NARANG, R. L. & AGARWAL, A. K. (1971) Depression across cultures. *British Journal of Psychiatry,* **119**, 253.

THASE, M. E. (1989) Comparison between seasonal affective disorder and other forms of recurrent depression. In *Seasonal Affective Disorders and Phototherapy* (eds N. E. Rosenthal & M. C. Blehar), pp. 64–78. New York, London: Guilford Press.

THEBAUD, E. & RIGAMER, E. F. (1972) *Some Considerations of Students Mental Health in Liberia. Proceedings of the Third Pan African Conference.* Nigeria: Abeokuta.

THUVE, I. (1974) Genetic factors in puerperal psychosis. *British Journal of Psychiatry,* **125**, 378–385.

TONGYOUT, J. (1972) Depression in Thailand in the perspective of comparative transcultural psychiatry. *Psychiatric Association of Thailand,* **16**, 337–344.

TOONE, B. K. & RON, M. (1977) A study of predictive factors in depressive disorders of poor outcome. *British Journal of Psychiatry,* **131**, 587–591.

VAHIA, N. S., DONGAJI, D. R. & JESTE, D. V. (1975) Value of Patanjali's concepts in the treatment of psychoneurosis. In *New Dimensions in Psychiatry* (eds S. Arieti & G. Chrzanowski). New York: John Wiley & Sons.

VARMA, V. K. & GHOSH, A. (1976) Psychotherapy as practised by Indian Psychiatrists. *Indian Journal of Psychiatry,* **18**, 177.

VENKOBA RAO, A. (1978) Epidemiology of depression. *Indian Journal of Psychological Medicine,* **1**, 37.

—— (1984) Depressive illness in India. *Indian Journal of Psychiatry,* **26**, 301–311.

—— (1986) *Depressive Disease.* New Delhi: Indian Council of Medical Research.

——, RAWLIN CHINNIAN, R. & HARIHARAN, G. (1974) Epilepsy and suicide behaviour. In *International Congress of Physiological Sciences.* Abstracts. New Delhi.

—— & NAMMALVAR, N. (1976) Life events and depressive disease. *Indian Journal of Psychiatry,* **18**, 293.

—— & —— (1977) The course and outcome in depressive illness. *British Journal of Psychiatry,* **130**, 392.

VERGHESE, A., BEIG, A., SENSEMAN, L. A., *et al* (1973) A social and psychiatric study of a representative group of families in Vellore Town, India. *Indian Journal of Medical Research,* **61**, 608.

VYAS, J. N. (1992) Mood Disorders. In *Postgraduate Psychiatry* (eds J. N. Vyas & Niraj Ahuja), pp. 50–70. New Delhi: Churchill Livingstone.

WATSON, S. J., RICHARD, C. W., CIARANELLO, R. D., *et al* (1980) Interaction of opiate peptides and noradrenaline system. *Peptides,* **1**, 23.

WEISSMAN, M. M. & PAYKEL, E. (1974) *The Depressed Woman: A Study of Social Relationships.* Chicago: University of Chicago.

—— (1979) The psychological treatment of depression: research evidence for the efficacy of psychotherapy alone, in comparison and in combination with pharmacotherapy. *Archives of General Psychiatry,* **36**, 1261.

——, PRUSOFF, B. A., DIMASCIO, A., *et al* (1979) The efficacy of drugs and psychotherapy in the treatment of acute depressive episodes. *American Journal of Psychiatry,* **136**, 555.

—— & MYERS, J. K. (1978) Affective disorders in a US urban community; the use of research diagnostic criteria in an epidemiologic survey. *Archives of General Psychiatry,* **35**, 1304–1311.

——, LEAF, P. J., BRUCE, M. L., *et al* (1988) The epidemiology of dysthymia in the community: rates risks, comorbidity and treatment. *American Journal of Psychiatry,* **145**, 815–819.

WHYBROW, P. C., PRANGE, A. J. & TREADWAY, C. R. (1969) Mental changes accompanying thyroid gland dysfunction. *Archives of General Psychiatry,* **29,** 48–63.

WIG, N. N., VARMA, H. D. & SHAH, D. K. (1969) Parental deprivation and mental illness: a study of incidence of parental death in childhood in 2000 psychiatric patients. *Indian Journal of Psychiatry,* **11,** 1.

—— (1984) Psychiatric research in India. In *Psychiatry in India* (eds A. DeSouza & D. A. DeSouza). Bombay: Bhilani.

WINOKUR, G., CLAYTON, P. & REICH, T. (1969) *Manic Depressive Illness.* St Louis: Mosby.

WOODRUFF, R. A., MURPHY, G. E., HERJANIC, M. (1967) The natural history of affective disorders – I. Symptoms of 72 patients at the time of index hospital admission. *Journal of Psychiatric Research,* **5,** 255–263.

WORLD HEALTH ORGANIZATION (1992) *The Tenth Revision of the Classification of Mental and Behavioural Disorders. Clinical Descriptions and Diagnostic Guidelines (ICD–10).* Geneva: WHO.

ZUBER, T. & KELLY, J. (1984) Pseudocyesis. *American Family Physician,* **5,** 131–134.

11 Epilepsy

STEPHEN W. BROWN

Definition and epidemiology

Epilepsy refers to a tendency to have recurrent seizures. Hughlings Jackson described it as 'occasional, sudden, excessive, rapid and local discharges of grey matter', though as this could be over-embracing, he also stated that 'a sneeze is a kind of healthy epilepsy' (Reynolds, 1986). This was of course written before the advent of the electroencephalograph (EEG). Today we would want to include in the definition an acknowledgement that true epileptic seizures have a characteristic EEG accompaniment. Since EEG electrodes are rarely in place when someone has a seizure, and even if they are it may be impossible to record from the precise relevant brain area, epilepsy remains primarily a clinical diagnosis.

Epileptic seizures reflect synchronised bursts of firing affecting massive populations of neurones. These lie at the basis of the spike discharge seen in the EEG. Deafferented neurones fire continually in a paroxysmal manner and may recruit other partially deafferented cells depending on incidental traffic (Lockard & Ward, 1980), so that in some cases damaged nerve cells may lie at the heart of an epileptic focus. However, large scale paroxysmal discharges can also occur in the absence of epilepsy or brain damage, as Hughlings Jackson implied. For example, the Senegalese baboon *Papio papio* shows a convulsive EEG response to photic stimulation. This is maximal in females between 6 months and 4 years, and in those found in the dense forest of southwest Senegal, and much less common in those found in the north-eastern savannah where there is more exposure to direct sunlight. The age and gender distribution mirrors that of the photoconvulsive response in humans without epilepsy, and it has been suggested that the ability to generate these discharges plays a part in the maturation of the reproductive system via the effect of light on the pineal body, especially where natural sunlight is relatively low. The photoconvulsive response in humans is markedly increased in the Northern Hemisphere and is low in Africans in Nigeria (Danesi & Oni, 1983a; Danesi, 1988). Stevens (1986) suggests that the spike discharge conveys an imperative message that can override background nervous system noise. If this becomes excessively propagated, an epileptic seizure may occur.

Recent interest has focused on the role of amino-acid neurotransmitters in epilepsy, especially glutamate and other excitatory transmitters in the spread of epileptic discharges, and gamma-amino butyric acid (GABA) in inhibiting the spread. Excess extracellular glutamate can also damage neurones, an observation which stimulates debate regarding possible pathological sequelae of seizures (Manev *et al*, 1990; Concas *et al*, 1992; Dunn *et al*, 1992; Gale, 1992; Engelsen, 1992; Fisher *et al*, 1992; Joy *et al*, 1992; Nakanishi, 1992). A microdialysis study in humans with temporal lobe epilepsy suggested that focal seizures may be precipitated by a rise in extracellular glutamate, and that the concentrations reached may cause cell death, while GABA concentrations rise later, following the rise in glutamate (During & Spencer, 1993). This emerging neurochemical understanding of epilepsy has paralleled the development of new antiepileptic drugs which limit glutamate release or enhance the actions of GABA (Cheung *et al*, 1992; Benmenachem *et al*, 1993).

Epidemiological considerations

It is customary to consider that the occurrence of febrile convulsions or anoxic seizures do not necessarily indicate an epileptic condition. It is not clearly agreed whether seizures provoked by alcohol or drugs are included in the epidemiological definition of epilepsy. Although most would agree such events may not contribute to a clinical diagnosis, they may still be included in population studies, and it is difficult to define the cut-off clearly for research purposes. Isolated seizures without obvious provocation seem to be followed by other seizures in 30–70% of cases (Hopkins, 1987).

Incidence and prevalence in different cultures

The incidence of epilepsy is usually expressed as the number of cases per 100 000 of the population diagnosed per year, and prevalence as the number of people with epilepsy per 1000 of the population at any given time (Zielinski, 1988).

Case ascertainment for epidemiological research poses obvious difficulties. For example, incidence and prevalence rates based on perusal of medical records are usually lower than those obtained from field surveys (e.g. Stanhope *et al*, 1972) but are sometimes greater (e.g. Maremmani *et al*, 1991). One study from Australia showed that approximately one quarter of people known to have epilepsy denied this when completing a research questionnaire (Beran *et al*, 1985). Diagnosis is not always straightforward, and people with syncopal episodes or with non-epileptic seizures (pseudoseizures or hysterical seizures) may be inadvertently included. Criteria used for diagnosis in epidemiological studies vary and are not always clearly specified in reports. One African study used the following criteria (Osuntokun *et al*, 1987): a) if untreated, at least two afebrile seizures, at least one of which occurred within the last two years; b) if being treated for epilepsy, at least two afebrile seizures in the last five years, at least one of which occurred in the last three years; c) seizures used to fulfil the above criteria should not be related to any acute metabolic insult, such as alcohol consumption or withdrawal; d) at least one seizure must be observed by a reliable eyewitness. Other studies have used both more and less stringent criteria.

Despite these problems there are some findings which remain more or less constant. The incidence of epilepsy varies according to age. In North America it seems that between the ages of 20 and 60 the annual incidence is between 20 and 40 per 100 000 with a sharp rise either side of this age group, the greatest peak being in the first year of life. By the age of 80 the lifetime risk of having acquired a diagnosis of epilepsy is more than 3% (Hauser *et al*, 1983). A similar age distribution has been described in China (Li & Schoenberg, 1987). Most reports suggest that epilepsy is slightly more common in men than women, in both developing and Western countries. The reasons for this are not clear.

The prevalence of epilepsy varies from 6–8 cases per 1000 population in developed countries to between 10–20 per 1000 in developing countries (WHO, 1979; Placencia *et al*, 1992), though some areas seem to show very much higher rates. One Panamanian study (Gracia *et al*, 1990) found a prevalence of 57 per 1000 among Guaymi Indians living in banana plantations, the most important risk factor being a positive family history of epilepsy, and concluded that this high prevalence rate was probably an underestimate.

Nevertheless, when incidence and prevalence rates are taken together the evidence implies that epilepsy is a condition which in many, perhaps the majority of cases is short lived (Sander & Shorvon, 1987).

Classification

Approximately 40 different types of epileptic seizures are recognised. More than one seizure type may occur in the same patient. The classification of seizure types together with other clinical features constitutes a vocabulary which may be used to describe epileptic syndromes.

By international convention (Commission on Classification and Terminology of the International League Against Epilepsy, 1981), seizures are described in terms of clinical and EEG findings and are regarded as generalised, or partial (focal), though the classification also allows for a third category of unclassified seizures (Table 11.1).

TABLE 11.1
Classification of epileptic seizures

Partial (focal)
  Simple
    Motor
    Sensory
    Autonomic
    Psychic
  Complex
    Simple partial onset
    Consciousness impaired from onset
    Partial evolving to secondarily generalised

Generalised
  Absence
    Typical
    Atypical
  Myoclonic
  Tonic–clonic (grand mal)
  Atonic (drop attacks)

Unclassified

A short note on the EEG

Epilepsy is a clinical diagnosis. The EEG may have a role in defining seizure type and in syndrome diagnosis. Because the international classification is partly based on EEG findings it is appropriate to consider some EEG phenomena here. Although the availability of EEG technology may not yet be high in many developing countries, the technique is certainly used and is important. In epidemiological studies in Nigeria and Ethiopia, EEG has been of value in assigning subcategories of epilepsy (Osuntokun *et al*, 1987). A full account is obviously beyond the scope of this chapter, but the interested reader is referred to a textbook such as Hughes (1982).

The scalp EEG records fluctuations in potential difference which reflect summated synaptic potentials of underlying cortical cells. The rhythms seen are divided into four wavebands: *alpha* (8–13 Hz) is the normal background resting rhythm of the waking adult brain, usually maximal over the posterior region; *beta* (>13 Hz) occurs frontally and centrally in light sleep, in some waking adults who are tense or anxious, and in people taking some drugs such as barbiturates or benzodiazepines; *theta* (4–7 Hz) and *delta* (<4 Hz) are slower rhythms found in normal sleep but which may signify abnormality if found in waking adults. Abnormal slow waves are associated with damaged or malfunctioning nerve cells.

In a typical recording, electrodes are placed according to a convention called the '10–20 system' where each position is determined by taking the head circumference and nasion-inion length and measuring units of 10 or 20% of these. A recording is usually made with the subject resting with eyes open and then with eyes closed. Flashing light and overbreathing are used as activation techniques which may precipitate abnormal discharges in subjects so predisposed. The EEG taken between seizures may appear quite normal in a person with epilepsy, especially in partial epilepsy. However, certain types of abnormal discharge, referred to as epileptiform discharges, may occur which tend to be associated with epilepsy. These include the spike (a wave of duration 20–70 msecs with a pointed peak and a mainly negative component) and the spike-wave complex (a spike followed by a slow wave). A sharp wave is a pointed negative wave with a duration of 70–200 msecs and is less significant than a spike. Spikes occur in normal subjects under some conditions, and spike-wave complexes may be seen in the unaffected relatives of people with certain types of seizure disorders. Paroxysmal slow waves, such as runs of *theta*, may be associated with some epileptic phenomena. Epileptiform discharges may be focal or generalised, and this observation may assist in diagnosis.

Partial (focal) seizures

Partial seizures are defined as having an onset from a restricted area of one cerebral hemisphere, and tend to follow a stereotyped course in each patient. They are formally classified as simple or complex depending on whether consciousness is retained or lost. Both simple and complex partial seizures may become secondarily generalised. Unfortunately difficulties arise over the definition of consciousness, and this has provoked some debate which remains as yet unresolved. In any partial seizure impairment of consciousness increases with the degree of spread of the discharge. Any separation of this continuum into two categories is bound to be subjective. Also, some epileptologists contend that even the distinction between partial and generalised seizures is not as clear as it may seem (for a discussion of the issues see Parsonage, (1986, 1988)).

Simple partial seizures

These are usually brief, lasting under a minute and often only a few seconds. They may occur at the onset of secondary generalised seizures, or serve as a warning of the onset of a secondary generalised seizure, in which case the partial seizure is also referred to as an aura. They may be divided into motor, sensory, autonomic, and psychic.

Motor seizures. These arise from precentral cortex. Theoretically the precise area of cortex from which the seizure discharge commences should define the seizure phenomenology. For example, a seizure commencing in the motor strip of the precentral gyrus causes jerking in the appropriate contralateral part of the body. If this spreads to recruit adjacent parts of the cortex, the jerking spreads too, giving the classic Jacksonian march. The areas most commonly involved are those with the greatest cortical representation, the hand and the face. Spread is usually ipsilateral in the first instance. Partial motor seizures may very rarely occur continuously and this is referred to as epilepsia partialis continua or Kojewnikow's syndrome. Versive seizures involve turning the eyes and head to one side (often, but not exclusively, away from the side of the discharge), and they arise from the frontal cortex anterior to the precentral gyrus. In postural seizures arising from the supplementary motor area the hand may be raised as the head turns and a statuesque position may be adopted. Phonatory seizures may consist of either a forced vocalisation or of transient speech arrest. The vocalisation may be a simple sound or a complex stereotyped utterance (speech automatism). Transient speech arrest is a typical feature of dominant hemisphere seizures, while speech automatism is said to be more likely to occur with non-dominant temporal lobe lesions.

Sensory seizures arise from postcentral cortex. They include somatosensory experiences such as tingling sensations starting in one hand, often spreading in a Jacksonian sensory march, and also include sensations of bodily distortion and negative phenomena where a body part is sensed to be absent. Sensory seizures can also be accompanied by focal pain or burning sensations, which may arise subcortically. Visual seizures originating in the occipital region consist of transient scotomata or simple visual phenomena such as spots, flashes of light or colour, often confined to the appropriate half of the visual field. Temporal lobe seizures can cause stereotyped hallucinatory experiences in almost any sensory modality; brief olfactory and gustatory sensations, usually unpleasant, are very common, while some patients experience complex visual and/or auditory phenomena. That these phenomena can occur in seizures where the subject retains contact with what is going on serves to illustrate the difficulty in distinguishing 'simple' from 'complex' partial events. The stereotyped nature of these experiences means that the patient often becomes aware of their significance when they occur, which technically brings them into the category of 'pseudo-hallucinations'.

Autonomic seizures. One of the commonest partial seizure experiences is an unpleasant sensation in the abdomen which may rise towards the throat. This is the epigastric aura, and may be associated with other autonomic features such as sweating, tachycardia, and dilatation of the pupils. It characteristically occurs in temporal lobe epilepsy of limbic system origin. Such experiences may be accompanied by a feeling of fear, though whether this is due to the occurrence of the other autonomic sensations or whether the fearful sensation is a separate ictal phenomenon is not always clear.

Psychic seizures. Distortions of thought processes can occur as a consequence of seizure activity in the limbic system. Such activity tends to be associated with impairment of consciousness and therefore with complex partial events, and only occasionally occurs as an isolated simple partial seizure. The most well-known is an intense sensation of *déjà vu*, of having experienced the present moment before. *Déjà vu* is of course a normal phenomenon which occurs in a mild form without seizure manifestations in most people from time to time. However, in an intense, stereotyped repetitive form of sudden onset and cessation, it can represent an epileptic event. It is phenomenologically related to other experiences which may be ictal events, such as a sense of unfamiliarity in familiar surroundings (*jamais vu*). Forced thinking is the sudden intrusion of stereotyped thoughts, often words, phrases or snatches of poetry or literature, into the person's mind. Typically, the intrusion stops suddenly after a few seconds. Another of these phenomena is the sudden rapid recollection of past events, sometimes called panoramic vision.

Complex partial seizures

By definition consciousness is impaired in complex partial seizures (CPS). This may be so from the beginning of the seizure, but in some there is a simple partial onset followed by impairment of consciousness. CPS may consist of a period of blankness only, resembling an absence seizure (see below), except that they are often followed by a period of confusion. Often however they also contain a component of automatism.

An automatism may be defined as "a state of clouding of consciousness which occurs during or immediately after a seizure, during which the individual retains control of posture and muscle tone but performs simple or complex movements without being aware of what is happening. The impairment of awareness varies. A variety of initial phenomena before the interruption of consciousness and the onset of automatic behaviour may occur" (Fenton, 1972). Ictal automatisms are said to occur when there are bilateral discharges in amygdalal–hippocampal structures. It is customary to regard three stages: *initial*, e.g. lipsmacking; *mid-portion*, e.g. picking movements, fumbling with hands; and *terminal* where more semi-purposive acts may merge into normal activity. Most automatisms last less than five minutes. Figure 11.1 shows a series of events which may occur in a CPS. It is quite common for the terminal part of an automatism to include exiting behaviour, such as leaving through a door or climbing out of a window. The person is unlikely subsequently to recollect this behaviour.

Most CPS are considered to start in the temporal lobe. Temporal lobe seizures often show a mixture of 'simple' and 'complex' features. Extensive depth electrode

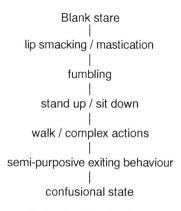

Blank stare
|
lip smacking / mastication
|
fumbling
|
stand up / sit down
|
walk / complex actions
|
semi-purposive exiting behaviour
|
confusional state

Fig. 11.1. Complex partial seizure.

recording studies by Weiser (1987) have shown four major types of temporal lobe seizure onset:

1) *Mesiobasal limbic seizures,* the commonest type, frequently associated with auras of *déjà vu,* epigastric sensations or memory flashbacks. If the seizure spreads bilaterally consciousness is lost and oro-alimentary automatisms may occur, with more complex automatisms sometimes occurring later. This seizure could terminate in a tonic–clonic event.
2) *Temporal polar seizures,* which are similar to mesiobasal seizures but autonomic changes and oro-alimentary automatisms are prominent and occur earlier.
3) *Opercular seizures* cause focal motor activity in the face and upper limbs with auditory hallucinations as the discharge spreads to Heschl's gyrus.
4) *Posterior temporal neocortical seizures,* which are associated with vestibular symptoms and complex visual hallucinations, usually with rapid spread to other regions.

Generalised seizures

Generalised seizures are those in which clinical and EEG evidence points to involvement of both cerebral hemispheres from the onset. They include absence seizures, myoclonic seizures, tonic–clonic (grand mal) seizures and atonic seizures (drop attacks).

Absences. These are episodes of loss of consciousness without loss of posture, and constitute an interruption in the usual flow of behaviour, of which the person may or may not be aware. 'Typical' or 'classical' absences are usually of short (a few seconds) duration, and in untreated cases occur many times per day. They are accompanied by a generalised and regular three per second spike-wave EEG discharge which starts suddenly and ceases abruptly. Typical absences probably represent a type of genetically acquired epileptic diathesis, and are not particularly associated with brain damage. 'Atypical absences' are associated with slower (c. 2–2.5/sec), irregular spike-wave EEG discharges, and usually signify an encephalopathic process or the presence of brain disease. They are usually of longer duration than typical absences, with a more gradual onset and resolution. There is sometimes partial awareness.

Myoclonic seizures. Single or multiple myoclonic jerks may be accompanied by a polyspike and wave or sometimes just spike-wave or sharp and slow wave EEG discharges. They occur in some childhood syndromes which reflect severe cerebral disturbance, but also in some more benign conditions.

Generalised tonic–clonic ('grand mal') seizures (GTCS). These consist of a period of muscle stiffening with loss of consciousness lasting a few seconds, the *tonic* phase, and a period of jerking which may last up to a few minutes, the *clonic* phase. The jerking subsides to leave the person unconscious with reduced muscle tone. Recovery may be rapid but often follows a period of post-ictal sleep and confusion. The seizure may be associated with incontinence of urine with or without incontinence of faeces, and tongue biting. This constitutes what most non-medical people would recognise as an epileptic seizure. During the clonic phase slow waves intrude in the EEG, representing periods of muscle relaxation between the periods of stiffening which are associated with faster, high amplitude discharges. One or other phase may clinically predominate, and hence the classification allows for tonic seizures and clonic seizures. GTCS seizures often represent secondarily generalised events from both simple and complex partial seizures.

Atonic seizures. These consist of a sudden loss of muscle tone and posture so that the person falls to the ground and then recovers very rapidly, and are also known as 'drop attacks'. They tend to be associated with polyspike and wave on the EEG. Clinically they must be distinguished from tonic seizures or certain myoclonic seizures which may cause someone to fall to the ground and get up again quickly.

Status epilepticus

Status epilepticus refers to a condition where a series of seizures occur without recovery in between. Mention has already been made of epilepsia partialis continua, which is rare. More common and significant are generalised convulsive and nonconvulsive status.

Generalised convulsive status. Continuous GTCS constitute a medical emergency. Brain damage may be likely to occur after an hour or more of continuous convulsions, while the average length of time in convulsive status of patients who die is about 13 hours (Swartz & Delgado-Escueta, 1987). Convulsive status epilepticus is commonly symptomatic of an underlying metabolic toxic or infective condition, and may therefore be seen in people without previously established epilepsy. In people with established and treated epilepsy it is unusual, but not unknown for the seizure disorder itself to be so unstable as to cause episodes of status without other obvious provocation. Intercurrent infection may precipitate status in some patients. One of the commonest causes in people with established epilepsy is abrupt withdrawal of anticonvulsant medication. The differential diagnosis includes non-epileptic seizure disorder (hysterical or pseudostatus epilepticus), which is discussed later.

Nonconvulsive status epilepticus. Continuous epileptic activity causing clinical changes but not continuous GTCS is often misdiagnosed as a behavioural or other psychiatric condition. There is a theoretical division into absence or complex partial status, although the distinction is not always totally clear clinically. Both these conditions are almost certainly underdiagnosed and much more common than is usually appreciated (Tomson *et al*, 1992; Cascino, 1993). Careful mental state examination will usually reveal obvious organic features if the patient is accessible enough. Psychotic features may appear, and the episode may conclude with a tonic–clonic seizure if not aborted pharmacologically. In absence status the patient will show clouding of consciousness which can vary in severity over a period of hours or even days. Clinical features vary from stupor to quite subtle changes in behaviour which can only be detected by people who know the patient well. It is usually seen in young patients with a history of generalised epilepsy, but cases have been described in middle-aged people with no previous seizure history (Ellis & Lee, 1978) where overt psychotic symptoms may be more prominent. Complex partial status is said to be characterised by repeated stereotyped episodes of behaviour occurring against a background confusional state. The stereotypies represent the automatism of the seizure, e.g. lip-smacking or fumbling movements. The patient may appear to be psychotic with or without clouding of consciousness and sometimes the repetitive nature of the behaviour only becomes apparent with careful observation. Nonconvulsive status epilepticus may occur in people with learning disability, where clouding of consciousness can be difficult to define in the presence of communication disorders (Brodtkorb *et al*, 1993; Staufenberg & Brown, 1994).

Clinical picture of epileptic syndromes and relationship to psychiatry

Epileptic syndromes

Clinical features that characteristically occur together constitute syndromes. The international classification (Commission on Classification and Terminology, International League against Epilepsy, 1985, 1989) divides epileptic syndromes into those with only generalised seizures and those with focal seizures, the latter being referred to as 'localisation-related' epilepsies. Both these groups are further subdivided into idiopathic, where there may be an underlying genetic predisposition but there is thought to be no other underlying cause; symptomatic, which are related to a central nervous system disorder; and cryptogenic, which are presumed to be symptomatic but the aetiology is still unknown. The classification of idiopathic and cryptogenic syndromes is age-related. Many epileptic syndromes have been recognised, and only a few of the more relevant ones can be further described here.

Localisation-related epilepsies

The most important of these are temporal lobe epilepsy and frontal lobe epilepsy, which are both symptomatic epilepsies. Mention should also be made of the idiopathic syndrome of benign childhood epilepsy with centrotemporal spikes.

Temporal lobe epilepsy. Up to 80% of CPS are of temporal lobe origin. Temporal lobe epilepsy is characterised by simple and/or complex partial seizures with or without secondary generalisation. The seizure types have been described above. The interictal scalp EEG may show no abnormality, or slight asymmetry of the background rhythms, or temporal epileptiform discharges. There is often a history of febrile convulsions in early childhood, and the patient may have a demonstrable discrete memory deficit.

Frontal lobe epilepsy. Simple and/or partial complex seizures with or without secondary generalisation are also features of frontal lobe epilepsy, and on occasions the distinction from temporal lobe epilepsy may be clinically unclear. Frontal lobe seizures may occur several times a day, and are often nocturnal. There is often a motor component, and focal features may be briefly present at the onset because rapid generalisation is common. They may be accompanied by rather strange automatisms and be misdiagnosed as non-epileptic (pseudo-) seizures. They may be brief, and secondary generalisation may be rapid. Some types of frontal lobe seizures were described above. Both generalised and partial status epilepticus are relatively common.

Benign childhood epilepsy with centrotemporal spikes. About one fifth of epilepsies occurring in children in developed countries fall into this category (Aicardi, 1986). There is a peak onset at about 10 years of age, and recovery usually occurs in the mid teens. Seizures are often mainly nocturnal and typically consist of partial hemifacial motor events which may evolve to GTCS. Despite the benign outcome there is a tendency to treat this syndrome. Most patients show no other clinical features, but some atypical cases have additional neurological abnormality, and detailed EEG analysis can differentiate the two groups by topographical analysis of the spike discharge (Wong *et al*, 1989).

Idiopathic generalised epilepsies

In these disorders the seizures are generalised from the onset. Associated neurological conditions or mental impairment are not characteristic features of these syndromes.

Childhood absence epilepsy (pyknolepsy) is characterised by typical absence seizures accompanied by generalised 3 Hz spike-wave on EEG. The peak age of onset is about seven years, with girls being more frequently affected than boys. There is often a family history of absence seizures. GTCS may occur at or after puberty, and the absences frequently remit by early adult life. This syndrome may be less common in Africa than in the West (Osuntokun *et al*, 1974).

Juvenile myoclonic epilepsy is a common cause of seizures presenting in adolescence. Myoclonic seizures tend to occur on awakening and may usher in GTCS. Classical absence seizures may also occur. This syndrome is similar to (and may not be clearly delineated from) *epilepsy with grand mal on awakening*, in which seizures mainly occur on or shortly after awakening as the name implies, but some may occur in the evening during a period of relaxation. Occasionally absence or myoclonic seizures may also occur. There may be a reflex element to seizure precipitation, such as sleep deprivation, and EEG often shows a positive photoconvulsive response. Some cases show a positive family history.

Cryptogenic or symptomatic generalised epilepsies

These may be associated with neurological or mental impairment.

West syndrome presents before the age of one year with psychomotor developmental arrest, infantile spasms (including so-called 'Salaam attacks'), which probably represent varieties of myoclonic jerks in this age group, and a characteristic EEG picture of high voltage irregular slow waves interspersed with spikes without constant synchrony, called hypsarrhythmia. In some cases (the symptomatic group) there is evidence of previous brain insult, while in others there is not (the cryptogenic group). West syndrome often leads on to a condition of severe developmental delay and learning difficulties, in which severe epilepsy may occur, such as the Lennox–Gastaut syndrome.

Lennox–Gastaut syndrome usually has its onset between the age of 1 to 5, though new cases may occur up to the age of 8 or 9. Tonic seizures affecting the axial muscles which especially occur during sleep, together with atonic seizures and atypical absences constitute the most characteristic seizure types, but myoclonic seizures, GTCS and even CPS may also occur (Beaumanoir, 1985). Nonconvulsive status epilepticus is common. The interictal EEG may show generalised slow spike-wave together with a number of other epileptiform features against a slowed background rhythm. In a number of cases the onset of epilepsy is preceded by a history of neurological illness, which has led to speculation of a viral or immune deficiency aetiology, but this has never been adequately shown. Many cases have a more obvious history of perinatal hypoxia or other cerebral insult, which is regarded as aetiological. Severe learning difficulties with progressive loss of intellectual skills is typical although a small number stay within the average range of ability. The seizures tend to persist into adult life but become less severe, while the learning and behavioural difficulties may become more significant.

Syndromes undetermined whether focal or generalised

Landau–Kleffner syndrome, also called *acquired epileptic aphasia* is a condition in which an acquired aphasia occurs in childhood with an EEG picture of multifocal spike and spike-wave discharges. Only about two-thirds of patients actually have clinical seizures, usually GTCS or focal motor, and these are infrequent. Loss of spontaneous speech occurs with verbal and auditory agnosia. There is often associated severe behaviour disorder or apparent psychosis. The seizures and EEG changes tend to remit before the age of 15.

Epilepsy with continuous spike-waves during slow-wave sleep, also sometimes known as Tassinari's syndrome (Tassinari *et al*, 1985; Yasuhara *et al*, 1991) is a rare but fascinating cause of intellectual and behavioural deterioration in children which may be completely unrecognised as an epileptic syndrome. A child of previously normal development may apparently become psychotic with the appearance of a mild or infrequent epilepsy. Only sleep EEG will show that almost the whole of slow-wave sleep is taken up by continuous spike-wave activity. This electrical status may last for years, but be only observable on the sleep EEG. The status tends to remit eventually, often with some recovery of function. Recognition of the underlying epilepsy may assist in choosing the appropriate treatment.

It has been observed that electrical status in sleep can occur as part of the picture of Landau–Kleffner syndrome, and the nosology of these two interesting, but fortunately uncommon, conditions remains undetermined (Genton *et al*, 1992; Paquier *et al*, 1992; Tassinari *et al*, 1992; Feekery *et al*, 1993).

Epilepsy and psychiatry

It is often stated that there is an increased rate of psychiatric disorder in people with epilepsy compared with the population as a whole. The evidence from this largely comes from studies of groups of patients with active or continuing epilepsy, and it has been pointed out that the high prevalence of psychiatric disorder might be partly accounted for by excluding patients whose epilepsy is in remission (Reynolds, 1989). Nevertheless, population studies in the United Kingdom have shown that nearly one-third of all identified patients with epilepsy have had a previous psychiatric referral (Pond & Bidwell, 1960; Edeh & Toone, 1987) while interview with a standard questionnaire increased the rate of 'caseness' to nearly one half (Edeh & Toone, 1987). It has been customary to classify the psychiatric disorders of epilepsy into three groups (Pond, 1957):

(1) *Those caused by the brain disease that also causes the fits.* Further consideration of this is beyond the scope of this chapter.
(2) *Those directly related to seizures.* These may be pre-ictal, ictal or post-ictal. A pre-ictal prodromal mood or behavioural change is very common, perhaps especially in partial epilepsy, and patients and their carers may be very aware of this. The mood change is usually depressive or irritable, and may last from a few minutes to a few days. It is usually terminated by a seizure, often generalised tonic–clonic in type, but may occasionally pass off without an obvious clinical event. Ictal events causing psychiatric symptoms have been mentioned above, and include the perceptual and affective changes during partial seizures, ictal automatisms, and nonconvulsive status. Post-ictal confusional states are extremely common and often strangely unrecognised; it may take from a few minutes to a few days to fully regain awareness, although the patient may superficially appear to have recovered. Prolonged post-ictal confusional states with wandering are sometimes called post-ictal fugues. In patients with focal epilepsy a discrete cognitive deficit may persist for several days after a seizure. The phenomenon of post-ictal psychosis is considered below with the other psychoses of epilepsy.
(3) *Those unrelated in time to seizure occurrence.* These include non-epileptic seizures (pseudoseizures), other neurotic conditions, the psychoses of epilepsy, and other personality and behavioural changes including the sexual disorders of epilepsy.

Repeated head injury due to seizures may also contribute to psychiatric morbidity, as may the effects of some antiepileptic drugs on mood and cognition.

Non-epileptic seizures

Up to 20% of patients referred to specialist epilepsy services in developing countries have seizures which are not epileptic, and this also represents a significant diagnostic and therapeutic problem in developing countries (Shorvon *et al*, 1991). These phenomena are variously referred to as pseudoseizures, psychogenic seizures, hystero-epilepsy or hysterical seizures. There is a current trend to use the terms 'non-epileptic seizures' (NES) or 'non-epileptic attack disorder' (NEAD), which are considered to be less judgemental (Betts, 1990). It is usually stated that NES are very unlikely to occur in people who have not experienced true epilepsy (Lesser, 1985; Fenwick, 1987*a*). In one recent study nearly 40% of admissions to a specialist epilepsy unit had NES, and of these about half also had a proven diagnosis of true epilepsy (McDade & Brown, 1990). There has been a tendency to regard these as hysterical conversion phenomena. Certainly it is fruitful to remember that these attacks are real to the patient, and there is absolutely no point in making accusations of malingering, although this happens all too often in some primary care facilities. In Britain a significant number of cases of status epilepticus admitted to hospital are actually pseudo-status epilepticus (Howell *et al*, 1989), and the patient may suffer iatrogenic damage from overzealous treatment (Anonymous, 1989).

The clinical distinction from true epilepsy may not always be obvious. NES do not occur when the patient is truly asleep, and do not often occur when the patient is alone. It is often stated that injury is uncommon, but since injuries can occur during NES this is not always a useful observation. Conscious malingering is actually quite rare, but some people who do malinger may present with self-inflicted burns or abrasions which they claim to be the result of seizures unobserved by others. The patient's movements during NES may be obviously unusual for a true epileptic seizure, with varying amplitude and frequency of clonic movements. Back arching is probably more common in NES but can also occur in true epilepsy. Pelvic thrusting is particularly more likely to occur in NES, but may form part of the automatism associated with a complex partial seizure. In patients who have a history of true epilepsy the NES may mimic the initial phase of the person's true seizure experience.

During a non-epileptic seizure neurological reflexes should be unaltered; plantar responses will therefore be downward (if that is the patient's usual condition), and conjunctival reflexes will be normal. In fact, attempts to examine the pupils or conjunctivae may be met with resistance by screwing up the eyes. During true major epileptic seizures the plantar response tends to become upward, the conjunctival reflex is lost, and it is usually possible for the examiner to open the patient's eyelids. During post-ictal sleep after a true seizure, raising the patient's arm above the face and letting go will result in the arm falling onto the face, whereas after NES this manoeuvre nearly always results in the arm falling away from the patient's face.

It might be thought that an ictal EEG recording would assist diagnosis, and although this may be true, the EEG needs to be interpreted skilfully. Muscle jerking in NES may cause artefacts which can look surprisingly 'epileptiform' while some true simple partial seizures may have little or no scalp EEG accompaniment. Simultaneous video-EEG is helpful in some cases, but also needs skilled interpretation for the same reasons, and of course it is an investigation unlikely to be available in everyday practice. True epileptic seizures often commence with an abrupt tachycardia, while NES may show a preceding build-up of heart rate over a period of time.

True GTCS are associated with a rise in plasma prolactin, which peaks about 20 minutes after the onset of the fit, usually reaching a level of greater than 800 IU/ml. A less spectacular, but significant, peak is often seen after complex partial seizures where the majority show a rise to above 500 IU/ml (Dana-Haeri *et al*, 1983). If the pituitary stores are depleted by frequent true seizures, the rise is less marked or absent. It is important to compare with a baseline measure to confirm a genuine increase above that person's normal level.

Betts (1990) has proposed a useful working classification of non-epileptic seizures. Non-organic seizures are divided into those which represent psychiatric disorders that have been mistaken for epilepsy (panic attacks, hyperventilation, anxiety with depersonalisation phenomena, episodic dyscontrol syndrome), and emotionally-based attacks, which he further classifies as 'swoons' (cut-off behaviour), 'tantrums' (immature displays of emotion), 'abreaction' (symbolic attacks) and deliberate simulation. In one type of abreactive attack seen in women the convulsions may consist of back arching and pelvic thrusting, which is said to suggest a history of sexual abuse.

In some patients with NES it is difficult to establish any more formal psychiatric diagnosis. However, attention should be paid to the possible presence of affective disorder (Roy, 1977). There may sometimes be a history of sexual abuse. The presence of the hysterical personality is not necessary for NES to occur. In some cases NES may represent a form of learned behaviour and become manifest when the true epileptic seizures are successfully treated.

Patients with NES seen in specialist units have often had some kind of confrontational experience with the medical profession regarding diagnosis before, and this has often been non-therapeutic. On the other hand an honest factual explanation delivered after a good therapeutic alliance has been established has a high rate of success (McDade & Brown, 1990). It is important never to be accusatory, to acknowledge that the patient's seizures are very real to the patient, and to emphasise an expectation of good outcome. Appropriate psychotherapeutic support needs to be offered if the patient wishes it, and of course coexisting psychiatric illness must be properly treated.

Depression and epilepsy

In Western countries a diagnosis of epilepsy is associated with a substantially increased risk of deliberate self-harm and at least five times the rate of suicide compared to the general population. In temporal lobe epilepsy the suicide risk appears to rise to 25 times the expected rate (MacKay, 1979; Barraclough, 1981; Robertson & Trimble, 1983).

Although social factors undoubtedly play a part, the increase in temporal lobe epilepsy does raise the intriguing possibility of a biological disposition to affective disorder. Higher rates of depression than expected have been reported in patients with temporal lobe epilepsy (Rodin *et al*, 1965; Dikman *et al*, 1983). Most often, depressive illness is said to be associated with a decrease in seizure frequency (displaying the same relationship that is exploited in electroconvulsive therapy), but it may also occur in the context of deterioration in seizure control, the reasons for these two courses being unclear (Flor-Henry, 1969; Betts, 1988). There are generally no special features which distinguish depression occurring in epilepsy from that occurring in the absence of epilepsy, although Betts (1981) has reported that the mood state may show a relatively abrupt onset and fluctuation.

Psychoses of epilepsy

Episodic or intermittent psychoses. Mention has already been made of absence and complex partial status, and of ictal automatisms. In *post-ictal psychosis* (Logsdail & Toone, 1988) a cluster of seizures may be followed by apparently normal recovery, after which there is an abrupt onset within one week of a florid psychotic state, in which visual and auditory hallucinations, paranoid delusions and marked mood disorder may occur. The seizures are usually tonic–clonic but the patient typically has a localisation-related epilepsy, and cases have been described following complex partial seizures (Barczak *et al*, 1988). Disorientation may be present, but the abnormal phenomena can occur in clear consciousness. The clinical picture may resemble schizophrenia, mixed affective psychosis, mania or paranoid psychosis. The psychosis tends to settle over a few days but may last up to three months. The seizure recovery phase may merge directly into the psychotic stage without a clinically obvious latent interval. Post-ictal psychosis is said to be more common in men, and seems to be more likely to occur in patients with localisation-related epilepsies. A family history of functional psychosis tends to be absent. However, at least some of these patients eventually go on to develop chronic interictal psychoses. Post-ictal *twilight states* are acute confusional states marked by psychomotor retardation, hallucinations and disorientation which settle over hours or days and probably represent a continuation of epileptic activity causing abnormalities of subjective experience (Lishman, 1987).

Chronic psychoses. It is generally accepted from a number of lines of evidence that a chronic interictal psychosis occurs more commonly in association with epilepsy than would be expected by chance. This seems to be particularly related to temporal lobe epilepsy, and may be related to a dominant hemisphere focus. The psychosis usually appears some years after the onset of seizures. The picture is generally that of a schizophrenia-like illness, with an insidious onset of delusions which may have a religious or mystical content. Visual and auditory hallucinations may occur, along with passivity phenomena and thought disorder. Catatonic phenomena, however, seem to be infrequent. Despite earlier reports that the personality might be better preserved in this condition than in schizophrenia (Slater *et al*, 1963), recent work suggests that there is no consistent phenomenological difference (Toone *et al*, 1981; Perez *et al*, 1985). Reviews of current concepts are given by Toone (1991) and Trimble (1991).

Behavioural and personality disorders

It has been postulated that episodic disorders of behaviour can arise from paroxysmal subcortical EEG discharges (Monroe, 1970), although whether these discharges are a cause or a consequence of the behavioural change is not clear. One study of adults who demonstrated episodic dyscontrol showed that 30% had a history of complex partial seizures (Elliot, 1982). Since epilepsy may be associated with brain damage, behavioural disorders may occur which are related to the brain damage itself rather than to the epilepsy.

Damage to the orbitofrontal region of the frontal lobe is associated with disinhibited impulsive behaviour, the so-called 'pseudopsychopathic syndrome', in which cognitive impairment may not be a feature, while a more extensive lesion involving the dorsolateral frontal lobe may produce profound slowing of thought and action with difficulty in initiating intentional action, distinguished from retarded depressive illness only by the lack of the characteristic mood change, the 'pseudodepressed syndrome'. Both syndromes may coexist.

There has been a great deal of speculation about the effects of temporal lobe dysfunction on personality and behaviour, in particular the inter-ictal personality characteristics found in temporal lobe epilepsy. Some authors refer to a syndrome of personality change caused by excessive discharges in the limbic system, the 'temporo-limbic syndrome' (Bear & Fedio, 1977; Brown, 1982; Roberts, 1984), which contains most of the elements of the 'epileptic personality' described by 19th and early 20th century authors, such as emotional lability, hyposexuality and a tendency to adhere to each thought feeling and action, so-called 'thought viscosity'. The latter would obviously affect cognitive processes. Unfortunately it is not easy to tease out the relative contributions of seizures, subclinical seizure discharges or associated brain damage from the psychosocial effects of a seizure disorder, and of course all these factors may interact with chronic anticonvulsant effects.

Epileptic dementia

Epilepsy is often included in lists of possible causes of dementia shown in textbooks, though little is written about the precise nature of such associated chronic cognitive deterioration.

Patients with frequent generalised seizures, or with some types of partial seizures may fall on their heads. The orbitofrontal region and temporal lobes are especially vulnerable to closed head injury, and it is well-recognised that damage here may lead to subtle personality and attentional difficulties. Head injury in children may lead to subtle cognitive deficits which may persist after other neurological sequelae have disappeared so that the origin of the cognitive deficit may be unclear to later observers (Solomons *et al*, 1963; Chadwick *et al*, 1981). It is not absolutely clear whether this could also be the case in adults, although there is some evidence that recovery of function is less complete in adults than in children (Mahoney *et al*, 1983). Repeated head trauma can lead to a dementia-like syndrome with dysarthria, ataxia, concreteness of thinking, circumlocution and memory problems.

Cognitive impairment may also be related to drugs. Many studies have been carried out using sophisticated computerised cognitive testing, with serum level monitoring, of both normal volunteers and patients with epilepsy on single drug therapy and before and after reduction of polypharmacy (e.g. Thompson *et al*, 1981; Thompson & Trimble, 1981, 1982, 1983; Tomlinson *et al*, 1982; Andrewes *et al*,

1984). There is an overwhelming consensus that polytherapy is associated with greater cognitive impairment than monotherapy, and that phenytoin is associated with greater cognitive impairment than carbamazepine. This should be borne in mind when choosing treatment in a newly diagnosed patient.

Finally, recent evidence suggests that a small number of people with temporal lobe epilepsy may develop a behavioural change at or after puberty with or without aggression and paranoid ideation, which either continues as a condition with features of the temporo-limbic syndrome, paranoid ideation and a moderate loss of learning ability, or develops into a picture with more marked clinical frontal lobe impairment such as slowness and perseveration, in which the paranoid ideation ceases to be obvious. The clinical features may by this stage include the appearance of sequelae of repeated head injury, but these cannot explain the total picture (Brown & Vaughan 1988, 1990; Brown, 1989).

Sexual dysfunction

Many patients with epilepsy suffer a decline in libido, and in some impotence has been described (Gastaut & Collomb, 1954; Hierons & Saunders, 1966; Taylor, 1969). This may be related to social isolation, low self-esteem and the fear of sexual behaviour causing a seizure, but the rather higher rate of dysfunction found in temporal lobe epilepsy suggests a link with the temporo-limbic syndrome. There have also been observations of lowered free testosterone levels in men taking anticonvulsants (Toone *et al*, 1983), and this may be related to a direct effect on the testes.

One recent Egyptian study (Demerdash *et al*, 1991) specifically addressed the issue of sexual dysfunction in women. Nearly one-fifth of an out-patient population had psychosexual disorders (CPS). CPS were more common than expected in the sample. There was a predominance of sexually coloured prodromata of seizures, and menstrual problems were over-represented. The most frequent disorders were hyposexuality and exhibitionism.

Differential diagnosis

Epilepsy has to be differentiated from any other cause of transient impairment of consciousness or transient behavioural change (Table 11.2). Some of these are discussed below.

Syncope

Straightforward fainting attacks can be distinguished from epilepsy by their precipitants (standing around, pain, heat), by their slow and gradual onset and especially 'seeing stars' or greying out of vision before consciousness is lost. There may be a brief clonic convulsion at the depth of a syncopal attack. Lombroso & Lerman (1967) first drew attention to the cyanotic and pallid subtypes of breath-holding attacks in children aged between 18–24 months. The *cyanotic* type is the result of a valsalva manoeuvre, often induced by emotion. Brief clonic jerkings

TABLE 11.2
Some non-epileptic paroxysmal disorders

Syncope
  Fainting
  Pallid and cyanotic breath-holding attacks
  Cough and micturition syncope
  Cardiac (Ward–Romano syndrome, ischaemic and rheumatic heart
    disease, aortic stenosis, cardiomyopathies)
Migraine
Transient ischaemic attacks
Transient global amnesia
Sleep disorders
  Narcolepsy
  Night terrors
Hypoglycaemia
Dystonic reactions
Menière's disease

may occur. The *pallid* attack is due to vagally mediated cardiac asystole and may follow an unexpected stimulus, including a blow to the head. If asystole is prolonged this may provoke a generalised tonic–clonic seizure, though this is rare. Other reflex phenomena which may be confused with epilepsy include cough and micturition syncope.

Both tachycardias and bradycardias may cause syncopal events. These may be a result of rheumatic heart disease, which is common in many parts of the world. The Ward–Romano syndrome is an hereditary prolongation of the Q-T interval of the electrocardiogram, and can present with symptoms resembling epilepsy. Appropriate treatment of the dysrrhythmia can prevent sudden death (Gospe & Choy, 1989).

Migraine

Headaches in epilepsy tend to be bilateral and post-ictal. The visual phenomena of some epileptic auras are very short-lived and well-formed. Focal epileptic symptoms spread rapidly but tend to remain bilateral if consciousness is retained. Epileptic events as a whole are short-lived. Classical migraine attacks on the other hand consist of a throbbing unilateral headache which occurs during, not after the event (though the headache of common migraine is bilateral). Visual phenomena are disorganised and of longer duration. Focal symptoms such as paraesthesiae spread slowly and may be bilateral. Migraine attacks generally last longer than epileptic seizures.

Basilar migraine may present with episodes of transient bilateral visual disturbance with cerebellar or brainstem symptoms such as dysarthria and ataxia, leading to loss of consciousness followed by occipital headache, and needs to be carefully distinguished from partial epilepsy.

Both epilepsy and migraine are common conditions, so they often coexist. In patients with both conditions, the two types of phenomena need to be distinguished from each other when assessing the results of therapy.

Transient ischaemic attacks (TIAs)

TIAs in carotid artery territory may present in a number of ways with transient phenomena including blindness or homonymous hemianopia, aphasia, unilateral paraesthesiae and paresis. The aphasic presentation may be particularly difficult to distinguish from epilepsy. TIAs never involve a march of symptoms, and tend to be shorter lived than epileptic events.

Transient global amnesia is now regarded as a consequence of temporary ischaemia in limbic structures. An attack consists of disorientation and perplexity with perseverative behaviour due to the sudden marked short-term memory deficit. There is a gradual return to normal memory function with persistent amnesia for the attack. Most patients seem to have only one attack, though a few cases with two or more episodes have been described (e.g. Lou, 1968).

Sleep disorders

These include night terrors in children, and narcolepsy. In *night terrors* a sleeping child may suddenly utter a cry, sit up and appear frightened. If awoken the child is confused, and the next day is amnesic for the event. The events occur during deeper stages of slow-wave sleep, and are therefore different to nightmares which occur during rapid eye movement (REM) sleep. Night terrors are benign phenomena.

Narcolepsy is a sleep disorder with four main symptoms, by no means all of which occur in all patients. These are: a) sudden attacks of daytime sleepiness; b) cataplexy (sudden loss of muscle tone and inability to move provoked by emotion, such as laughter); c) sleep paralysis, a temporary inability to move on waking up from sleep while retaining awareness; and d) hypnogogic hallucinations, which may be extremely vivid and resemble some states associated with temporal lobe epilepsy. Diagnostic uncertainty may occur in some cases where cataplexy occurs without the other features, but the retention of consciousness throughout the attack will suggest a non-epileptic cause. In all narcoleptic phenomena there is no post-event confusion.

Other causes

Hypoglycaemia severe enough to cause changes in consciousness is most likely to be seen in patients with insulinoma or in insulin-dependent diabetics, or in alcoholics after a heavy drinking bout. Alterations in consciousness and confusion may occur, and in some cases tonic–clonic seizures may be provoked. 'Reactive hypoglycaemia' may be a cause of alterations in consciousness, palpitations and mood swings following ingestion of carbohydrate, and could possibly be confused with partial epilepsy.

Dystonic reactions caused by phenothiazines have been mistaken for seizure phenomena as they cause paroxysmal episodes of muscle stiffening. Consciousness is usually retained through these episodes.

Menière's disease causes attacks of severe vertigo which might be confused with partial seizures. Epileptic events of this nature are short-lived and of rapid onset and resolution. The vertigo of Menière's disease almost always occurs against a history of tinnitus and progressive hearing impairment, and the attacks may last for hours.

Aetiology

The synchronised discharges of epilepsy represent part of the available repertoire of behaviour of neural tissue under certain circumstances. The ability to have seizures is present in all people. Aetiological factors in epilepsy are reasons why seizures may occur at inappropriate or inconvenient times. The seizure threshold may be lowered by genetic predisposition, by certain intercurrent toxic infective or metabolic conditions, or may be a consequence of a specific lesion in the brain or may follow head injury. Epilepsy therefore has a firm pathophysiological basis. However, social and psychological factors, as well as biological influences, may play a part in its course and prognosis. Consideration of aetiology may direct efforts to finding a treatable cause.

A list of some aetiological factors for seizures is given in Table 11.3. Certain important ones are briefly discussed below.

Febrile convulsions have a peak onset between 9–18 months of age and are extremely common. The convulsions, if prolonged, can cause mesial temporal lobe damage with cell loss and sclerosis. This may form a focus for the possible development of temporal lobe epilepsy later in life (Sagar & Oxbury, 1987).

Space occupying lesions such as intracranial tumours which give rise to epilepsy tend not to be rapidly growing. A slow growing glioma may not be easy to differentiate histologically from a hamartoma. Intracranial abscess, especially frontal, has a high likelihood of causing seizures. Subdural haematoma may cause seizures in association with clouding of consciousness; the original head trauma however may have been unobserved.

Infections. Neurosyphilis can cause seizures, psychosis and dementia, as can chronic tuberculous meningitis. Tuberculous granuloma may be an important cause of seizures in some developing countries (e.g. Yaqub *et al*, 1987). Seizures may occur as part of the acute presentation of bacterial meningitis. Viral encephalitis (e.g. herpes simplex) causes seizures in the acute phase, and may be an important cause of chronic epilepsy with learning difficulties. Congenital toxoplasmosis causes epilepsy in association with severe learning difficulties, upper motor neurone lesions and often microcephaly or hydrocephalus. Patients with seizures due to cysticercosis often have intracranial calcification with parenchymal cysts. Acute cerebral malaria may be associated with convulsions as coma and hyperpyrexia develop, but seizures are not a feature of the chronic illness. A thorough review of epilepsy and central nervous system parasitosis is given by Bittencourt *et al* (1988).

TABLE 11.3
Aetiological factors in epilepsy

Febrile convulsions and mesial temporal sclerosis

Infections

  Meningitis, especially tuberculous, but also including
    H. influenzae, Pneumococcus, Meningococcus
  Tuberculous granuloma
  Herpes simplex encephalitis
  Toxoplasmosis
  Neurosyphilis
  Cerebral cysticercosis
  Note possible predisposition by HIV

Progressive focal encephalitis
Head injury, especially if dura is penetrated

Space occupying lesions
  Intracranial tumour
  Hamartoma
  Intracranial abscess, especially frontal
  Angioma
  Chronic subdural haematoma

Congenital abnormalities (e.g. cerebral palsy)
  Storage disorders
  Leukodystrophies
  Tuberose sclerosis
  Neurofibromatosis
  Pick's disease
  Alzheimer's disease
  Creutzfeldt–Jakob disease
  Cerebral atheroma
  Hypertensive encephalopathy
  Cerebral lupus erythematosis

It should be remembered that infection with human immunodeficiency virus (HIV), besides sometimes causing a progressive subacute encephalopathy in its own right, can also predispose to neoplasms, to viral and bacterial meningitides, including tuberculous infection, and may even provoke a more aggressive course for neurosyphilis (Johns *et al*, 1987).

Assessment and treatment of an acute episode

Initial assessment

The occurrence of a seizure may cause great distress to the patient and the family, perhaps fearing some inappropriate association such as madness, possession, contagion or approaching death. There may therefore be a tendency to deny the existence of the symptom, or else to make the initial presentation to a traditional healer. All this should be borne in mind by the doctor, nurse or village health worker who first comes into contact with the family. The process of history taking and indeed the whole conduct of the initial consultation should be regarded as an important part of the treatment, with the opportunity to explain, comfort and reassure. This may be very difficult. Osuntokun (1979) has drawn attention to the initial history being 'not infrequently unhelpful and distorted by cultural taboos and by disregard and contempt for details and temporal sequence'.

History and examination

Since people with epilepsy are often unconscious during their seizures, an accurate eye-witness account is vital. The history taker will seek to define the precise events associated with the first seizure, the frequency of subsequent seizures, and the number of seizure types that the patient has experienced. Careful attention should be paid to possible precipitants such as alcohol or other drugs, recent head injury, etc. The time of day and relationship to eating should be noted. The patient will explain if there was any subjective aura, but observers may have noted a pre-ictal behavioural change of which the patient was unaware, but which might be useful in predicting further episodes. A careful note should be made of the quality and speed of recovery after the seizure. Physical examination, including the central nervous system should be carried out with special regard for identifiable and treatable aetiological factors.

The diagnosis of epilepsy with GTCS is usually fairly straightforward as witnesses will describe the person going stiff, falling to the ground, shaking all four limbs and convulsing, with or without tongue biting and incontinence of urine. Occasionally nocturnal seizures may only present as nocturnal enuresis, or the person may feel exceptionally exhausted in the morning and wake with a sore tongue, but often someone will have overheard the seizure. More difficulty may be found with other seizure types; absences in children may be regarded as daydreaming, and the subsequent inattention attributed to laziness or wilful misbehaviour, and the organic nature of complex partial seizures may not be obvious.

Investigations

Since epilepsy is a clinical diagnosis, the most important investigation is the history. Physical examination and mental state assessment may reveal potential causes of seizures, such as intercurrent infection, trauma or substance abuse. Other investigations will be appropriately directed to the various treatable aetiological factors, such as tuberculosis, but these will not be further considered here. A single seizure occurring in an otherwise healthy person would merit enquiry into precipitating factors, such as sleep deprivation or heavy alcohol intake, but need not lead to further investigation unless a second episode occurs. After a second episode, the EEG, where available, has a role in differentiating localisation, related from generalised epileptic syndromes, as this may have treatment consequences as well as point to aetiology. However, an EEG needs to be appropriately requested, carried out, and reported, to be meaningful.

Treatment

It goes without saying that where a treatable underlying cause for an isolated seizure is found, this should be appropriately addressed. Most epileptologists would agree that specific anti-epileptic treatment should be recommended if someone has had two unprovoked seizures in one year, or one episode of status epilepticus. The mainstays of initial treatment are drugs and appropriate social support.

Drugs in initial treatment

Rational prescribing in developing countries has been a matter of intense debate (Richards, 1986; Shorvon, 1986), where clinical effectiveness, safety and lack of side-effects for any agent have to be balanced against cost and availability. The World Health Organization (WHO, 1989) has produced a list of essential drugs in epilepsy which goes some way to acknowledging these problems. It is recommended that initial treatment should always be with a single drug. The importance of continuing with medication even though seizures may have ceased should be emphasised, and account taken of the continuity of drug supplies. The general principle is to start with a small dose and gradually increase (usually at not more than two-weekly intervals) until seizures stop or signs of dose-related toxicity such as ataxia, appear. If a drug is ineffective and a second agent is added which proves effective, the first drug should be slowly withdrawn. Generally anticonvulsants should never be abruptly withdrawn, as this precipitates withdrawal seizures or status epilepticus. This effect is especially notable with phenobarbitone. A list of WHO essential drugs, with indications, typical doses and side-effects is given in Table 11.4. It is possible to manage epilepsy effectively without recourse to frequent serum drug level monitoring provided these principles are followed. However, the pharmacokinetics of phenytoin in particular are such that small dose increments can make large changes to the serum level, causing toxicity, and for this reason serum level monitoring may be helpful. This is less true of carbamazepine, but access to serum monitoring can be helpful, while monitoring of sodium valproate is largely unnecessary. To assist compliance, a once or twice daily medication regime should be used. Compliance aids, such as boxes for pills divided into sections for different doses, may be helpful.

Long-term treatment needs and rehabilitation

Management of chronic epilepsy

Reynolds (1989) argues that epilepsy should be viewed as a process which is influenced by the promptness of appropriate treatment, and which may otherwise become more difficult to control. Where seizures continue in the face of monotherapy with the correct dose of the correct drug, a reappraisal of the diagnosis should be sought, in particular the emergence of non-epileptic seizures or a misclassification of seizure type may have occurred, leading to apparent treatment failure. Focal seizures related to a structural brain lesion

TABLE 11.4
Antiepileptic drugs (after WHO, 1989)

Drug	Seizure type(s)	Typical dose range	Side-effects
Carbamazepine	Partial seizures, including those with secondary generalisation	Begin at 50–100 mg twice daily. Maintenance range usually 800–1200 mg/day (adults) or 10–20 mg/kg/day (children)	About 4% show allergic rash. Dose related diplopia, ataxia, dryness of mouth. Neutropenia may occur
Diazepam	Given intravenously or rectally for convulsive and nonconvulsive status epilepticus and serial seizures	10–20 mg as single dose	Respiratory depression rarely significant unless pre-existing pulmonary problem
Ethosuximide	Typical (classical) absences	Begin at 250 mg twice daily. Maintenance dose usually 20–30 mg/kg/day	Gastro-intestinal disturbances. Rarely may precipitate psychotic state
Phenobarbitone	As carbamazepine	2 mg/kg/day up to a maximum of 6 mg/kg/day in one or two doses	Sedation, memory problems, may precipitate hyperactivity in children, contra-indicated in acute intermittent porphyria
Phenytoin	As carbamazepine	Begin at 4–5 mg/kg/day, increase by 25 mg steps up to a maximum of 8 mg/kg/day	Dose related; diplopia, ataxia, sedation, confusion. Chronic effects may include gum hyperplasia, acne, hirsutes, osteomalacia/rickets
Valproic acid (also supplied as sodium valproate)	Generalised seizures, including absences akinetic and tonic–clonic. Also active against partial seizures	15 mg/kg/day up to a maximum of 30 mg/kg/day	Weight gain, alopecia. Interacts with phenobarbitone (raising phenobarbitone levels)

may be particularly difficult to control. Treatments for refractory epilepsy may include further drug manipulations, dietary approaches, psychological treatments, and surgery.

Drugs

If seizures persist despite appropriate investigations and treatment as outlined in the previous section, the following options are available.

Change of main drug. An alternative major anticonvulsant may be introduced, for example sodium valproate in place of carbamazepine. It is recommended that the new agent is added to the first and gradually built up into the normal dose range and its efficacy assessed. If it is successful, the first anticonvulsant could be withdrawn; if it does not work, the new drug should be withdrawn. Pharmacokinetic changes during withdrawal are usually settled within a week of stopping an agent, with the exception of phenobarbitone (Duncan *et al*, 1991). Generally sodium valproate can be withdrawn fairly quickly from a regime, phenytoin and carbamazepine less so and phenobarbitone should be withdrawn very slowly (e.g. 15 mg per month). The risk is of withdrawal seizures. Where an increase in seizure frequency occurs after withdrawal, this may take several weeks to settle. Change of main drug is also an option where unacceptable side-effects occur with the first treatment.

Adjunctive treatments. If seizures continue at an unacceptable rate, some degree of improvement may be gained by using an additional drug which would not usually be given as monotherapy. Adjunctive treatments include acetozolamide and clobazam. Both are associated with the development of tolerance, and clobazam is expensive. Acetozolamide is a carbonic anhydrase inhibitor. A typical adult dose is 250 mg twice daily. Some patients with very frequent partial seizures show a dramatic decrease if this is added but the effect frequently wears off after a few weeks. Occasionally, a persistent remission is obtained. Clobazam, a 1,5-benzodiazepine, has been shown to be a highly successful adjunctive agent in an adult dose of 20–40 mg/day (Callaghan & Goggin, 1989). Side-effects are uncommon. Tolerance may develop after weeks or months, with breakthrough of seizures. With both clobazam and acetozolamide, tolerance may be reversed if the drug is tailed off and temporarily discontinued, with a further period of remission after reintroduction. Some patients may benefit from taking intermittent courses of adjunctive therapy, knowing that during these periods there will be relief from seizures, while understanding that during the period off the adjunct, seizures will return. Clonazepam, a 1,4-benzodiazepine, is a more sedative alternative to clobazam, which is occasionally used as monotherapy. Its side-effect profile would not recommend it as a first line agent. Epilepsy with perimenstrual exacerbation (catamenial epilepsy), may respond to adjunctive clobazam taken only during the few days when seizure could be predicted to be likely to occur. There may also be a response to using didrogesterone, or progesterone pessaries, or pyridoxine in low doses, for one week premenstrually besides continual main drug treatment.

Drug holiday. Occasionally lack of response to treatment with or without unacceptable side-effects leads to consideration of not using drugs at all, or at least of having periods without treatment. This should be considered as an option which, if handled correctly, carries relatively few increased risks over continuing with drugs. The main problem is an increase in seizure frequency and the risk of precipitating status during and after withdrawal. These factors need to be discussed with the patient so that an informed decision can be made. Sometimes patients are no better off with regard to their seizures, but feel better for not having drug side-effects.

New drugs. At the time of writing four new drugs have been licensed in some European countries for epilepsy (vigabatrin, oxcarbazepine, lamotrigine and gabapentin), and several others are under investigation. As time passes these are likely to become relevant in developing countries. *Vigabatrin* seems particularly useful in partial seizures but there have been reports of it causing psychosis, which must make it a second-line treatment for the time being. *Oxcarbazepine* is chemically related to carbamazepine, but seems to have fewer side-effects and is less likely to precipitate an allergic reaction. *Lamotrigine* is effective against both partial and generalised seizures, and may play a part in treating refractory atonic seizures and atypical absences, as in

Lennox–Gastaut syndrome. It has a rate of allergy probably comparable with carbamazepine, though this may be reduced by using a slowly escalating dose regime. Concomitant valproate inhibits the excretion of lamotrigine, which therefore requires a much lower dose regime, while enzyme inducers such as phenytoin and carbamazepine effectively lower lamotrigine levels, requiring a higher dose regime. *Gabapentin* seems most effective against partial onset seizures, and is well tolerated and doesn't interact with other antiepileptic drugs.

Figure 11.2 shows a flow sheet with a treatment strategy for partial seizures which fail to respond to first-line treatment with valproate.

Diet

In some children, and to a lesser extent some adults, a degree of remission of seizures may be obtained if the diet contains a very high proportion of lipid which induces ketosis, the ketogenic diet. This may be achieved with expensive and unpalatable long chain fats taking up to 80% of the diet, or by a modification

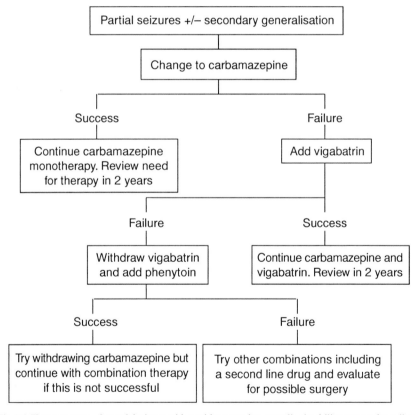

Fig. 11.2. Treatment strategy for partial seizures with or without secondary generalisation failing to respond to sodium valproate.

using medium chain triglycerides in a special oil together with 30% dietary long chain fats (Schwartz *et al*, 1983). Most patients find the regime unpleasant, and remissions are often only temporary, but the technique is still sometimes useful.

Surgery

Intractable temporal lobe epilepsy arising from one damaged hippocampus may be susceptible to temporal lobectomy, or to the more recently introduced selective amygdalohippocampectomy. Atonic seizures unresponsive to medical treatment may be greatly modified by partial section of the corpus callosum. Intractable seizures arising from one damaged hemisphere in children with a dense hemiplegia or those with a progressive focal encephalitis may be helped by a larger scale procedure such as hemispherectomy. Assessment of patients must always be carried out by a specialist team with experience in this particular field. The presurgical evaluation should involve detailed neurophysiological and neuropsychological testing. Further discussion is beyond the scope of this chapter, but the interested reader is referred to one of the recent detailed texts by Engel (1987) or Spencer & Spencer (1991).

Psychological treatments

It has always been known that seizures can be precipitated in some patients by certain external stimuli, such as visual patterns or particular noises. These are known as 'evoked seizures'. Besides this, some patients find that they are able to trigger seizures by a direct act of will, while others may report seizure precipitation associated with carrying out a specific mental activity without deliberate intent to provoke a seizure. These are therefore true psychogenic seizures. The word 'psychogenic' has also been used to describe non-epileptic seizures, but here it will be used to describe true epileptic seizures triggered by an act of will or specific function of the mind, as proposed by Fenwick & Brown (1989).

If seizures can be psychogenically provoked, the possibility should be entertained that they could be psychogenically inhibited. Some early work has been carried out in this area using behavioural techniques such as covert desensitisation and cue-controlled arousal (Dahl *et al*, 1985; Brown, 1987; Brown & Fenwick, 1989; Marcano & Brown, 1990). Behavioural techniques may continue to play an important part in the treatment of refractory epilepsy.

Even if seizures may not be completely suppressed, the ability to postpone them returns a degree of control to the patient which enhances psychological wellbeing.

Management of psychiatric complications

This does not substantially differ from the orthodox management of psychiatric conditions in the absence of epilepsy. Issues in treating non-epileptic seizures have been discussed above. For affective and psychotic disorders the question of choice of drugs arises, since some may precipitate seizures in people without epilepsy. In fact, where epilepsy is treated with anticonvulsants, the prescription of tricyclics or neuroleptics rarely causes a clinically significant relapse of the epilepsy. It has been proposed however that the effectiveness of antipsychotics in such cases may be related to the lowering of seizure threshold (Trimble, 1985). The suggestion is that butyrophenones (e.g. haloperidol) or thioxanthines are less likely to affect seizure threshold than phenothiazines such as chlorpromazine or thioridazine.

Follow-up

Ideally, an initial treatment plan should be drawn up by a medical practitioner. Long-term follow-up can be carried out by a primary health care worker with a doctor supervising where possible. Further medical consultation needs be organised only if complications or failure of therapy occur. Epilepsy care could be incorporated into the remit of mobile clinics run by psychiatrists or physicians, or even senior health care workers. Doctors have a responsibility to include epilepsy in the continuing education of primary health workers.

Primary health workers live in the community and therefore play a part in the education of the community as a whole, not only breaking down stigma but also assisting in early recognition of cases. They may be able to undertake home visits, and are in a unique position to provide long-term support and follow-up. This is crucial because the long-term compliance for anti-epileptic treatment in developing countries is notoriously poor. Indeed, an apparent low rate of haematological side-effects has been attributed to this factor (Akinsete & Danesi, 1988) which of course has to be balanced against the possibility of being able to obtain regular supplies of medication. The actual choice of maintenance therapy will be influenced by such local factors as availability and likelihood of continuing supply.

Nevertheless, Senanayake (1987) and Senanayake & Meinardi (1989) have shown how a community project aimed at disseminating information and raising awareness at a grassroots level in Kandy District, Sri Lanka, achieved its aims and has the potential to be incorporated into any primary health care programme. This included preparing health education materials appropriate to the culture of the population, and setting up special training courses for health workers and preschool teachers.

Any community project has to take into account the status of traditional healers. Shorvon *et al* (1991) point out that Western views regarding aetiology and treatment need not be contradictory to traditional beliefs, but could be complementary. A spiritual as well as a biological perspective may be important to the patient.

Forensic aspects

In some countries epilepsy may be allowed as grounds for divorce. Compulsory sterilisation of people with epilepsy has apparently been practised in the past in some Western countries (Fenwick, 1987*b*). However, it seems that these sorts of legal prejudices are disappearing. The law regarding driving motor vehicles varies enormously from country to country. Mani & Hedge (1989) show how the blanket disqualification applied to driving with epilepsy in India is actually counter-productive since this causes the law to be widely flouted. The position in most Western countries is that people with epilepsy may drive if they have been seizure-free for a determined period of time (currently two years in the UK) whether or not they are still taking medication. It is possible that European Community law may become standardised in this respect.

People with epilepsy may be prone to periods of confused behaviour associated with seizures. This may bring them directly into contact with the law. Violence as an ictally-related phenomenon is actually quite rare, but cases do occur. In countries where the McNaughten rules apply, a legal distinction may be made between sane and insane automatisms. Sane automatism is regarded as due to a cause extrinsic to the mind, and a person acting due to this could plead not guilty to any crime apparently committed during one, for example a confusional state due to an infective illness. Insane automatism is regarded as due to a disease of the mind, and if offered as a defence will bring the special McNaughten verdict of 'not guilty by reason of insanity', which in most countries results in compulsory committal to a mental hospital. In the UK, until 1991, epileptic states were regarded as insane automatisms, but this was changed after pressure and publicity from within the legal and medical professions. A doctor going to court to give evidence where epilepsy is being used as a defence should check the following (after Fenwick, 1987*b*):

(1) The patient should be known to suffer from epilepsy
(2) The act should be out of character and inappropriate to the circumstances
(3) There should be no evidence of premeditation or concealment
(4) If a witness is available they should report a disorder of consciousness at the time of the act (e.g. staring eyes, stereotyped movements, etc.)
(5) Memory for the act should be impaired
(6) Remember epilepsy is a clinical diagnosis.

Advice to family and to the patient

This will include making sure that a proper explanation of the condition is given to the patient and if appropriate the whole family, and if necessary counselling should be ongoing to assess attitude and preconceptions. Patients should be encouraged to keep a record of their seizures to assist health workers in assessing progress of treatment, and it may be helpful to keep a record card of medication to show new health workers who may become involved. Ways of doing this should take into account the degree of literacy of the family. The record card may be initially written by the doctor who first sets up the treatment programme. The usually favourable outcome should be explained along with the necessity of continuing treatment. It may be possible to identify and avoid precipitating factors for seizures, such as alcohol or sleep deprivation. Epilepsy is compatible with a normal lifestyle in the vast majority of cases.

In the absence of any other more specialist knowledge, families will fall back on what is widely believed in their own culture about epilepsy. Fear of contagion may mean that if a person falls into a fire during a fit, assistance will not be forthcoming because of fear by others of catching the disease, while elsewhere relatives may rub pepper into the eyes of a person in a post-ictal state in an attempt at resuscitation (WHO, 1979). Familial and cultural attitudes may force the patient to become a social recluse, missing school, employment and social contact. An Indian study (Nadkarni, 1980) showed that overprotectiveness was more common than rejection within families. Counselling the family therefore involves being aware of the cultural expectations of the person with epilepsy and raising the level of factual knowledge of the subject. First aid for individual seizures should be taught; for example it is not necessary to put anything in the patient's mouth during a seizure. It should be stressed that individual seizures cease spontaneously, and that most people get complete control of seizures if they take their medication regularly. Epilepsy is not contagious, is not in itself a form of mental illness, and is not commonly hereditary.

An important development is the movement to forming self-help groups which may form part of the network of a national organisation (Loeber, 1987). Patients should be put in touch with the relevant local or national organisation affiliated to the International Bureau for Epilepsy, for example the Kenya Association for the Welfare of Epileptics (KAWE). These groups have a supportive and information providing role as well as being pressure groups for changing social attitudes. National organisations dedicated to work in the social sphere may be affiliated to the International Bureau for Epilepsy (current address of the secretariat is c/o Instituut voor Epilepsiebestrijding, Heemstede, The Netherlands).

Most people with epilepsy are able to ride bicycles safely, though if seizures are not completely controlled they should be accompanied and should avoid busy roads. Swimming is usually quite safe so long as a person still subject to seizures is accompanied by someone with first aid or life-saving knowledge. Alcohol need not be totally avoided, although seizures may occur as a withdrawal phenomenon after a bout of heavy drinking. With all activities the person with epilepsy should be allowed to take responsibility for the decision after discussion of relative risks involved, and it is important to remember that in the vast majority of cases there is little or no reason to curtail normal activities.

Pregnancy

Recent evidence suggests that there is no increased rate of obstetric complications in women with epilepsy, although there is a tendency to a lower birth weight in the offspring of mothers with epilepsy. The risk of foetal malformation in the children of mothers with epilepsy seems to be two or three times greater than expected in Western countries (Cleland & Espir, 1988). Sodium valproate may be associated with neural tube defects, and while phenytoin causes cleft palate in mice, whether it does so in humans is less certain. A 'foetal hydantoin syndrome' has been described (Hanson & Smith, 1975), with features of growth retardation and craniofacial and digital changes, but the interpretation of observations is subjective. There has been little evidence yet to implicate carbamazepine.

Outcome

Outcome of seizures

Between 60–80% of patients will enter a long remission if treated with the appropriate drug in monotherapy as outlined in the above section. The chance of achieving lasting remission falls dramatically if seizures continue after the first one or two years, perhaps emphasising the importance of early treatment (Annegers *et al*, 1979; Reynolds *et al*, 1983). Compliance is a problem in developing countries, and this may explain some of the lower figures of good outcome for prognosis which have been described. Another factor may be the higher incidence of symptomatic epilepsies. Danesi (1983*b*), in a three-year follow-up in Nigeria, found that only 37% of cases were seizure-free, although no improvement was only found in 13%. The prognosis was worse in those who had been to traditional healers prior to hospital, perhaps because of delay in starting treatment. Once started, treatment should ideally be continued until a two-year period free of any epileptic event has been achieved. After this, a slow withdrawal of anticonvulsant may be attempted if the patient so wishes. In the United Kingdom a large study of drug withdrawal has shown that two years after discontinuation of medication 59% of patients were still seizure-free. Factors affecting the risk of recurrence were previous anticonvulsant polytherapy, and a history of tonic–clonic seizures. The latter is probably accounted for by the inclusion of patients with juvenile myoclonic epilepsy who get good control with treatment but have a particularly high likelihood of relapse on discontinuation of therapy. The most important predictor of good outcome was the length of seizure-free period (Anonymous, 1991). A Uruguayan study showed that the risk factors for relapse after withdrawal included having large number of seizures (>10) or long duration of epilepsy (>5 years) prior to remission, with a non-significant trend towards juvenile myoclonic epilepsy being more likely to relapse, and childhood absence epilepsy less likely to do so (Gerstle de Pasquet *et al*, 1989).

Mortality

It seems that there is a small, but demonstrable, excess mortality associated with a diagnosis of epilepsy. Hauser & Kirland (1975) and Hauser *et al* (1980) have suggested that the risk of mortality is highest in the first ten years after diagnosis, and especially so in the first two years. It holds even if the seizure disorder is apparently in remission. The presence of tonic–clonic seizures increases the risk, and patients with absence seizures alone display no increased risk. Possible causes of excess mortality include suicide, accident, convulsive status epilepticus, true asphyxia and sudden unexpected death (SUD). Suicide has been mentioned above, as has status epilepticus. True asphyxia due to inhalation of gastric contents during a GTCS is possible, but in our personal experience relatively uncommon. SUD during or after a seizure is probably more common than asphyxia. SUD may be related to autonomically mediated cardiac dysrhythmia, and may be predisposed to by poor medication compliance (Jay & Leestma, 1981; Oppenheimer 1990). This phenomenon needs to be seen in context against the overall rate of sudden unexpected death in the population without epilepsy.

Prevention

In up to 70% of cases of epilepsy no cause can be identified, and most symptomatic cases are difficult to prevent (Shorvon *et al*, 1991). However, there is scope for attending to certain causes such as poor perinatal care, infectious diseases, dehydration, febrile convulsions, and head injury.

It should be possible to identify risk factors in each community by appropriate epidemiological studies. Li & Schoenberg (1987), reporting on work carried out in China stress the importance of the following factors: being aged below 10 or over 50, poor health care in the perinatal period, head trauma, low socioeconomic class, having a first degree relative with epilepsy, having another neurological illness, febrile convulsions, and illnesses during pregnancy. In Nigeria, Danesi (1983*a*) reports major factors as being childhood febrile convulsions, head injury, birth injury, central nervous system infections, cerebrovascular disease and sickle cell disease. From Kenya, Telang & Hettiaratchi (1981) have especially stressed the importance of head injury. The last two studies were based on clinic attenders.

Since the genetics of epilepsy remain ill understood, genetic counselling has a relatively small part to play in primary prevention. Prompt attention to febrile convulsions, both by appropriate treatment of the infection and the use of antipyretics will probably reduce the risk of subsequent epilepsy. Vaccination programmes and other public health measures aimed at parasitic and infectious diseases will obviously reduce the incidence of epilepsy due to these causes, and anti-smoking campaigns may reduce the amount of cerebrovascular disease. The rate of head injury may be affected by increasing public awareness of the risks, by attention to road safety and industrial practice, with appropriate use of helmets and safety belts.

Secondary and tertiary prevention rely upon the availability of primary health care in a society where there is awareness of the medical nature of epilepsy and benefits of treatment. This therefore requires work to raise public consciousness using voluntary organisations as well as programmes from professionals, and it requires sensitivity to the role of traditional systems of medicine, so that the old and the new can work side by side.

References

AICARDI, J. (1986) Some epileptic syndromes in infancy and childhood and their relevance to the definition of epilepsy. In *What is Epilepsy? The Clinical and Scientific Basis of Epilepsy* (eds M. R. Trimble & E. H. Reynolds), pp. 21–29. Edinburgh: Churchill Livingstone.

AKINSETE, I. & DANESI, M. A. (1988) Long term use of phenytoin: effects on haematological parameters in Nigerian epileptics. *Central African Journal of Medicine*, **34**, 28–30.

ANDREWES, D. G., TOMLINSON, L. L., ELWES, R. D. C., *et al* (1984) The influence of carbamazepine and phenytoin on memory and other aspects of cognitive function in new referrals with epilepsy. *Acta Neurologica Scandinavica*, **69**, 23–30.

ANNEGERS, J. F., HAUSER, W. A. & ELVEBACK, L. R. (1979) Remission of seizures and relapse in patients with epilepsy. *Epilepsia*, **20**, 729–737.

ANONYMOUS (1989) Pseudostatus epilepticus. *Lancet*, ii, 485.

——— (1991) Antiepileptic drug withdrawal – hawks or doves? *Lancet*, **337**, 1193–1194.

AWARITEFE, A., LONGE, A. C. & AWARITEFE, M. (1985) Epilepsy and psychosis, a comparison of societal attitudes. *Epilepsia*, **26**, 1–9.

BARCZAK, P., EDMONDS, E. & BETTS, T. (1988) Hypomania following complex partial seizures. *British Journal of Psychiatry*, **152**, 137–139.

BARRACLOUGH, B. (1981) Suicide and epilepsy. In *Epilepsy and Psychiatry* (eds E. H. Reynolds & M. R. Trimble), pp. 72–76. Edinburgh: Churchill Livingstone.

BEAR, D. & FEDIO, P. (1977) Quantitative analysis of interictal behaviour in temporal lobe epilepsy. *Archives of Neurology*, **34**, 454–467.

BEAUMANOIR, A. (1985) The Lennox-Gastaut syndrome. In *Epileptic Syndromes in Infancy, Childhood and Adolescence* (eds J. Roger, C. Dravet, M. Bureau, *et al*), pp. 88–99. London: John Libbey.

BENMENACHEM, E., HAMBERGER, A. & MUMFORD, J. (1993) Effect of long-term vigabatrin therapy on GABA and other amino acid concentrations in the central nervous system: a case study. *Epilepsy Research*, **16**, 241–243.

BERAN, R. G., MICHELAZZI, J., HALL, L., *et al* (1985) False-negative response rate in epidemiologic studies to define prevalence ratios of epilepsy. *Neuroepidemiology*, **4**, 82–85.

BETTS, T. A. (1981) Depression, anxiety and epilepsy. In *Epilepsy and Psychiatry* (eds E. H. Reynolds & M. R. Trimble), pp. 60–71. Edinburgh: Churchill Livingstone.

——— (1988) Epilepsy and behaviour. In *A Textbook of Epilepsy* (eds J. Laidlaw, A. Richens & J. Oxley), pp. 350–385. Edinburgh: Churchill Livingstone.

——— (1990) Pseudoseizures: seizures that are not epilepsy. *Lancet*, **336**, 163–164.

BITTENCOURT, P. R. M., GRACIA, C. M. & LORENZANA, P. (1988) Epilepsy and parasitosis of the central nervous system. In *Recent Advances in Epilepsy* (Vol. 4) (eds T. Pedley & B. S. Meldrum), pp. 123–60. Edinburgh: Churchill Livingstone.

BRODTKORB, E., SAND, T., KRISTIANSEN, A., *et al* (1993) Non-convulsive status epilepticus in the adult mentally retarded. Classification and role of benzodiazepines. *Seizure*, **2**, 115–123.

BROWN, S. W. (1982) Epilepsy and psychotherapy. In *Progressos Em Terapeutica Psiquiàtrica* (ed. G. Lopes), pp. 131–160. Porto: Biblioteca do Hospital do Conde de Ferreira.

——— (1987) Psychological treatments. In *Epilepsy* (ed. A. Hopkins), pp. 328–337. London: Chapman & Hall.

——— (1989) Cognitive impairment in epilepsy. *Educational and Child Psychology*, **6**, 25–32.

——— & FENWICK, P. B. C. (1989) Evoked and psychogenic seizures. II: Inhibition. *Acta Neurologica Scandinavica*, **80**, 541–547.

——— & VAUGHAN, M. (1988) Dementia in epileptic patients. In *Epilepsy, Behaviour and Cognitive Function* (eds M. R. Trimble & E. H. Reynolds), pp. 177–188. Chichester: John Wiley & Sons.

——— & ——— (1990) The nature of cognitive changes in people with chronic epilepsy. *Acta Neurologica Scandinavica, Supplementum 133*, **82**, 13.

CALLAGHAN, N. & GOGGIN, T. (1989) Adjunctive therapy in resistant epilepsy. In *Chronic Epilepsy. Its Prognosis and Treatment* (ed. M. R. Trimble), pp. 166–176. Chichester: John Wiley & Sons.

CASCINO, G. D. (1992) Nonconvulsive status epilepticus in adults and children. *Epilepsia*, **34**, S21–S28.

CHADWICK, D., RUTTER, M. & BROWN, G. (1981) A prospective study of children with head injuries. II: Cognitive sequelae. *Psychological Medicine*, **11**, 49–61.

CHEUNG, H., KAMP, D. & HARRIS, E. (1992) An *in vitro* investigation of the action of lamotrigine on neuronal voltage-activated sodium channels. *Epilepsy Research*, **13**, 107–112.

CLELAND, P. G. & ESPIR, M. L. E. (1988) Some aspects of epilepsy in women. In *A Textbook of Epilepsy* (eds J. Laidlaw, A. Richens & J. Oxley), pp. 539–560. Edinburgh: Churchill Livingstone.

COMMISSION ON CLASSIFICATION AND TERMINOLOGY OF THE INTERNATIONAL LEAGUE AGAINST EPILEPSY (1981) Proposal for revised clinical and electroencephalographic classification of epileptic seizures. *Epilepsia*, **22**, 489–501.

——— (1985) Proposal for classification of epilepsies and epileptic syndromes. *Epilepsia*, **26**, 268–269.

——— (1989) Proposal for revised classification of epilepsies and epileptic syndromes. *Epilepsia*, **30**, 389–399.

CONCAS, A., SERRA, M., SANNA, E., *et al* (1992) Involvement of GABA-dependent chloride channel in the action of anticonvulsant and convulsant drugs. *Epilepsy Research*, **15**, 77–85.

DAHL, J., MELIN, L., BRORSON, L. O., *et al* (1985) Effects of a broad spectrum behaviour modification treatment program on children with refractory epileptic seizures. *Epilepsia*, **26**, 303–309.

DANA-HAERI, J., TRIMBLE, M. R. & OXLEY, J. (1983) Prolactin and gonadotrophin changes following generalised and partial seizures. *Journal of Neurology, Neurosurgery and Psychiatry*, **46**, 331–335.

DANESI, M. A. (1983*a*) Acquired aetiological factors in 370 Nigerian epileptics. *Tropical and Geographical Medicine*, **35**, 293–297.

—— (1983*b*) Prognosis of seizures in medically treated adolescent and adult Nigerian epileptics. *Tropical and Geographical Medicine*, **35**, 395–399.

—— (1988) Seasonal variation in the incidence of photoparoxysmal response to photic stimulation among photosensitive epileptic patients: evidence from repeated EEG recordings. *Journal of Neurology, Neurosurgery and Psychiatry*, **51**, 875–877.

—— & —— (1983*a*) Photosensitive epilepsy and photoconvulsive responses to photic stimulation in Africans. *Epilepsia*, **24**, 455–458.

—— & —— (1983*b*) Profile of epilepsy in Lagos, Nigeria. *Tropical and Geographical Medicine*, **35**, 9–13.

DEMERDASH, A., SHAALAN, M., MIDANI, A., *et al* (1991) Sexual behaviour of a sample of females with epilepsy. *Epilepsia*. **32**, 82–85.

DIKMAN, S., HERMAN, B., WILENSKY, A., *et al* (1983) Validity of the Minnesota Multiphasic Personality Inventory (MMPI) to psychopathology in patients with epilepsy. *Journal of Nervous and Mental Disease*, **171**, 114–122.

DUNCAN, J. S., PATSALOS, P. N. & SHORVON, S. D. (1991) Effects of discontinuation of phenytoin, carbamazepine, and valproate on concomitant antiepileptic medication. *Epilepsia*, **32**, 101–115.

DUNN, R. W. & CORBETT, R. (1992) Yohimbine-induced seizures involve NMDA and GABAergic transmission. *Neuropharmacology*, **31**, 389–395.

DURING, M. J. & SPENCER, D. D. (1993) Extracellular hippocampal glutamate and spontaneous seizure in the conscious human brain. *Lancet*, **341** (8861), 1607–1610.

EDEH, J. & TOONE, B. (1987) Relationship between interictal psychopathology and the type of epilepsy. Results of a survey in general practice. *British Journal of Psychiatry*, **151**, 95–101.

ELLIOT, F. (1982) Neurological findings in adult minimal brain dysfunction and the dyscontrol syndrome. *Journal of Nervous and Mental Disease*, **170**, 680–687.

ELLIS, J. M. & LEE, S. I. (1978) Acute prolonged confusion in later life as an ictal state. *Epilepsia*, **19**, 119–128.

ENGEL, J. Jr. (ed.) (1987) *Surgical Treatment of the Epilepsies*. New York: Raven Press.

ENGELSEN, B. A., FONNUM, F. & FURSET, K. (1992) Changes in the levels of glutamate and related amino acids in the intact and decorticated rat neostriatum during various conditions associated with convulsions. *Epilepsy Research*, **15**, 211–217.

FEEKERY, C. J., PARRY-FIELDER, B. & HOPKINS, I. J. (1993) Landau–Kleffner syndrome: six patients including discordant monozygotic twins. *Pediatric Neurology*, **9**, 49–53.

FENTON, G. W. (1972) Epilepsy and automatism. *British Journal of Hospital Medicine*, **7**, 57–64.

FENWICK, P. B. C. (1987*a*) Epilepsy and psychiatric disorders. In *Epilepsy* (ed. A. Hopkins), pp. 511–552. London: Chapman & Hall Medical.

—— (1987*b*) Epilepsy and the law. In *Epilepsy* (ed. A. Hopkins), pp. 553–562. London: Chapman & Hall Medical.

—— & BROWN, S. W. (1989) Evoked and psychogenic seizures. I: Precipitation. *Acta Neurologica Scandinavica*, **80**, 535–540.

—— & FENWICK, E. (eds) (1985) *Epilepsy and the Law – a Medical Symposium on the Current Law*. International Congress and Symposium Series No. 81. London: Royal Society of Medicine.

FISHER, R. S., COLE, A. E., PUMAIN, R., *et al* (1992) Apparent desensitization to glutamate: possible role in epilepsy. *Epilepsy Research*, **15**, 197–201.

FLOR-HENRY, P. (1969) Psychosis and temporal lobe epilepsy. *Epilepsia*, **10**, 363–395.

GALE, K. (1992) GABA and epilepsy: basic concepts from preclinical research. *Epilepsia*, **33**, 3–12.

GASTAUT, H. & COLLOMB, H. (1954) Etude du comportement sexuel chez les épileptiques psychomoteurs. *Annales Medico-Psychologiques*, **112**, 657–696.

GENTON, P., MATON, B., OGIHARA, M., *et al* (1992) Continuous focal spikes during REM sleep in a case of acquired aphasia (Landau–Kleffner syndrome). *Sleep*, **15**, 454–460.

GERSTLE DE PASQUET, E., BONNEVAUX DE TOMA, S., SCARAMELLI, A., *et al* (1989) Discontinuation of antiepileptic drugs after remission of seizures and risks of relapse: a prospective study. In *Advances in Epileptology: XVIIth International Symposium*, pp. 323–326. New York: Raven Press.

GOSPE, S. M. & CHOY, M. (1989) Hereditary long Q-T syndrome presenting as epilepsy: electroencephalography laboratory diagnosis. *Annals of Neurology*, **25**, 514–516.

GRACIA, F. LAO, S. L., CASTILLO, L., *et al* (1990) Epidemiology of epilepsy in Guaymi Indians from Bocas del Toro Province, Republic of Panama. *Epilepsia*, **31**, 718–723.

GRAM, L. (1990) Epileptic seizures and syndromes. *Lancet,* **336,** 161-163.

HANSON, J. W. & SMITH, D. W. (1975) The fetal hydantoin syndrome. *Journal of Pediatrics,* **87,** 285-290.

HAUSER, W. A., ANNEGERS, J. F., ELVEBACK, L. R. (1980) Mortality in patients with epilepsy. *Epilepsia,* **21,** 399-412.

—— & KIRKLAND, L. T. (1975) The epidemiology of epilepsy in Rochester, Minnesota, 1935 through 1967. *Epilepsia,* **16,** 1-66.

——, ANNEGERS, J. F. & ANDERSON, V. E. (1983) Epidemiology and the genetics of epilepsy. In *Epilepsy* (eds A. A. Ward, J. K. Penry, *et al*). New York: Raven Press.

HIERONS, R. & SAUNDERS, M. (1966) Impotence in patients with temporal lobe lesions. *Lancet,* ii, 761-762.

HOPKINS, A. (1987) Definitions and epidemiology of epilepsy. In *Epilepsy* (ed. A. Hopkins), pp. 1-18. London: Chapman & Hall.

HOWELL, S. J. L., OWEN, L. & CHADWICK, D. W. (1989) Pseudostatus epilepticus. *Quarterly Journal of Medicine,* **7,** 509-519.

HUGHES, J. R. (1982) *EEG in Clinical Practice.* Boston: Butterworths.

JAY, G. W. & LEESTMA, J. E. (1981) Sudden death in epilepsy. *Acta Neurologica Scandinavica, Supplementum* **82, 63**.

JOHNS, D. F., TIERNEY, M. & FELSENSTEIN, D. (1987) Alterations in the natural history of neurosyphilis by concurrent infection with human immunodeficiency virus. *New England Journal of Medicine,* **316,** 1569-1589.

JOY, R. M., ALBERTSON, T. E. & TICKU, M. K. (1992) *In vivo* assessment of the importance of GABA in convulsant and anticonvulsant drug action. *Epilepsy Research,* **15,** 63-75.

KAMPHUIS, W., MONYER, H., DeRIJK, T. C., *et al* (1992) Hippocampal kindling increases the expression of glutamate receptor-A flip and -B flip mRNA in dentate granule cells. *Neuroscience Letters,* **148,** 51-54.

LESSER, R. P. (1985) Psychogenic seizures. In *Recent Advances in Epilepsy, Vol. 2* (eds T. Pedley & B. Meldrum), pp. 273-296. Edinburgh: Churchill Livingstone.

LI, S.-C. & SCHOENBERG, B. S. (1987) Risk factors for epilepsy in China and other developing countries. *Chinese Medical Journal,* **100,** 813-815.

LISHMAN, W. A. (1987) *Organic Psychiatry* (2nd edn). Oxford: Blackwell.

LOCKARD, J. S. & WARD, A. A. (1980) *Epilepsy: a Window to the Brain Mechanisms.* New York: Raven Press.

LOEBER, J. N. (1987) Epilepsy self-help groups: an international perspective. In *Advances in Epileptology XVIth International Symposium,* pp. 639-645 New York: Raven Press.

LOGSDAIL, S. J. & TOONE, B. K. (1988) Post-ictal psychoses. *British Journal of Psychiatry,* **152,** 246-52.

LOMBROSO, C. T. & LERMAN, P. (1967) Breath-holding spells (cyanotic and pallid infantile syncope). *Pediatrics,* **39,** 563-581.

LOU, H. O. (1968) Repeated episodes of transient global amnesia. *Acta Neurologica Scandinavica,* **44,** 612-618.

MACKAY, A. (1979) Self-poisoning-a complication of epilepsy. *British Journal of Psychiatry,* **134,** 277-82.

MAHONEY, W. J., D'SOUZA, B. J., HALLER, J. A., *et al* (1983) Long term outcome of children with severe head trauma and prolonged coma. *Pediatrics,* **71,** 756-762.

MANEV, H., BERTOLINO, M. & DEERAUSQUIN, G. (1990) Amiloride blocks glutamate-operated cationic channels and protects neurons in culture from glutamate-induced death. *Neuropharmacology,* **29,** 1103-1110.

MANI, K. S. & HEDGE, N. S. (1989) Epilepsy and the law: position in India. In *Advances in Epileptology XVIIth International Symposium,* pp. 428-431. New York: Raven Press.

MARCANO, J. L. & BROWN, S. W. (1990) Affective precipitatory factors and behavioural strategies in seizure control. *Acta Neurologica Scandinavica Supplementum 133,* **82,** 54.

MAREMMANI, C., ROSSI, G., BONUCCELLI, U., *et al* (1991) Descriptive epidemiological study of epilepsy syndromes in a district of Northwest Tuscany, Italy. *Epilepsia,* **32,** 294-298.

McDADE, G. & BROWN, S. W. (1990) The multidisciplinary approach to treating pseudoseizures – an audit. *Acta Neurologica Scandinavica Supplementum 133,* **82,** 17.

MONROE, R. (1970) *Episodic Behavioural Disorders.* Boston: Harvard University Press.

NADKARNI, V. V. (1980) Having epilepsy is a problem regardless of geographical location. *Advances in Epileptology XIth International Symposium,* pp. 209-221. New York: Raven Press.

NAKANISHI, S. (1992) Molecular diversity of glutamate receptor and implications for brain function. *Science,* **258,** 597-603.

OPPENHEIMER, S. (1990) Cardiac dysfunction during seizures and the sudden epileptic death syndrome. *Journal of the Royal Society of Medicine,* **83,** 134-135.

OSUNTOKUN, B. O. (1979) Management of epilepsy in developing countries. *Nigerian Medical Journal*, **9**, 1–11.

——, ADEUJA, A. O. G., NOTTIDGE, V. A., *et al* (1987) Prevalence of the epilepsies in Nigerian Africans: a community-based study. *Epilepsia*, **23**, 272–279.

——, BADEMOSI, O., FAMILUSI, J. B., *et al* (1974) Electroencephalographic correlates of epilepsy in Nigerian children. *Developmental Medicine and Child Neurology*, **12**, 659–663.

PAQUIER, P. F., VAN, D. & LOONEN, M. (1992) The Landau–Kleffner syndrome or acquired aphasia with convulsive disorder: long-term follow-up of six children, and review of the recent literature. *Archives of Neurology*, **49**, 354–359.

PARSONAGE, M. (1986) Problems in the classification of paroxysmal seizures. In *What is Epilepsy? The Clinical and Scientific Basis of Epilepsy* (eds M. R. Trimble & E. H. Reynolds), pp. 8–20. Edinburgh: Churchill Livingstone.

—— (1988) Classification of the epileptic seizures: part two. In *A Textbook of Epilepsy* (eds J. Laidlaw, A. Richens & J. Oxley), pp. 8–14. Edinburgh: Churchill Livingstone.

PEREZ, M., TRIMBLE, M. R., MURRAY, N. M. F., *et al* (1985) Epileptic psychosis: an evaluation of present state examination profiles. *British Journal of Psychiatry*, **146**, 155–163.

PLACENCIA, M., SHORVON, S. D., PAREDES, V., *et al* (1992) Epileptic seizures in an Andean region of Ecuador – incidence and prevalence and regional variation. *Brain*, **115**, 771–782.

POND, D. A. (1957) Psychiatric aspects of epilepsy. *Journal of the Indian Medical Profession*, **3**, 1441–1451.

—— & BIDWELL, B. H. (1960) A survey of epilepsy in 14 general practices. II: Social and psychological aspects. *Epilepsia*, **1**, 285–299.

REYNOLDS, E. H. (1986) The clinical concept of epilepsy: a historical perspective. In *What is Epilepsy? The Clinical and Scientific Basis of Epilepsy* (eds M. R. Trimble & E. H. Reynolds), pp. 1–7. Edinburgh: Churchill Livingstone.

—— (1989) The prognosis of epilepsy: is chronic epilepsy preventable? In *Chronic Epilepsy, Its Prognosis and Management* (ed. M. R. Trimble), pp. 13–20. Chichester: Wiley.

——, ELWES, R. D. C. & SHORVON, S. D. (1983) Why does epilepsy become intractable? Prevention of chronic epilepsy. *Lancet*, **ii**, 952–954.

RICHARDS, T. (1986) Drugs in the developing countries: inching towards rational policies. *British Medical Journal*, **292**, 1347–1348.

RICHENS, A. & PERUCCA, E. (1994) Clinical pharmacology and medical treatment. In *A Textbook of Epilepsy* (4th edn) (eds J. Laidlaw, A. Richens & D. Chadwick). Edinburgh: Churchill Livingstone.

ROBERTS, J. K. A. (1984) *Differential Diagnosis in Neuropsychiatry*. Chichester: Wiley.

ROBERTSON, M. & TRIMBLE, M. R. (1983) Depressive illness in patients with epilepsy: a review. *Epilepsia*, **24**, S109–S116.

RODIN, E., RHODES, R. & VELARDE, N. (1965) The prognosis for patients with epilepsy. *Journal of Occupational Medicine*, **7**, 560–563.

ROY, A. (1977) Hysterical fits previously diagnosed as epilepsy. *Psychological Medicine*, **7**, 271–273.

SAGAR, H. J. & OXBURY, J. M. (1987) Hippocampal neurone loss in temporal lobe epilepsy: correlations with early childhood convulsions. *Annals of Neurology*, **22**, 334–340.

SANDER, J. W. A. S. & SHORVON, S. D. (1987) Incidence and prevalence studies in epilepsy and their methodological problems: a review. *Journal of Neurology, Neurosurgery and Psychiatry*, **50**, 829–839.

SCHWARTZ, R. H., EATON, J., AYNSLEY-GREEN, A. & BOWER, B. D. (1983) Ketogenic diets in the management of epilepsy. In *Research Progress in Epilepsy* (ed. F. C. Rose), pp. 326–332. London: Pitman.

SENANAYAKE, N. (1987) Epilepsy control in a developing country – the challenge of tomorrow. *Ceylon Medical Journal*, **32**, 181–199.

—— & MEINARDI, H. (1989) Improvement in the care of people with epilepsy in rural areas of a developing country. *Advances in Epileptology XVIIth International Symposium*, pp. 441–444.

SHORVON, S. D. (1986) Drugs in developing countries (letter). *British Medical Journal*, **292**, 1666–1667.

——, HART, Y. M., SANDER, J. W. A. S., *et al* (1991) *Management of epilepsy in developing countries: An 'ICEBERG' manual*. International Congress and Symposium Series No. 175. London: Royal Society of Medicine.

SLATER, E., BEARD, A. W. & GLITHEROE, E. (1963) The schizophrenia-like psychosis of epilepsy. *British Journal of Psychiatry*, **109**, 95–150.

SOLOMONS, G., HOLDEN, R. H. & DENHOFF, E. (1963) The changing picture of cerebral dysfunction in early childhood. *Journal of Paediatrics*, **63**, 113–120.

SPENCER, S. S. & SPENCER, D. D. (eds) (1991) *Surgery for Epilepsy*. Oxford: Blackwell Scientific Publications.

STANHOPE, J. M., BRODY, J. A. & BRINK, E. (1972) Convulsions among the Chamorro people of Guam, Mariana Island. *American Journal of Epidemiology*, **95**, 292–298.

STAUFENBERG, E. F. & BROWN, S. W. (1994) Some issues in non-convulsive status epilepticus in children and adolescents with learning difficulties. *Seizure*, **3**, 95–105.

STEVENS, J. R. (1986) All that spikes is not fits: epilogue and update 1985. In *What is Epilepsy? The Clinical and Scientific Basis of Epilepsy* (eds M. R. Trimble & E. H. Reynolds), pp. 109–115. Edinburgh: Churchill Livingstone.

SWARTZ, B. E. & DELGADO-ESCUETA, A. V. (1987) The management of status epilepticus. In *Epilepsy* (ed. A. Hopkins), pp. 417–442. London: Chapman & Hall.

TALLIS, R. (1990) Epilepsy in old age. *Lancet*, **336**, 295–296.

TASSINARI, C. A., BUREAU, M., DRAVET, C., DALLA BERNARDINA, B. & ROGER, J. (1985) Epilepsy with continuous spike-wave during slow sleep. In *Epileptic Syndromes in Infancy Childhood and Adolescence* (eds J. Roger, C. Dravet, M. Bureau, *et al*), pp. 194–204. London: John Libbey.

———, MICHELUCCI, R., FORTI, A., *et al* (1992) The electrical status epilepticus syndrome. *Epilepsy Research*, **15**, 111–115.

TAYLOR, D. C. (1969) Sexual behaviour and temporal lobe epilepsy. *Archives of Neurology*, **21**, 510–516.

TELANG, B. & HETTIARATCHI, E. S. (1981) Patterns of epilepsy in Kenya: a clinical analysis of 115 cases. *East African Medical Journal*, **58**, 437–444.

THOMPSON, P. J., HUPPERT, F. A. & TRIMBLE, M. R. (1981) Phenytoin and cognitive function: effects on normal volunteers and implications for epilepsy. *British Journal of Clinical Psychology*, **20**, 155–162.

——— & TRIMBLE, M. R. (1981) Sodium valproate and cognitive functioning in normal volunteers. *British Journal of Clinical Pharmacology*, **12**, 819–824.

——— & ——— (1982) Anticonvulsant drugs and cognitive function. *Epilepsia*, **23**, 531–554.

——— & ——— (1983) The effect of anticonvulsant drugs on cognitive function: relation to serum levels. *Journal of Neurology, Neurosurgery and Psychiatry*, **46**, 227–233.

TOMSON, T., LINDBOM, U. & NILSSON, B. Y. (1992) Nonconvulsive status epilepticus in adults: 32 consecutive patients from a general hospital population. *Epilepsia*, **33**, 829–835.

TOMLINSON, L. L., ANDREWES, D. G., MERRIFIELD, E., *et al* (1982) The effect of anticonvulsant drugs on cognitive and motor functions. *British Journal of Clinical Practice*, **18**, 177–183.

TOONE, B. K. (1991) The psychoses of epilepsy. *Journal of the Royal Society of Medicine*, **84**, 457–459.

———, FENWICK, P. B. C., EDEH, J., *et al* (1983) Sex hormones, sexual activity and plasma anticonvulsant levels in male epileptics. *Journal of Neurology, Neurosurgery and Psychiatry*, **46**, 824–826.

———, GARRALDA, M. E. & RON, M. A. (1981) The psychoses of epilepsy and the functional psychoses: a clinical and phenomenological comparison. *British Journal of Psychiatry*, **141**, 256–261.

TRIMBLE, M. R. (1985) The psychoses of epilepsy and their treatment. In *The Psychopharmacology of Epilepsy* (ed. M. R. Trimble), pp. 83–94. Chichester: Wiley.

——— (1991) *The Psychoses of Epilepsy*. New York: Raven Press.

WEISER, H. G. (1987) The phenomenology of limbic seizures. In *Current Problems in Epilepsy. 3. The Epileptic Focus* (eds H. G. Weiser, E.-J. Speckman & J. Engel), pp. 113–116. London: Libbey.

——— (1979) Epilepsy in the developing countries. *WHO Chronicles*, **33**, 183–186.

WORLD HEALTH ORGANIZATION (1989) Drugs in Epilepsy. *WHO Drug Information*, **33**, 28–39.

WONG, P. K. H., BENCIVENGA, R. & GREGORY, D. (1989) Statistical classification of spikes in benign rolandic epilepsy. *Brain Topography*, **1**, 123–130.

YAQUB, B. A., PANAYIOTOPOULOS, C. P., AL NOZHA, M., *et al* (1987) Causes of late onset epilepsy in Saudi Arabia: the role of cerebral granuloma. *Journal of Neurology, Neurosurgery and Psychiatry*, **50**, 90–92.

YASUHARA, A. Y., YOSHIDA, H., HATANAKA, T., *et al* (1991) Epilepsy with continuous spike-waves during slow sleep and its treatment. *Epilepsia*, **32**, 59–62.

ZIELINSKI, J. J. (1988) Epidemiology. In *A Textbook of Epilepsy* (eds J. Laidlaw, A. Richens & J. Oxley), pp. 21–48. Edinburgh: Churchill Livingstone.

12 Mental retardation

TOM FRYERS

In the early years of promoting primary health care in the developing countries, the needs of disabled children and adults, and the potential for prevention, were almost totally ignored. Priority was given to early mortality, communicable diseases and nutrition. However, the International Year of the Disabled Person, 1981, had a major impact and placed disability permanently on the agenda.

Mental retardation has since received increasing attention. It is generally accepted that acute illness cannot be separated from its long-term sequelae, that mental retardation imposes serious burdens on individuals, families and communities, and that many syndromes are preventable. In many countries, health priorities are still concerned with the control of communicable diseases, improved nutrition, and the equitable provision of health care through a primary health care infrastructure. These priorities are inextricably intertwined with general socioeconomic development, universal primary education, technical training, communications, and political stability. They were European priorities a hundred years ago, and are directly relevant to mental retardation. The biological causes of mental retardation in Western countries are the same as those present in developing countries, where their impact on communities may be even greater. Infections and undernutrition, inadequate health care and lack of technical knowledge reduce the capacity of individuals, families and communities to cope with the problems, and conspire to hide them from official view.

Where infant mortality is high most children with serious abnormalities die early. Decreasing birth rates usually lead to fewer impairments, as women and children get more resources and better care. However, as infant mortality decreases, so the survival of children with impairments and disabilities is likely to increase, and as educational demands increase, so those who cannot live up to expectations are likely to be exposed as failures.

These are dynamic processes, reflecting many aspects of development, and are very variable and difficult to predict. Key indicators of development include low infant mortality, a comprehensive primary health care infrastructure, and universal primary education. In areas where these factors indicate significant progress, mental retardation is likely to become a significant issue of concern, whether officially recognised or not. On the other hand, communities with high rates of infant mortality and little health care or education are likely to have few severely impaired children surviving, and are unlikely to recognise mildly impaired children as significantly 'different'.

Concepts, classifications, terms and labels

Research into mental retardation has suffered from confusion of concepts, inconsistency of classification and variety of terminology, but a coherent taxonomic structure is now available and is presented in detail elsewhere (Fryers, 1984*a*; 1987; 1991; 1993*a*), where it is related to and discussed in the context of ICD–9 (World Health Organization, 1978) DSM–III (American Psychiatric Association, 1980) and the classification of the American Association on Mental Deficiency.

Concepts arising from different professional and scientific perspectives are difficult to reconcile. They include restricted genetic potential, aetiological diagnosis, brain damage and disorder, low measured intelligence, social maladaptation and personal dependency. Each poses problems of classification and measurement. Moreover, terms are used not only for scientific study and professional practice, but also as legal categories and social labels, perpetuating stereotyping, stigma and prejudice. In this situation, no one concept or set of categories can serve all purposes. We need a variety of taxonomies, categories and terms, carefully specified and defined according to the purpose to be served.

The World Health Organization's *International Classification of Impairments, Disabilities and Handicaps* (1980) provides a basic structure. Impairment is a fault in an organ or body system; disability is loss of function; handicap is social disadvantage. In the field of mental retardation, global categories define the whole group; partial categories define groups not exclusive to mental retardation (Table 12.1).

Careful definition and measurement can be applied to the categories shown in Table 12.1, but in everyday professional practice, terms and categories are used much more loosely. Research categories serve different purposes from administrative and professional categories which are used for the organisation, planning and monitoring of services. Medical diagnoses, that is aetiological categories, though important to inform preventive action, seldom fit wholly into one category of intellectual impairment or learning disability. Individual needs cannot be assumed from any categories or labels, but require thorough individual assessment.

The only well established convention offering some consistency between communities, cultures and periods of time is the use of IQ < 50 as the *sole essential criterion* for severe intellectual impairment (but called many names including severe mental handicap, severe mental retardation, and severe learning disability; it encompasses profound, severe and moderate categories in the WHO's classification of mental retardation (1986)). This criterion may allow comparisons of prevalence and distribution, but only if IQ tests are standardised for the community tested, are rigorously applied by professionals, and are repeated for individuals to ensure reliability. These conditions seldom hold in well developed countries; they are very rare in developing countries.

With that exception, it should be recognised that calling an individual 'mentally retarded' is a function of social selection using a variety of criteria,

TABLE 12.1
Taxonomies in mental retardation

Global categories

Intellectual impairment
  Criteria: intellectual.
  Measures: intelligence or developmental tests.
  Main categories: Severe impairment, IQ < 50; Mild impairment, IQ 50–69.

Generalised learning disability
  Criteria: educational.
  Measures: mostly proxies of learning achievement (rather than learning process) such as memory
    recall, reading, number, problem solving, etc.
  Main categories: 'severe', 'moderate', and 'mild' are generally used but in non-standard ways;
    often ill-defined.

General dependence handicap – related to intellectual impairment
(Mental handicap or handicap due to retardation).
  Criteria: social – highly variable in different societies.
  Measures: scales of dependency or maladaptation.
  Main categories: 'severe' (or severe and profound combined), commonly limited to IQ < 50,
    and therefore co-extensive with severe intellectual impairment. 'Mild', used with very variable
    criteria of social selection.

Partial categories

Physical impairments
  Criteria: commonly pathological or aetiological diagnosis.
  Measures: usually clinical and laboratory.
  Main categories: diagnostic groups.

Specific disabilities
  Criteria: functional.
  Measures: standardised assessments where available.
  Main categories: few named syndromes; mostly specific motor, sensory, intellectual, emotional
    and behavioural dysfunctions.

Individual handicaps
  Criteria: social disadvantage.
  Measures: very few standard measures available.
  Main categories: income, housing, employment, education.

(After Fryers, 1991; 1993*a*; 1993*b*).

often not explicit. There are no standard, consistent definitions because reasons
for selection as 'retarded' vary with legal, political, professional, organisational,
social, economic, environmental and cultural factors (Table 12.2). To investigate
these factors in different countries in relation to the disabilities and handicaps
experienced by individuals selected is an interesting challenge to current
research.

For example, in many developing countries where there is no expectation that
all children will go to school, mildly retarded children will not generally be
identified. Indeed, the concept may have no currency in cultures with value
systems and conventions of language which are significantly different from
those of 'Western' models of education, vocation and social function (Serpell *et
al*, 1993). Similarly, in many developed countries where adults who cannot cope
with employment or independent living are referred for help to social welfare
rather than medical agencies, they may never be perceived as retarded or
considered to belong to a specific group. There may be confusion with mental

TABLE 12.2
Factors affecting selection as mentally retarded

Legislation: criminal, health, education, social welfare, and employment law all relevant.
Service structures and traditions: in education, health, social welfare, etc.
Professional cultures: concepts, perceptions, expectations, labelling, etc.
Patterns of employment and unemployment: work and training opportunities.
Social class and social attitudes: cultural expectations, deprivation, discrimination, etc.
Family support: structures and security of families.
Historical service patterns: older clients inherited from earlier situations; e.g. in institutional care.
Perceived low intelligence: with or without additional factors, e.g. antisocial behaviour, mental illness, motor, sensory or communication disabilities, multiple disabilities.

illness, though this probably applies mostly to adults. In some cultures the shame of having an overtly abnormal child leads to their being hidden from all authorities; in others, such children are brought early by parents for help. Nevertheless, in most countries, children with obvious serious developmental delay will generally be known, and given some distinguishing label.

Epidemiology

Mental retardation is not a medical diagnosis, but a scientific, professional or administrative category. Many syndromes contribute to it, their contributions varying between countries. Whatever criteria are used to define the group, the prevalence of mental retardation at any age is determined by the inception rate of each syndrome, the mortality of each syndrome and the effectiveness of identification. Both the inception of syndromes associated with retardation and the death of affected individuals may occur before, during and after birth, depending on the syndrome. Identification improves with age. Prevalence *rates*, that is numbers related to the population from which cases derive, depend also upon differential migration.

The basic facts about the prevalence and distribution of severe intellectual impairment (IQ < 50) can be generalised and presented simply (Table 12.3; Fryers, 1993a). Mild mental retardation however, having no consistent definition even in research, provides no comparative or generalisable statistics from anywhere.

Given this situation, what can we say about the epidemiology of retardation in developing countries? Prevalence studies in poor countries cannot be justified for the pursuit of scientific curiosity alone; potential benefits to those communities would be too remote to have validity for them. However, four objectives might be served:

1. to offer practical assistance to those identified as disabled within the community;
2. to identify specific preventable causes in that community;
3. to raise the client group and their needs to 'visibility' with governments, community leaders, professionals, and the people;
4. to provide estimates of community need to those in local or national government, national or international agencies, who might plan services and provide resources.

TABLE 12.3

Basic epidemiology of severe intellectual impairment. Prevalence in developed countries

There is geographical variation within similar birth cohorts
Range at least 1.62–7.34/1000

There is temporal variation in successive birth cohorts in the same community
e.g. 1.98–5.54/1000 in Salford children aged 5–9, 1961–1971

There has been a similar pattern of temporal change in many developed countries
Low prevalence for children born in the early 1950s
High prevalence for the children born in the early 1960s

There is variation by age due to variations between birth cohorts in incidence and mortality
Currently the highest prevalence ratios are in the age group 25–30 years

There is increased survival at all ages and into old age
There are more clients aged >45 than aged <15

There is probably a social class gradient in both incidence and mortality
There are excesses in lower socioeconomic groups

There are usually more males than females
But there are no consistent patterns in the sex ratio

These features are typical of developed countries. They will be true to varying extents for communities in developing countries depending upon development and economic status, demographic characteristics, vital statistics, and many other social indicators (see text)

Such studies will not usually provide statistics susceptible to international comparison, but there have, of course, been studies which do. Methodological problems are generally the same as in developed countries, but may be harder to solve. Physical communications may be difficult and expensive, but linguistic and cultural translation of concepts and questions, and interviewer reliability, may pose even greater difficulties. High rates of acceptance and compliance may be difficult to achieve in communities not used to strangers asking apparently irrelevant questions, while lack of local information may preclude satisfactory resolution of technical issues of sample size, representativeness of samples, and precise knowledge of population denominators. Relating observations of child development to age norms is a special problem in those cultures who place no value on knowing the age of a child so that it is neither recorded nor recalled.

The evidence we do have suggests that there is greater epidemiological variation in developing than in developed countries because environments, cultures and development status are more variable. For example, Table 12.4 shows prevalence rates from one developing country, China, taken from several studies (Tao Kuo-Tai, 1988).

For *severe* intellectual impairment, the range derived from six independent studies, 1.27–4.8/1000 (all but one all-age prevalence) is similar to that found in Western countries. Rural rates were consistently higher than urban rates, double on average, though with much variation. The 1988 multi-centre study of children aged 0–12 (Tao Kuo Tai, 1990), produced four rates between 3.05 and 3.89, but two very high rates for the severe group, of 13.51 and 15.79/1000. The first of these is from a remote 'minority' area, where nutrition, medical care and education may be inadequate, but also where cultural differences may prejudice testing (12% of children in this area were categorised 'retarded'). The second is

TABLE 12.4
Mental retardation in China: prevalence per 1000 total population

	Age range	'Severe'	All 'Retarded'
Independent studies			
Sichuan (1973–1974)	all	2.56	5.36
Shanghai (1978)	all	1.27	–
Nanjing (1980)	all	1.52	3.36
'12 Districts' (1982)	all	3.00	—
Beijing (1982)	0–14	2.94	7.84
'14 Areas' (1988)	all	4.80	12.00
National Collaborative Study (1988); Children aged 0–12			
Nanjing		3.43	21.87
Xiamen		3.05	4.58
Baimzang minority		13.51	122.34
Shanxi (i)		15.79	46.44
Shanxi (ii)		3.89	11.67
Anhui		3.33	57.98
Mean		5.52	34.47

(After Tao Kuo Tai, 1988; 1990).

from an iodine deficient area with no iodine supplementation programme at the time, so must be related to endemic cretinism. In contrast, two iodine deficient areas with supplementation programmes produced figures of 3.33 and 3.89/1000.

These studies are probably as reliable as many in Western countries, and it is important to explore possible reasons for variation. Some are clear. In iodine deficient areas, cretinism can affect more than 10% of the population, and perpetual consanguinity in isolated communities can produce high rates of recessive genetic disorders. Down's syndrome varies with family size and is likely to be more prevalent in ethnic minorities where the 'one child' policy is not applied. On the other hand, variations in infant mortality, generally low in China, are likely to lead to higher survival rates in urban than rural areas, especially for children with disabilities not obvious until well after birth. It may also be that children from remote, poorly resourced communities test badly with instruments prepared in urban settings by urban professionals in a different language and culture.

A very different study in ten locations in nine developing countries, the International Pilot Study of Severe Childhood Disability, gave a similar range for prevalence of 5–15/1000 for children aged 3–9 years with one exception in India. Positive and negative results of two screening questionnaires were validated by professional assessment (Belmont, 1984). The 'Ten Questions' (TQ) screening instrument developed and tested in that pilot study has now been used in full scale studies, and seems useful for a first stage before professional examination (Zaman *et al*, 1990; Durkin *et al*, 1991; WHO, 1992).

The high Indian figures in the above study are matched by the results of previous studies in rural communities around Bangalore. Narayanan (1981) identified 12/1000 in children, and 30/1000 in 14–19-year-olds. He explained the latter in terms of migration; young men go to the city for work or training, young women to marry, but retarded youngsters remain. However, rural communities do not always have an excess of retarded people; Saunders (1982) in a thorough survey of 6000 children under the age of 16 years in Plateau State, northern Nigeria, found urban rates for 'severe mental handicap' (3.32/1000) twice those of rural communities (1.5/1000). As he was well aware, the numbers are very small for statistical reliability. He found no children with Down's syndrome; in communities where they survive, prevalence would be greater. Interestingly, he was aware that he was recording 'handicap' rather than 'disability', justifying this as essential if the social and cultural context of mental retardation was to be accommodated.

In association with the Zambia Campaign to Reach Disabled Children, Desai (1986) assembled national statistics which gave essentially similar figures to Saunders. She estimated 1.12 and 4.93/1000 for rural and urban populations. Serpell (1993) considers the latter figure especially to be an overestimate as it contains some children in mainstream schools who are unlikely to be severely affected.

These statistics illustrate the variety of prevalence rates obtained from studies aspiring to scientific validity (Fryers, 1984*b*). It is clear that results cannot be applied from one community to another, and prevalence studies in developing countries are futile unless they serve the four objectives listed above: identification of individuals in need, informing preventive programmes, raising visibility, and justifying resourcing. As Serpell points out, unless the statistics used, especially if drawn from developed countries, are limited to those children likely to benefit from being identified as mentally retarded, they will overestimate the problem and mislead governments and professionals alike. And such children are, in most developing countries, likely to be only those we would recognise as 'severely' mentally retarded.

Biological causes: aetiological diagnosis

The syndromes contributing to severe mental retardation are numerous but can be summarised within three main groups. *Pure primary disorders* are present at conception, an autosome or sex chromosome aberration in one gamete resulting in an abnormal karyotype. The most important are trisomy 21 (Down's syndrome) and fragile X syndrome. *Primary disorders with secondary neurological damage* have a genetically determined specific defect which affects development, with or without environmental provocation. The commonest are phenylketonuria, and sporadic hypothyroidism. *Pure secondary disorders* arise from an environmental insult to a normal zygote, before, during or after birth. Among the most important are iodine deficiency disorders, various communicable diseases and trauma.

Table 12.5 shows many syndromes contributing to mental retardation, but most are rare. Many factors affect the cause of each syndrome, and it is wise always to think in terms of causal processes. Cause in individuals must be considered differently from cause in populations. For an individual case, one asks what factors contributed to the damage or disorder observed; for a population, one asks what factors contribute to the prevalence in that population. This is particularly important when planning preventive interventions; we may not be able directly to intervene in the causal process, but we may be able to influence factors which

TABLE 12.5
Summary of main organic aetiologies related to mental retardation (frequencies are approximate and sometimes insecure)

A. Primary disorders (Chromosome aberrations which are present at conception)

Down's syndrome:
Trisomy 21 (94% of all Down's): refer to text for birth prevalence
Trisomy mosaics (1–3%): birth prevalence 0.03/1000
Translocation (3–5%): birth prevalence 0.03/1000
All retarded but for some mosaics

Other autosomal anomalies: birth prevalence 2–4/1000
Patau's, Edward's, cri-du-chat syndromes
Occasionally severely or mildly retarded

Sex chromosome disorders: birth prevalence 2–3/1000
Occasionally severely or mildly retarded

Non-specific disorders associated with intellectual impairment
Recessive: birth prevalence ?0.5/1000
X-linked: birth prevalence 1/1000 – most boys but few girls retarded: see text

Doubtful aetiology: De Lange and hypercalcaemia syndromes

B. Primary disorders with secondary neurological damage

Defects of protein metabolism: all retarded if untreated
Phenylketonuria (PKU): birth prevalence 0.05–0.2/1000
At least five others: birth prevalence 0.1/1000

Defects of carbohydrate metabolism: all retarded if untreated
Galactosaemia: birth prevalence 0.02/1000

Defects of lipid metabolism: all retarded and die early
Tay–Sach's disease: birth prevalence 0.04/1000 in Ashkenazi Jewish communities; rarely elsewhere
Batten's disease: frequency uncertain

Defects of mucopolysaccharide metabolism: all retarded
Hurler's syndrome: birth prevalence 0.03/1000

Defects of hormone system: retarded unless treated early
Sporadic congenital: hypothyroidism: birth prevalence 0.1–2.0/1000

Mechanism not clear: retardation very variable
Epiloia (tuberous sclerosis): birth prevalence 0.01/1000
Neurofibromatosis (von Recklinghausen's disease): birth prevalence 0.33/1000
Some cases of microcephaly

C. Secondary disorders (damaged after conception)

Antenatal factors:
Iodine deficiency disorders: frequency of severe retardation (cretinism) very variable: see text
Neural tube defects: birth prevalence 1–8/1000, possibly 10% retarded
Rhesus incompatibility: frequency of retardation varied
Communicable diseases: very varied frequency of infection and of brain damage after infection; see Table 12.6 and text
Alcohol: foetal alcohol syndrome varied; many cases retarded
Drugs; irradiation; heavy metals; no satisfactory data

Perinatal factors, including gross trauma, hypoxia, hypoglycaemia, and cerebral thrombosis.
Definitions problematic and frequency of damage virtually unmeasurable
Often associated with cerebral palsy and epilepsy

Postnatal factors: all very variable in frequency
Physical trauma; accidents
Communicable diseases; meningitis and encephalitis or encephalopathies; see Table 12.6 and text
Chemical agents: lead may reduce intelligence
Nutritional/metabolic: high solute baby feeds combined with fever

(After Fryers, 1991).

reduce prevalence. For example, we do not know the underlying cause of non-disjunction in Down's syndrome and cannot intervene but if maternal age is reduced, birth prevalence will decrease.

It is important to realise that, however 'biological' the known causes of neurological impairment, there are social and environmental factors which increase or decrease their frequency in populations. Down's syndrome is influenced by age of marriage, family size, attitudes to contraception, economic circumstances, education, religion and law. Recessive genetic disorders are determined by consanguinity, religion, and isolation. Foetal alcohol syndrome depends upon attitudes to alcohol consumption in pregnancy, to cultural traditions, and to government tax policies. Perinatal damage reflects early nutrition of girls, traditions of child birth, and distribution of services. Similarly accidents, infectious diseases, neural tube defects, iodine deficiency disorders, and so on, are determined by environments, traditions, attitudes, government policies, and many other factors.

Neurological damage has little potential for healing or treatment, and, though some problems patients face are susceptible to medical treatment, management of cases is not mainly a medical matter, and is little influenced by the diagnosis. But opportunities for prevention may be specific to diagnostic groups, and are largely dependent upon manipulating social factors to reduce incidence.

Nevertheless, there are general issues concerning prevention. In some, mental retardation is only one of many justifications for social action; for example in reducing road traffic, industrial and home accidents, all common in developing countries. General economic and social development is important, and within this, the situation of women, their economic status and roles within the family are crucial. A comprehensive, efficient service infrastructure is probably more important than the level of technological sophistication, but an appreciation of scientific issues in policy makers is helpful. Both the prevention of mental retardation and the development of rehabilitation services are dependent on social and political stability.

Specific aetiological groups – causal processes, treatment and prevention of the most important syndromes

Down's syndrome

Down's syndrome is a universally common cause of intellectual impairment. Most affected individuals are severely intellectually impaired, IQs being mostly within the range 20–55. About 94% are associated with trisomy 21, due to non-disjunction, for which prevalence at birth increases with maternal age: about 0.5/1000 at age 20; 1/1000 at 30; 2.5/1000 at 35; 10/1000 at 40; 40/1000 at 45; and > 150/1000 at 50. The most efficient strategy for prevention is to reduce births in older women, effected in many countries by the advent of the contraceptive pill. Family size may reduce after economic improvement, but major family planning programmes in poor countries have had limited success.

Foetal diagnosis by amniocentesis, followed by abortion, are available in some centres, usually only for older women. Pre-screening samples of maternal blood can now reduce amniocentesis and its attendant risks if restricted to older women, but if offered to all women will increase the total of amniocentesis procedures required. Moreover, the ethical issues must be faced for all women offered the blood test: are they willing to undergo abortion if the tests prove positive?

For some years, cytogenetic analysis has shown that in 75–85% of cases, Down's syndrome is of maternal origin, but recent DNA polymorphic analysis suggests that this may have to be revised to about 95%. Most non-disjunctions occur at the first meiotic division, during the mother's foetal life, remote from fertilisation, and not susceptible to intervention. The most favoured explanations of the increased incidence with maternal age rely on assumptions about aging gametes within the ovary. Those incidences of paternal origin could arise just prior to fertilisation; recent research suggests the possible relevance of occupational exposures to toxins, but we do not yet know enough to intervene. Non-disjunctions show mosaicism in 1–3% of cases, with a mixture of normal and abnormal cells and a variable picture of features, impairments and disabilities. This probably explains the rare reports of a person with Down's syndrome of normal intelligence and achievements. Three to 5% of Down's syndrome are familial, due to genetic translocation.

Down's children have increased vulnerability to infectious diseases, which must be treated vigorously; 25–40% have a serious heart defect, a major cause of early death. There was a 50% first-year mortality in Western European countries only 30–40 years ago, though now it is probably less than 10%. Mortality in many developing countries will still exceed 50%, but the situation is changing. Narayanan (1981) found many children but no adults with Down's syndrome in his village studies, probably reflecting improvements in survival. Hypothyroidism, leukaemia and diabetes are relatively common, and should be looked for clinically and treated early. Pre-senile dementia of Alzheimer type is common in those who reach middle age.

The typical features of Down's syndrome are recognisable in all races even at birth, though they may be missed by inexperienced people. The most obvious, especially in somewhat older children, are epicanthic folds over the eyes, a flattened upper nose, a narrowed cranium and a small mouth, often with a protruding tongue. Hands and fingers are short, with only one prominent skin crease. Chromosome diagnosis is generally not available in developing countries; its main benefit is to identify the rare familial cases for genetic counselling.

Early milestones may not be much delayed, but children gradually lose out compared with others during early school years. Many families find children with Down's syndrome warm and loving, and relatively easy to bring up. The most capable can learn basic self-care, limited reading and writing, and simple work, contributing to the community. Early intervention, continuing stimulation and education are important and may increase achievements at later ages. However, they will always be dependent upon others, and if their natural family breaks down, a substitute family will be needed.

Fragile X syndrome

Although the total prevalence at birth of this sex chromosome disorder is probably about 1/1000, and about 80% of affected boys have IQs below 70, a minority of boys, and virtually no girls are severely intellectually impaired.

About 30% of affected girls have mild intellectual impairment. Purely clinical diagnosis is not very reliable, but men with severe intellectual impairment show a variety of physical abnormalities, commonly including large testes and long ears. They may indulge in self-damaging behaviour such as hand biting, and show behavioural features similar to autism. The current debate on the possibilities and ethics of mass screening and counselling is unlikely to interest developing countries yet. However, it is a prominent feature of current research, and could be relevant in the future.

Inheritable metabolic disorders

Congenital hypothyroidism occurs sporadically in all countries (0.1–2.0/1000), unrelated to iodine deficiency, usually as a mutation. Thyroid failure leads to cretinism if not detected and treated with thyroxine before three months of age. Very early treatment (<1 month) will preserve the original intellectual potential in most children, but it is possible that irreversible brain damage sometimes occurs before birth. A simple blood spot screening test can be done soon after birth, but needs a laboratory for rapid analysis.

In most developed countries the test for hypothyroidism has taken advantage of the long established screening programme for phenylketonuria (0.05–0.2/1000 births) and several other very rare enzyme disorders. In these, a defective gene leads to an enzyme deficiency and accumulation of toxic by-products from normal constitutents of diet, resulting in progressive brain damage and severe intellectual impairment. If identified soon after birth, a special diet can prevent serious damage and allow children to develop with a normal range of intelligence. The diet is not easy to obtain or take, must be continued at least into late childhood, and reinstated during pregnancy.

Some developing countries with good laboratories and primary health care systems, or where most births are in hospital, have instituted screening programmes. In developed countries it is demonstrably cost beneficial, but this may not be true in developing countries with different economies and different expectations for severely retarded children.

Recessive genetic abnormalities in general

Specific syndromes are rare, but collectively they are important. Physical anomalies often predominate and may be susceptible to surgical correction. There may be any degree of intellectual impairment or none. They are thought to be mostly mutations but in communities which exhibit a high degree of consanguinity, a substantial proportion may be familial. Consanguinity may be an intrinsic part of the culture, such as some communities in South India, or a product of geographical isolation (e.g. remote mountain or island communities), social isolation (e.g. elite groups or those marginalised by poverty), or cultural isolation (e.g. immigrant groups).

Isolation is rapidly diminishing in a world of all-pervading communications, development and mass migration, but long traditions of behaviour are not easily changed. In small, poor communities, adults with abnormalities may reproduce because there is little choice of partners; education may have little effect without socioeconomic development and wider inter-community contacts.

Because of the frequency of mutations, the avoidance of mutagenic factors in the environment could be important, especially in developing countries where protection of industrial workers and communities from chemical or radiation exposure is often inadequate. Pressure needs to be brought on employers, national and international, to improve protection to acceptable levels.

Neural tube defects

Neural tube defects (NDTs) may sometimes be associated with mental retardation. They show a notable geographical variation in incidence in many countries, and folate deficiency as a dietary aetiological factor is now established. Any supplement is required before conception, as damage is done before pregnancy. It is, therefore, feasible to prevent NDTs in second and subsequent babies, the risk being much higher after one NDT. Large scale studies are underway in Northern China and Hungary to see if incidence rates can be reduced for a whole community by changes in diet or specific folate supplementation, and official recommendations towards this have recently been published in the UK (Expert Advisory Group, 1992). Supplementation is cheap and easy to administer, so this could have important implications even for relatively poor communities at high risk.

Foetal alcohol syndrome

High incidence of this syndrome has been demonstrated in some communities, for example native Americans on 'reserves' with seriously prejudiced cultures and lack of employment and purpose. There are few good population studies in other developing communities, but there can be little doubt that it can occur both in identifiable subgroups and deviant individuals. It is not yet certain what dose of alcohol represents a calculable risk, and the best advice is still to avoid alcohol during pregnancy.

Iodine deficiency disorders (IDD)

Iodine deficiency is the commonest worldwide cause of mental retardation. Iodine is essential for the production of thyroxine, without which metabolism is slowed, and growth and development inhibited. Adults obtain the 150 micrograms a day they need mostly from water, but in many upland areas iodine has been leached from the soil and is insufficient. Children develop goitres and varying degrees of growth retardation, at worst frank 'cretinism'. More than 10% of a population can be affected. Variation in individual response is not understood, though other minerals in soils, goitrogenic toxins in food, and genetic factors may all have a part to play. Vast populations are at risk; possibly 400 million in China, 200 million in India, and many in other Himalayan, Asian, South American and African countries (*Lancet*, 1986). A WHO report estimated 6 million people with cretinism in the South East Asian region alone (WHO, 1985). This does not include China.

Endemic congenital hypothyroidism (cretinism) shows a variety of features which may appear in any degree and combination, especially severe intellectual impairment, stunting, hearing and speech deficits, and neuromuscular disorders.

The severest, neurological form comprises severe intellectual impairment, deaf-mutism, strabismus and spastic diplegia. Prevention is the only really effective intervention. Treatment generally produces no clinical or intellectual improvement, although rehabilitation can improve quality of life.

Prevention is technically simple and very cheap, but is not always logistically or culturally easy to introduce and maintain (Hetzel, 1989). To introduce iodine, preferably iodates for stability, into the diet of the whole community, the commonest vehicle is salt, used by everyone throughout the year. When the number of sources is limited, supplies can be controlled at costs around US$20–40/1000 people/year (1988). However, poor quality control, distribution delays, lack of acceptance and presence of alternative sources threaten the effectiveness of many programmes.

More recently, injections of iodised oil have been used. This is logistically more demanding and expensive, but is more certain, and is especially suitable for remote communities. One injection can be effective for several years, there are few side-effects, and no cold chain (maintenance of refrigeration in transit, as for many vaccines) is required. Oral iodised oil is also effective; it enters body fat stores from which iodine is slowly released. There is less experience yet but it is likely to be practicable on a one to three yearly basis depending upon circumstances (Hetzel, 1989). A few cases of drinking water supplementation have been successful. Bread and common sauces have occasionally been used, and in some communities oral potassium iodide tablets may be appropriate.

Most programmes serve whole communities, but oil may be targeted on women of reproductive age, including those who are pregnant, and children. However, it is important to include men whose improved productivity and quality of life will help persuade communities to accept it. Iodised oil is better avoided in those over 45 because of a risk of precipitating hyperthyroidism.

The prevention of iodine deficiency needs political and professional will for success. Every country with IDD should have a firm campaign to eradicate it. It will, of course, be a generation before cretinism disappears from a community, but very few years will bring tangible benefits, and in the long run, a successful programme will pay off abundantly.

General nutrition

Although many have asserted that gross maternal or early infant under-nutrition can damage the central nervous system and cause irreversible intellectual deterioration, this is not supported by the evidence. The known pattern of early brain development offers ready explanation of both foetal and infant protection. The second period of brain growth, from 20 weeks of foetal life to two years of postnatal life, permits repair of any spongioblast damage up to that age (Stein *et al*, 1975; Dobbing, 1984; Fryers, 1990).

It is likely, however, that generalised malnutrition contributes to increased foetal and infant vulnerability to other damaging factors such as communicable diseases. It may also contribute significantly to poor intellectual performance and consequent delayed development from which recovery is possible with a good diet. This issue may be especially important in developing countries, and was well addressed by Clarke & Clarke (1981). In some communities, especially during conditions of war, famine and epidemic disease, there are children who experience severe prolonged malnutrition and grossly deviant social rearing, and who may present as mentally retarded but have the capacity to recover normal mental and social function.

It is very important to identify such children and treat them with food, stimulation and care. This is not always easy; children may be assumed to be permanently retarded, especially if in orphanages or other institutions without informed professional supervision. Most permanently retarded children can also develop far more than most professionals expect, with appropriate help. The important lesson is that all retarded children should be given good physical, mental and emotional care from the earliest age possible, to maximise their potential and minimise their dependence. Signs of unexpected progress should be actively re-investigated.

Perinatal factors

The birth process is a hazardous experience. During the perinatal period, a baby may experience anoxia, hypoglycaemia, thrombosis or trauma, but we rarely know its fitness for birth or the mother's preparedness for delivery. Many factors vary with the mother's age, parity, health and nutritional state. If a mother's nutrition as a child has restricted the growth of her pelvis, the baby is prejudiced, especially if well nourished itself. Improvements in communities may take a generation to work through to safer childbirth.

Perinatal brain trauma may lead to physical impairment such as cerebral palsy and epilepsy, as well as intellectual impairment, but many cases, particularly of cerebral palsy, previously attributed to the perinatal period on circumstantial clinical evidence, are now thought to arise earlier in pregnancy. Similar syndromes may also arise in infancy from meningitis and encephalitis. The relationship between healthy survival, damaged survival and death is dynamic. Communities with poor maternal nutrition and inadequate health care are also likely to have high perinatal and infant mortality. Where many babies are damaged, many also die. If conditions improve, fewer babies may be damaged but fewer damaged infants may die, so that prevalence in the community at subsequent ages will not necessarily be lower until mortality and morbidity in both the perinatal period and the first year of life are extremely low, as now in many European countries.

Although the scientific evidence is hard to evaluate, perinatal factors are undoubtedly important causes of intellectual impairment, cerebral palsy, epilepsy and mortality; all may be reduced in frequency by effective antenatal and obstetric care. This may mean increasing access to care, improving nutritional state, training traditional birth attendants, providing professional midwives, and building up the primary health care system. Where cerebral palsy and epilepsy occur, children need medical assessment, treatment and supervision to minimise the physical disabilities so that optimal development of intellectual abilities, of whatever level, can be promoted.

Communicable disease

Damage to the foetal or infant brain may arise occasionally in many infections, though relating the damage to the infection may not be easy. Table 12.6 lists the

TABLE 12.6
Principle infectious agents causing mental retardation

Intra-uterine	Postnatal[1]
Cytomegalovirus (CMV)	Bacterial meningitides
Rubella	Pneumococcal
Varicella zoster	Meningococcal
Herpes simplex	Tuberculosis
Listeriosis	*H. influenzae*
Syphilis	*B. pertussis*
Toxoplasmosis	Viral encephalitides
Malaria	Herpes simplex
Trypanosomiasis	Measles
Cysticercosis	Varicella
Cryptococcosis	Mumps
	Rubella
	Arboviruses A & B
	ECHO viruses
Perinatal	Coxsackie A & B
	Parasitic infections
Group B Streptococci	Malaria
Escherichia coli	Trypanosomiasis
Enteroviral infections	Cysticercosis
Herpes simplex	Cryptococcosis
Other gram -ve organisms	

1. Postnatal infection can trigger several different mechanisms to provoke brain damage, and some are better described as reactive encephalopathies rather than direct encephalitides. (After Dudgeon *et al*, 1985.)

main infections (Dudgeon *et al*, 1985). Endemic and epidemic variation precludes even guideline incidence rates, but if a particular disease is very prevalent, especially in a poor community, it is reasonable to assume that there are risks, especially of meningitis and encephalitis. Some regions, particularly in Africa, have especially high rates of meningitis.

Cytomegalovirus (CMV) is common, and may cause more damage, including intellectual impairment and deafness, than generally realised, but there are as yet no specific means of prevention. Rubella syndrome, preventable by immunisation, and congenital syphilis, preventable by early diagnosis and treatment, are better recognised, though intellectual impairment is rare. There is great hope for the future for widespread immunisation against meningitis and encephalitis of bacterial origin after the successful introduction of a new vaccine for meningitis caused by *Haemophylus influenzae* (type b). Bacterial meningitis may be susceptible to appropriate chemotherapy. Encephalitis from any cause during infancy carries a much higher risk of brain damage than in older children, and careful clinical handling may both determine individual outcome and prevent secondary cases. Cerebral palsy and epilepsy may also result.

Toxoplasma gondii is a common protozoal infection spread from animal faeces or inadequately cooked meat. Foetal infection is well established, but signs may appear late and are very variable, including any degree of intellectual impairment. Antibiotic treatment in pregnancy may help, but prevention relies on good hygiene. Risks are very difficult to calculate with confidence; the current situation has been well reviewed recently (MDWG, 1992). Malaria is an important factor increasing vulnerability to other infections, and may sometimes cause damage itself *in utero* or following cerebral malaria in infancy.

Prevention largely depends upon good public health measures, including control of water supplies and waste water treatment, control of vectors, general hygiene, case isolation, early diagnosis and effective treatment, and improved resistance through good nutrition. The most important direct means of control of communicable disease is immunisation. Although individual protection is valuable, it is far more effective to achieve herd immunity (levels of immunity in a population sufficient to inhibit passage of the infective agent) with immunisation rates of at least 90% and better 95% of the whole community, to restrict spread. The MMR vaccine, incorporating measles, mumps and rubella is very successful, but pertussis and tuberculosis are also important. Vaccine development is a very active field, and future developments – for example for other causes of meningitis – should be closely followed. The quality of primary health care will determine the effectiveness of immunisation and other preventive programmes.

Details are to be found in regularly updated handbooks of communicable diseases such as Benenson (1990).

Associated disorders

Certain disorders, though not an intrinsic part of mental retardation, however defined, are always prominent in groups of retarded people. Congenital abnormalities tend to occur together. Epilepsy and cerebral palsy commonly arise from the same aetiological process as intellectual impairment before, during or after birth. *Epilepsy* may be a specific component of tuberose sclerosis. Proportions inevitably vary with the way the retarded group is defined, and, presumably, with different social situations, but studies report epilepsy, mostly controllable with appropriate medication, in 20–50% of people with severe intellectual impairment (IQ < 50) (see also Chapter 11). *Cerebral palsy* is reported in 15–40% of those with severe intellectual impairment, serious visual problems in 10–30%, hearing problems in up to 5%, and serious problems with speech in 60–85%. There is no reason to expect substantially different ranges in developing countries, but we have few data.

Autistic syndromes may also be associated with intellectual impairment. Strictly defined autism probably only affects 2–4/10 000 of the child population in developed countries, 50–75% of which may be considered retarded. Autistic continuum disorders are more prevalent, and some, like Asperger's syndrome, are not associated with intellectual impairment.

There is little evidence of the situation in developing countries. Many studies have reported higher prevalence rates of psychiatric illness in those designated mentally retarded, but there are serious problems of interpretation when neither term is clearly or consistently defined. Non-psychotic disorder probably is common, related to brain disorder, experience of abnormal social and interpersonal environments or other impairments and disabilities commonly associated with mental retardation. Severely retarded people also tend to be subject to closer surveillance than the rest of the population, not least by psychiatrists, who thus have unusual opportunities to make diagnoses. The special status of such conditions, especially epilepsy, in different cultures must be recognised, and traditional explanations in terms of witchcraft, breaking of taboos, or contagion, for example, must be accommodated in service and treatment programmes (Giel, 1968; Orley, 1970; Lewis, 1975).

Behaviour disorders are not necessarily comparable phenomena in people with and without serious central nervous system impairment. On the other hand, anxiety and depression are almost certainly recognised less frequently than they should be in retarded individuals. About 1% of those called retarded may suffer from schizophrenia.

Problems arise not only on account of ambiguous definitions, but also because most of these associated disorders make examination, diagnosis and assessment more difficult. It should also be remembered that any concurrent disability, disease or deviant behaviour may render an individual more likely to be identified as 'retarded' by health workers, social workers, police or the courts. Although this is unlikely to affect the severely intellectually impaired group, where low intelligence is overtly a sufficiently serious problem alone to justify labelling, it will certainly affect the constitution of the mildly mentally retarded group, leading to substantial selectivity for all these disorders.

Identification and assessment of mentally retarded people

Mentally retarded children and adults may come to official attention in many ways. Where services for mothers, babies and young children are comprehensive, most should be identified through routine developmental examinations and/or mothers' observations. Even so, if there are no services available, professionals may fail to identify retarded children, deliberately or not, because there would seem to be no advantage in doing so, and parents may be unwilling to admit their anxieties, especially if it would mean exclusion from school. Only where primary schooling is widely available will retarded children be identified as 'drop outs' when they fail to meet standards. In most developing countries, obviously retarded children never start school.

Sometimes, the shame of bearing an obviously disabled child is so great that the child is hidden within the family, and officials may connive at non-recognition. In many communities the only services specifically for retarded children are organised by parents themselves, and theirs may be the only children identified. Screening programmes or surveys to identify unknown cases should only be undertaken if people identified can be offered some early tangible benefit (Fryers, 1986).

In developed countries many professionals share responsibility for assessment, treatment, rehabilitation and care: family doctors, paediatricians, psychiatrists, psychologists, nurses, social workers, teachers, physiotherapists, occupational therapists, speech therapists, and others. Each of these groups has its own professional orthodoxy and each has a range of conventional assessment techniques and instruments. In one sense all are important, but in developing countries most are rare and limited to urban centres. These professions may not perceive themselves as carrying any responsibilities in relation to mental retardation.

Parents may seek help from anyone who will listen to their problems. Health workers in primary care situations, teachers in local schools, and others should be trained in the recognition of mental retardation, in developmental and functional assessment, and in what can be done within the family and community. Where a psychiatrist or psychiatrically trained nurse or medical assistant is accessible, he or she is likely to be consulted about children and adults considered to be retarded. They should be familiar with a wide range of assessments, and trained in those needed to advise the family, promote appropriate activities, and refer to appropriate community facilities.

Assessment should not be used to exclude people from services, but as a starting point for action. It should include a careful description of a person's characteristics, strengths and weaknesses at a point in time, and a comparison of their performance with norms from a reference population, so as to predict or monitor progress. Assessment should include both formal testing and less structured observation in common environments. There are many scales, tests and checklists; some are suitable for population screening, others for individual assessment; Mittler's (1992) summary and annotation and Hogg & Raynes' (1987) critical review are both valuable. Few tests, however, are validated for developing country populations, and most must therefore be used with caution.

The 'Ten Questions' (TQ) test was piloted in ten countries and has proved useful in larger studies as a first level screen before professional examination (Belmont, 1984; Durkin *et al*, 1991; Stein *et al*, 1992). Although a 'coarse' screen, it is probably better than key informant methods (Durkin *et al*, 1990). Two recent books on disabled children in developing countries include practical guidance (Werner, 1987; Baine, 1988).

Physical impairments and concurrent illnesses are usually identified by medical examination, and thorough assessment of epilepsy, cerebral palsy and psychiatric illness should not be neglected. Standard protocols for diagnosis and assessment may be useful where fully trained doctors are not available. Unfortunately, doctors are generally poorly trained in the functional assessment of disabilities. The Disability Assessment Schedule (DAS; Holmes *et al*, 1983) provides short scales for self-care, mobility, speech and communication, seeing, hearing, problem behaviour, and social interaction. Detailed physical assessment is part of a very practical guide written for carers (Golding & Goldsmith, 1986).

Sensory assessment is important, as deafness and poor sight often prejudice the assessment of development and intelligence, but hearing tests need special equipment and training. It is also important to assess and emphasise abilities which represent positive resources for rehabilitation in the individual.

Intelligence tests giving Intelligence Quotients (IQs) can guide professionals on an individual's capacity especially for education, but few are standardised for specific non-industrialised populations. Their potential and problems are usefully discussed in Graham (1992). They are not independent of education, experience and culture, and should always be repeated, should include subscores and be accompanied by an interview report. There are shortened tests available for use by less trained workers. Development tests use age-related 'milestones' for young children (e.g. Gesell, Griffiths, Bayley), and checklists may be used to guide specific interventions as in the Portage system (see below). Serpell's (1993) comment (as a psychologist with a long experience in Africa) should be noted: "Given the key function of assessment as a guide to ameliorative action, most field workers in Africa find behaviour checklists to be much more useful instruments than intelligence tests".

Social adaptation is assessed to guide rehabilitation. There are several instruments. The American Adaptive Behaviour Scale examines personal independence and maladaptive behaviour, but is relatively complex, covering over 20 areas of social function such as self-direction, responsibility and socialisation. The Vineland Social Maturity Scale is simple but more used for research. The Progress Assessment Chart (Gunzberg, 1977) is successfully used in developing countries, providing a progressive visual record of mobility, self-care, practical skills, and communication. Others have been developed locally (e.g. Hughes, 1986, in Sri Lanka).

Handicaps, that is social disadvantages, can only be assessed in a specific cultural context, but it is often the handicaps which represent the greatest personal and family burdens and needs. An assessment might ask questions such as:

● What social roles should a person of this age and gender be fulfilling in this society?
● What social roles could this person be fulfilling even with his/her disabilities?
● What would help to increase independence now, and develop independence in the future?
● What activities would the person like to undertake in this particular social context?
● What activities would the family like him/her to share in this community?

Mentally retarded people in society

Mentally retarded people's human needs are primarily the same as other people's: love and parental care, family life, a range of relationships, and opportunities for valued activities. Like others, they need access to professional help – teachers, doctors and the like – but they may need more of it; for example; early stimulation, education and training, especially in self-care, practical literacy, social skills and vocational skills. They usually need extra encouragement and support in establishing and maintaining themselves in any aspect of normal community life.

The 'hierarchy of human needs' is a useful model (Fig. 12.1; Maslow, 1954). There is little value in aiming at upper levels of need if lower levels are not met, but the objective of services is to move progressively up the hierarchy toward self-realisation and full independence. In the planning of services, and their ethos in practice, a creative tension is required between pragmatic and idealistic objectives. Families must also be fully considered. They are usually the principal carers, and have substantial needs of their own. If families are not part of the service network, community-based care and rehabilitation may be impossible.

The common experience of retarded people in most societies is to be the subject of fear, ridicule and discrimination. Families feel shame and guilt, even

5. Self-
actualisation

4. Need for self-esteem

3. Social needs

2. Needs for safety and security

1. Basic physiological needs

Fig. 12.1. Hierarchy of human needs (After Maslow, 1954).

hiding their children and carrying the burdens alone. Conventional services often reflect and reinforce negative images and attitudes in society. Extreme examples have led to policies of elimination (the Nazis in Germany and the Khmer Rouge in Cambodia), but most countries have had examples of oppressive policies, providing minimal, grudging care, usually having people shut away in segregated, isolated institutions, sometimes in appalling and inhuman squalor.

Improvement of standards in conventional services are to be welcomed, but objectives must be changed to maximise development skills, and promote a satisfactory lifestyle, a range of relationships, integration into the community and participation in valued roles and activities. These processes are simplistically called 'normalisation' (see below). Only when retarded children and adults are accepted as part of society's everyday experience will stigma be seriously challenged, and their and their families rights to as fulfilling a life as lies within their capacity, begin to be realised.

Organisation of services for mentally retarded people

In the past, most developed countries built large, remote, residential institutions for retarded people, custodial in character, poorly resourced and hidden from public view. Over the last 25 years, most communities have been struggling to overcome this tragic inheritance, by developing humane, individualised, professional, community-based services with a rehabilitative orientation based on an 'ordinary life' model.

The same institutional model can be found in most developing countries, though usually on a smaller scale, and often combined with care for the destitute or mentally ill. However, almost everywhere, most retarded children and some adults are cared for at home by parents and families, and in some cultures, disabled children have always been accepted by the community, though technical assistance has rarely been available. Until recently, professionals and politicians have largely ignored the needs of retarded people and their families, and any initiative has often come from the parents themselves who have raised money and created organisations.

Throughout the world, the last decade has seen significant changes; the International Year of the Disabled Person, 1981, gave great encouragement to those campaigning for the ignored millions of disabled people in developing countries. Although situations vary greatly, the basic philosophy, principles and many elements of good practice are the same (Mittler & Serpell, 1985). There are two essentials: at the individual level, the objective of all services should be normalisation; at the organisational level services should be community-based.

Normalisation

The principles of *normalisation* (Table 12.7) declare that people designated as mentally retarded have the same human value as others and the same human rights. They are developing human beings with their own abilities, preferences and needs. They should be involved in decisions about their own lives wherever possible, should normally live with their own families or a substitute family, and should not be segregated from the rest of the community. The goals of all services should be to maximise independence, foster normal lifestyles and behaviour appropriate to age, gender and culture, and encourage the adoption of social roles and participation in community activities valued in their own culture. The principles apply to services for all individuals, though a very few with seriously challenging behaviour may defeat even the most imaginative and resourceful attempts to render their presence in the community meaningful.

These principles can be applied in all countries, though there will be many ways of achieving them, and different levels of resourcing. Developing countries must emphasise appropriate technology, though many developed communities could learn from them in this respect. Using locally available resources makes best use of scarce resources, but also ensures that something can be done for virtually all disabled people. It uses the experience and skills of local people who may know better how to achieve particular aims in rehabilitation than visiting professionals. Rehabilitation must be practical and realistic, yet those involved should not forget that both professionals and families have almost always underestimated the potential of retarded people in any situation.

TABLE 12.7
Principles of normalisation

Services should, as far as is possible, enable people to live *ordinary* lives by using means which are common, accepted and *valued* in their local community and culture.

Services should *enhance* the status of disabled people by both what they do and how they do it.

Services should acknowledge and respect disabled people as *individual* human beings with their own needs, preferences, abilities and social networks.

Services should work *with* disabled people, who retain, as far as possible, the initiative, choice and direction of their own habilitation and lives.

Disabled people should *not be segregated* from the rest of the community in housing, work, education or recreation.

Special services should be available to meet needs inadequately served by ordinary means; these should be local and accessible to all relevant clients in the community served.

Services should be *professional* in management and staffing, efficiently coordinated and subject to effective quality control.

Community-based services

Community-based services recognise that where clients live is where they have their natural networks of relationships, and that is where the focus of services should be, with distant and specialist resources in a supporting role. Conventional models of service provision are generally located in major centres, available only to urban or elite populations. They tend towards over-professionalisation, removing problems from the client, family and local community, emphasising technological solutions unavailable in local communities, and dependent upon specialists. They may also be segregated, stigmatising and prejudicial to successful rehabilitation in the client's home community. They are usually very expensive, and few countries can hope to provide for more than a tiny proportion of disabled people in this way. They are especially inappropriate to dispersed and rural communities.

Community-based rehabilitation

The alternative has become known as community-based rehabilitation (CBR). This is a comprehensive model; it considers community level to be the most important and the base of all services, but it encompasses all levels of provision, including secondary and specialist centres. The underlying motivation for CBR is the belief that most disabled people can be helped in their own community, by people in their own community, using locally available resources and simple, easily learnt techniques.

CBR aims to provide help appropriate to need and situation where the client and family can access it. The resources used are first those of the clients themselves; even severely retarded people usually have abilities, talents and qualities which can be nurtured, developed and used. The family is the main resource for many clients, which may need fostering, training and supporting. Other members of the community, including local professionals, can offer resources of great diversity and flexibility, often working through pre-existing community structures. Finally, specialists are needed, mostly to encourage, support, train and advise the others.

There is much in common between CBR and primary health care (PHC), but, sadly, there was no comprehension of the needs of disabled people in those who first promoted PHC, and early PHC literature largely ignored them. More recently there have been attempts to combine or link them (Kysela & Marfo, 1984).

In the last decade CBR projects have been set up in many developing countries, but most remain small scale, run by enthusiasts, often with foreign help. WHO, UNICEF, and other international agencies have sponsored many, some have been stimulated by governments, and others by local people. Thorough evaluation has proved difficult, but increasing experience is producing insights into the conditions for success (O'Toole, 1987). However, few have been able to expand to cover large populations, and few governments have programmed CBR on a large scale, though Mauritius is establishing a national programme, and Thailand is attempting to graft CBR onto a well organised national PHC system.

Not all CBR programmes encompass mentally retarded people, though many have done so successfully, and some have been solely concerned with them. In towns and cities, services tend to be developed piecemeal for specific client groups according to the interests and perceptions of those taking the initiative. Some countries make provision in government services, especially special schools or classes, but in many it is left to voluntary societies, often parents' societies, and development is likely to be *ad hoc*, pragmatic and opportunitist. In these situations, a CBR approach and overview may help to provide a rational structure for service development within which parents, professionals and government services can cooperate. But the elements of CBR are valid in their own terms, and can be promoted even without a comprehensive programme (WHO, 1985). Each major element in a programme should be monitored and evaluated with regard to effective fulfilment of objectives, satisfaction of clients, and efficiency of the service. Simple methods are most likely to be understood, accepted and undertaken systematically.

Elements of a comprehensive CBR programme

CBR materials

The WHO manual, *Training in the Community for People with Disabilities* (Helander *et al*, 1990) consists of many separate 'packages', to be copied and distributed to family members or local helpers as required, each one showing through simple pictures and text the procedures required for training a person with a particular defined disability. There are several 'packages' for people with learning disabilities, but many others, for example those concerned with mobility, seizures and 'strange behaviour', are also relevant. The book, *Disabled Village Children* (Werner, 1987) provides similar but wider advice in compact form which supplements the well established *Where There is no Doctor* (Werner, 1977).

These and many other publications also offer advice on how to design education and training programmes, and make simple aids using local resources: educational toys and games, walking aids from sticks to wheelchairs, physiotherapy aids, special furniture, and so on. Many aim to improve mobility and expand activities. Some provide instruction in particular techniques; for example, *A Manual of Appropriate Paper-based Technology* (Packer, 1989) and *Simple Aids for Daily Living* (Caston, 1989). A list of resources including books, pamphlets, periodicals, slide sets and videos, extensive but not comprehensive, is available from WHO (Fryers, 1989a). It includes a section on mental retardation. A practical journal, *CBR News* is available from AHRTAG, London. There is a great need for training videos; the medium is ideal for skills training in CBR, but few are available.

Educational and rehabilitation aids can often be made by family members in communities where skills are widespread, but there are usually local craftsmen who can, for example, make educational toys, adapt furniture or build wheelchairs. The publications above can work best by extending the repertory of ideas in the community, which can then be adapted to local materials and traditions. In many communities, workshops for disabled people have achieved this.

Support and training for parents, families and volunteers

The Portage system of home training for parents developed in the USA has been adapted and used in many countries (Thorburn, 1986; White & Cameron, 1988; Mariga & McConkey, 1989; Yamaguchi *et al*, 1990). It is currently being translated into Chinese. A home visitor, supported by a professional supervisor, assists parents in teaching their own children at home and in monitoring progress, using a package of materials including a development checklist, a Home Visitors' Manual, and an inventory of parent teaching behaviours. Portage acknowledges the educational role of parents, and supports and trains them in specific assessments and interventions. It may supplement or supplant special schooling, but it should not increase the parents' burden of responsibility without full professional support. CBR also places great emphasis on training parents, family members, or local volunteers to undertake education and rehabilitation programmes with individuals. In Zimbabwe, Zimcare have enrolled over 750 clients in a home-based teaching programme encompassing extensive training and independent evaluation (Mariga & McConkey, 1989). Recent mediation learning approaches to early intervention in Israel, Ethiopia and Nigeria are discussed by Serpell (1993).

Both support and training need a local CBR 'supervisor', who can be a local professional or a volunteer, but trained for the job, and equipped with a wide range of CBR materials. Training for supervisors (many titles are used, such as Community Rehabilitation Workers) has been varied and often *ad hoc*, but a number of courses are now available. A curriculum developed for Mauritius which might be a starting point for others, is now available from WHO (Fryers, 1989*b*). Volunteers are often parents or other relatives of disabled people, who bring a special experience and commitment.

A programme in the poorer quarters of Nairobi illustrates home training. Parents, or grandparents if parents were working, were taught, supervised and supported by trained school-leaver volunteers in a programme of assessment and step by step education. Families met weekly in a local centre to share problems and experiences and provide mutual support. This programme, starting as a small scale outreach from a local school, has faced the important question of 'going to scale' (Arnold, 1984). Similar programmes can be found in Sri Lanka, Nepal, Madagascar, Philippines, Guyana, Jamaica, Belize and elsewhere, sometimes also with access to specialist advice and specialist centres.

Parents' societies are always very important, and their formation and work should be positively encouraged. Help is available from the International League (Mittler, 1984). Even a small local group of families can sometimes achieve more than formal service organisations, as illustrated by Serpell (1993) from the Katete District in Zambia.

Living in your own home

Industrialised countries have had to rediscover the need and right of mentally retarded people to have their own homes. In developing countries those who survive have mostly lived at home, and the important issues are support for the family and daytime opportunities for education, work and leisure. In all communities children can lose parents, or families can break up; wherever possible the solution to such problems should adhere to the 'ordinary life' model, providing a substitute family, preferably within the same community, and certainly within the same culture. How easy it is to arrange will vary with cultural factors, such as family structures and attitudes to retarded children.

It may be necessary to create substitute homes, with paid carers if funding can be found. They should be kept of family size, should use similar accommodation to normal families in the area, and should be part of the same network of support as real families. It has to be acknowledged, however, that a few children are extremely difficult to manage at home, especially in poor families in subsistence cultures or areas of urban deprivation. Sometimes, the only help available is a residential institution, distant for many. Most such institutions around the world have been ill-resourced, poorly staffed, forgotten and squalid, but they need not be.

For professionals, community services may be something to work towards; meanwhile the institution can usually be improved. Human decency, privacy, good food and clothing, and a pleasant physical environment make good first objectives. Opening up to the community, involvement of families and community workers such as teachers and therapists, and establishing rehabilitation programmes do not necessarily require a lot more resources. A good example is what one occupational therapist achieved in a large institution in Mauritius, forming a 'day centre' with skills training programmes, self-help programmes, and leisure activities. Residents learnt to make their own clothes, and thus gained individuality and self-respect. They created a positive, relaxed and collaborative environment and learnt skills which could eventually take them back into the community.

Special education

In many communities, obviously retarded children are not accepted into ordinary schools, where classes may be large, buildings, books and equipment may be inadequate, or where teachers have only basic training. Whatever the theoretical argument for integration into ordinary schools, in these circumstances most parents welcome a special school or class for retarded children, preferably with specially trained teachers. However, special schools have only a short history even in industrialised countries, many starting as parents' initiatives in borrowed premises and with volunteer untrained teachers only 20–30 years ago.

This continues to happen in other countries. In Sfax, Tunisia, several schools started in this way, but have gained recognition for secondment of teachers from government service, and funding for new buildings through which they have gradually professionalised. As a part way to integration, many communities have established special classes in ordinary schools. For example, in Hefei, Anhui Province, China, where there was no special education, six schools developed special classes in little over a year as part of a rehabilitation project. A training course for teachers was created by the university. More formally, several large secondary schools in Manila have wide ranging 'special education centres' including particularly bright children as well as those with learning difficulties. Each child participates in ordinary classes with other children or in special classes as appropriate. In the absence of alternatives, schools may take on an additional role of providing vocational training, as has the parents' society school in Mauritius (also see Gardner, 1984).

Whatever schooling is created, it is important that it is located within the culture of the community, and that parents are involved, for the home remains a primary locus of learning. Wherever possible, parents should be partners with teachers and children in coordinated individual programmes. In many communities, for the foreseeable future, some of the most demanding children will be considered inappropriate to all schools and centres provided locally. For such children there may be a distant specialist educational institution, particularly for autistic children, or the only hope of help may be through a home teaching programme for the parents.

Training and work for adults

Most adults aspire to work and those who are mildly intellectually impaired will often be found doing the simpler jobs in many societies. For those who are less able or have multiple disabilities, economic work is problematic. Although programmes may be delivered in the home, most clients are better served in local centres which can provide occupation, leisure, further education, vocational training, sheltered work, job placement and support (King's Fund, 1984).

Basic education may concentrate on living skills to facilitate independence, such as simple cooking and finding the way round the community. Training in general work skills can be extended into true vocational training aimed at specific jobs identified in the local community. Whatever the orientation of a particular centre, social and communication skills should be fostered, and opportunities for leisure activities, with training where required, should not be neglected. Whatever formal programmes are offered, it is essential that a satisfying social environment is provided.

Centres may provide one of these programmes or a mixture of several, and staff require a variety of skills. As well as training skills, technical expertise is required in vocational training and sheltered workshops; for example in breaking down tasks into many small elements, and designing special jigs for a simple operation. Vocational training should aim at practical skills and experience required in the local community, and assistance with job finding should go with it. Employers may be willing to offer jobs only if some supervision and support is offered in combination. Some countries offer subsidies to employers to accept less efficient workers; others have legal employment quotas for disabled workers in larger firms, but these are seldom effective, especially for severely retarded people.

Separate workshops for mentally retarded people are often necessary, although it is preferable that they occupy similar premises in similar areas to other workshops. They can earn substantial reputations for high quality goods, as in Sfax, Tunisia, where the emphasis of the Parents Association on quality of environment, training and product helps to reinforce positive images of retarded people, and gain them acceptance in wider society, without letting commercial opportunities threaten the broader needs of their retarded clients. For example, an agricultural centre on the edge of the town provides a satisfactory sheltered work environment for many retarded workers, and incorporates small cooperative enterprises with a mixture of disabled and non-disabled workers, operating at a profit. In Anhui, a 'welfare' workshop changed its management, invited non-disabled people to work there alongside disabled workers, becoming integrated, non-stigmatising, and profitable.

Work programmes at home can also be successful, with training, supervision, supplies and sales centralised. Income generation is vital in very poor communities, if families are to survive with the extra demands of a disabled member. The CBR programme in Bacolod, Philippines, helps clients to establish small scale projects at home, providing a little capital, training in necessary skills, and supporting them and their families through the CBR volunteers. Examples include duck keeping, pig rearing, knitting, and soft drinks sales.

Medical treatment and special therapy

Many severely retarded people live in poor communities with little access to medical treatment. Parents' associations often gain the voluntary support of local family doctors or specialists. Prompt treatment of illness, mental disorder and epilepsy are essential for successful rehabilitation. Western trained psychiatrists are rarely available to remote rural communities, but some countries have trained a specialist cadre of primary health care workers in psychiatry to work alongside their conventional colleagues.

Epilepsy is a common associate of intellectual impairment and should be treated as thoroughly as resources permit in order to minimise the inhibiting effect of seizures on learning performance and social acceptance. Diagnosis of specific psychiatric illness is prejudiced by low intelligence and disordered behaviour, but physical treatment for schizophrenic syndromes and depressive illnesses should not be withheld if it is clearly indicated and available.

In the treatment of behaviour disorders, drugs have shown little success, and behaviour therapy techniques predominate, which may be learned by parents to assist them in managing their children at home, if an experienced teacher–therapist is available. Aversion techniques are less favoured currently than positive reinforcement alternatives. Autistic syndromes are likely to be ameliorated only by highly structured teaching and behavioural programmes.

Forensic issues arise mainly in two ways, criminal activity and false confession. People of low intelligence may be easily led into crime by others, and may not readily grasp the social significance of their actions or perceive the likely consequences. Most crime is petty, but arson seems relatively favoured. Sex offences are not uncommon, probably because of lack of opportunities for legitimate sexual expression afforded to more intelligent people in most societies, as well as the other factors above. Behaviour therapy may help, together with attention to social situation, lifestyle, opportunities for other sources of satisfaction, and, if necessary, a degree of social control in the community. False confession has become an issue in developed countries and probably occurs everywhere; intellectually impaired people may not understand the significance of questions, and may be over-anxious to please by giving the perceived desired answer. Health professionals need to educate police and courts and be aware of this issue if any clients are under accusation.

Many severely retarded people need help to improve bodily function in various ways. Physiotherapy can help to establish a more normal lifestyle and avoid serious problems in later life (Hardinge & Wilson, 1981; Golding & Goldsmith, 1986). In particular, the special needs of children with cerebral palsy should not be forgotten. Occupational therapy can direct many of the activities described above to therapeutic ends, their training being especially in relating the abilities and disabilities of clients to their specific social situation, and working with them to effect changes in living environments or life opportunities. Speech therapy, however desirable, is rarely available; training needs to be in the language of the clients. If available, these therapists may work best through teachers, supervisors, nurses, or family members, by training them in specific exercises activities.

Individual Programme Plan (IPP)

In recent years, individual plans based on systematic assessment, agreed with client, family and care staff, written down and monitored, have been widely adopted (Table 12.8). The idea draws elements from the 'nursing process', management 'goal setting', behaviour therapy, and task centred social work traditions, and assumes a developmental approach, asserting that even the most severely retarded person has potential for development.

An IPP system can be particularly helpful in coordinating the various elements of a CBR programme around the needs of individuals. It can be a simple process, but it fosters discipline in assessment and programming activities, and is especially needed where several staff members or centres serve one client. After assessment, precise short- and medium-term goals are agreed, trying to

TABLE 12.8
Individual programme planning

Features

Written assessments of an individual's developmental status, strengths, weaknesses, and needs.
In a structured format, through a structured process.
In consultation with the disabled person and others significant in his/her life.
Specifying agreed short- and long-term goals.
The means by which they will be tackled.
Who is responsible for action.
How performance will be monitored.
Identifying service deficiencies which prevent or restrict achievement of goals.

Strengths

Is an effective way of coordinating action by several people, facilities or agencies.
Promotes a view (and assessment) of the disabled person and his/her life as a whole.
Encourages a positive approach by emphasising strengths and realisable goals.
Encourages an individual approach to care and rehabilitation – a 'needs lead' service.
Ensures a strong voice for the 'consumer'.
Assigns clear accountability for action.
Helps those involved to recognise and measure progress.
Fosters an imaginative response to individual need.
Provides aggregated information on service deficiencies.

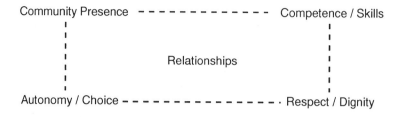

Fig. 12.2. *Framework of accomplishments for human services (After O'Brien & Tyne, 1982).*

build on positive qualities and abilities, then the steps and tasks by which these objectives will be reached, and the people responsible for each one.

Supervisory staff have an important role in managing regular review and updating, and defining the long-term goals. The *Framework of Accomplishments for Human Services* (Fig. 12.2; O'Brien & Tyne, 1981) offers a model with a strong philosophical base, but relationships, community presence, competencies, autonomy and respect are truly fundamental and should be considered within each particular cultural context. More pragmatic, and also useful, are checklists of 'needs', which ensure that important elements in a programme are not missed (Table 12.9).

Specialists and specialist centres

There is no doubt of the need for specialists within a CBR system to provide technical expertise, training and consultation for workers in the community (Serpell, 1986). The relationships are important. Specialists should be seen to support the community work through these activities, and this usually means being willing sometimes to travel to communities, and not be confined to a major centre. This is not easy. Specialists will almost always have higher status, salary and travel costs, but it is usually far harder for low paid community workers to travel.

Some balance must be maintained, and it is attitudes which matter most. Specialists must accept a teaching role, sharing their skills, as appropriate, with

TABLE 12.9
A needs check-list

1. Health/hygiene.
2. Physical appearance.
3. Social relations and contacts.
4. Activities and occupation.
5. Involvement in the community.
6. Self-care.
7. Domestic skills.
8. Daily living skills.
9. Communication.
10. Social adjustment.
11. Personal relationships.
12. Physical development.
13. Creative activities and spiritual life.

community workers. Teaching skills are important. Specialists should not usually take cases over, but should advise, guide and supervise as required. However, there will be some cases where it is appropriate to assess, treat or train in a specialist centre, for example people with concurrent mental illness, or severe challenging behaviour susceptible to therapy.

In towns, special training programmes can be in day centres, but for people in dispersed community settings residential training centres may be necessary to teach braille reading for the blind, manual communication for the deaf, and specific vocational skills for the mentally retarded people. They should offer discreet, time-limited programmes – like colleges for other students – and remember that rehabilitation can only be completed in the individuals' own community.

Training for CBR

Clearly there are many training issues implied by the needs and programmes described above, and few can be addressed here. Specialist centres offer distinct advantages and opportunities for formal training in technical aspects of rehabilitation and should be used wherever they are available. However, the principal locus of training for work in the community should be in the community. In Mauritius, there has been parallel development of CBR programmes in villages and training of community rehabilitation workers, though it is not easy for them to keep pace with each other (Fryers, 1989*b*). Training of workers should be as much as possible by clients – disabled people and their families are the most important teachers. Knowledge and skills are important, but attitudes at least equally so, so that selection may be as important as training. This is true whether rehabilitation is the responsibility of specific workers or that of certain community health, education or welfare staff already working in the community.

Community workers tend to be isolated in their daily work and need close support. A system of supervision and continuing training is essential if workers are to be retained for long. They must also have decent rates of pay, and recognition as professionals not inferior to hospital- and school-based staff. They also need a career structure: it must be possible for some to progress to supervisory and leadership posts, or they will remain a low status cadre. The corollary of this is that supervisors and eventually other senior staff should be required to have experience of working in community rehabilitation before gaining more senior posts.

Recommendations, with an outline curriculum, for training mid-level workers have recently appeared (WHO, 1992) which emphasise problem-solving approaches which are also appropriate to community workers. There is also a need for a close working relationship, whether within line management or not, between these generic rehabilitation workers and the various specialist therapists which may or may not be available in developing communities. Speech therapists, teachers of the deaf, physiotherapists and occupational therapists can be invaluable in both initial and continuing training, as well as recipients of referrals for more specialised treatment. But also, those therapists will benefit from the knowledge and experience of the community workers who see all disabled people and their families and social situations, not just the more complex cases in a specialist centre. In many CBR programmes, occupational therapists in particular have been prominent in encouraging, supporting and training.

Summary

An effective CBR programme would have community level programmes for individual retarded people and their families run by local rehabilitation workers and supervisors. Special school facilities and day centres would offer a variety of training, sheltered work and leisure opportunities. Specialist professionals from health centres, hospitals, colleges, and social welfare agencies would support the programmes with guidance, staff training and consultation, and provide access for occasional individuals to treatment or training in appropriate specialist centres. This model can be applied at many different levels of resourcing, but it always requires a certain level of infrastructure, organisational coordination, and professional and political commitment.

References and additional reading

AHRTAG (Periodical) *CBR News*. London: AHRTAG.

AMERICAN PSYCHIATRIC ASSOCIATION (1980) *Diagnostic and Statistical Manual of Mental Disorders* (3rd edn) (DSM–III). Washington, DC: APA.

ARNOLD, C. (1984) *Family/Parent Support Programmes – the Community Based Approach*. Nairobi: Action Aid.

BAINE, D. (1988) *Handicapped Children in Developing Countries*. Edmonton, Canada: Faculty of Education.

*BELMONT, L. (1981) Severe mental retardation across the world; epidemiological studies. *International Journal of Mental Health*, **10**.

—— (1984) *International Epidemiological Studies of Childhood Disability: Final Report*. Utrecht: Bishopp Becker Institute.

BENENSON, A. S. (ed.) (1990) *Control of Communicable Disease in Man* (15th edn). Washington: American Public Health Association.

CASTON, D. (1989) *Simple Aids for Daily Living*. London: ARHTAG.

CLARKE, A. M. & CLARKE, A. D. B. (1981) Problems of applying behavioural measures in assessing the incidence and prevalence of mental retardation in developing countries. *International Journal of Mental Health*, **10**, 76–84.

*——, —— & BERG, J. M. (eds) (1985) *Mental Deficiency: The Changing Outlook* (4th edn). London: Methuen.

*DOBBING, J. (ed.) (1984) *Scientific Studies in Mental Retardation*. London: Royal Society of Medicine/ Macmillan.

DUDGEON, J. A., PECKHAM, C. S., ROBINSON, R. O. (1985) Infectious agents in the aetiology of mental retardation (and commentary). In *Scientific Studies in Mental Retardation* (ed. J. Dobbing), pp. 203–232. London: Royal Society of Medicine/Macmillan.

DURKIN, M., DAVIDSON, L., HASAN, M., *et al* (1990) Screening for childhood disabilities in community settings. In *Practical Approaches to Childhood Disability in Developing Countries* (eds M. Thorburn & K. Marfo), pp. 179–197. Newfoundland: St. Johns.

——, ZAMAN, S., THORBURN, M., *et al* (1991) Population-based studies of childhood disability in developing countries. *International Journal of Mental Health*, **20**, 47–60.

EXPERT ADVISORY GROUP (1992) *Folic Acid and the Prevention of Neural Tube Defects*. London: Department of Health.

FRYERS, T. (1984a) *The Epidemiology of Severe Intellectual Impairment: The Dynamics of Prevalence*. London: Academic Press.

—— (1984b) Severe intellectual impairment in the developing world (Chapter 14). In *The Epidemi-

ology of Severe Intellectual Impairment: The Dynamics of Prevalence (T. Fryers), pp. 190–202. London: Academic Press.

——— (1986) Screening for developmental disabilities in developing countries: problems and perspectives. In *Childhood Disability in Developing Countries: Issues in Habilitation and Special Education* (eds K. Marfo, S. Walker & B. Charles), pp. 27–40. New York: Praeger.

——— (1989*a*) *List of Resources for Training Community Rehabilitation Workers.* Geneva: Rehabilitation Office WHO.

——— (1989*b*) *A Curriculum for Community Rehabilitation Workers,* Geneva: Rehabilitation Office WHO.

*——— (1990) Pre- and perinatal factors in the aetiology of mental retardation. In *Reproductive and Perinatal Epidemiology* (ed. M. Kiely). Florida: CRC Press.

*——— (1991) Public health approaches to mental retardation: handicap due to intellectual impairment. In *Oxford Textbook of Public Health* (2nd edn) (eds W. W. Holland, R. Detels & E. G. Knox), pp. 485–508. Oxford: OUP.

——— (1993) Epidemiological thinking in mental retardation: issues in taxonomy and population frequency. *International Review of Research in Mental Retardation,* **19**, 97–133.

GARDNER, R. (ed.) (1984) *Meeting Special Educational Needs in Developing Countries.* London: Institute of Education.

GIEL, R. (1968) The epileptic outcast. *East African Medical Journal,* **45**, 27–31.

GOLDING, R. & GOLDSMITH, L. (1986) *The Caring Person's Guide to Handling the Severely Multiply Handicapped.* London: Macmillan.

GRAHAM, P. & LANSDOWN, R. (1992) The uses and abuses of psychological tests in childhood. In *Assessment of People with Mental Retardation.* Geneva: World Health Organization.

GUNZBERG, H. C. (1977) *Progress Assessment Charts.* London: Royal MENCAP.

HARDINGE, E. & WILSON, P. (1981) *A Manual of Basic Physiotherapy for the Use of Nurses in Rural Hospitals.* London: Tear Fund.

HELANDER, E., NELSON, G., MENDIS, P., *et al* (1990) *Training in the Community for People with Disabilities.* Geneva: WHO.

HERON, A. & MYERS, M. (1983) *Intellectual Impairment: The Battle Against Handicap.* London: Academic Press.

HETZEL, B. S. (1989) *The Story of Iodine Deficiency.* Oxford: OUP.

HOGG, J. & RAYNES, N. (eds) (1987) *Assessment in Mental Handicap: A Guide to Assessment Practices, Tests and Checklists.* London: Croom Helm.

HOLMES, N., SHAH, A., WING, L. (1982) The Disability Assessment Schedule; A brief device for use with the mentally retarded. *Psychological Medicine,* **12**, 879–890.

HUGHES, J. M. (1986) The design of a basic assessment chart for use with the mentally retarded in Sri Lanka. In *Childhood Disability in Developing Countries: Issues in Habilitation and Special Education* (eds K. Marfo, S. Walker & B. Charles), pp. 147–164. New York: Praeger.

*KIELY, M. (ed.) (1990) *Reproductive and Perinatal Epidemiology.* Florida: CRC Press.

KING'S FUND (1984) *An Ordinary Working Life.* London: King's Fund.

KYSELA, G. & MARFO, K. (1984) Early handicapping conditions: detection and intervention in developing countries. In *Perspectives and Progress in Mental Retardation* (ed. J. Berg). Baltimore: University Park Press.

LANCET (1986) Prevention and control of iodine deficiency disorders. *Lancet,* **327**, 433–434.

LEWIS, D. (1975) *Knowledge of Illness in a Sepic Society.* LSE Monograph, 52. London: Athlone.

*MARFO, K., WALKER, S. & CHARLES, B. (eds) (1986) *Childhood Disability in Developing Countries: Issues in Habilitation and Special Education.* New York: Praeger.

MARIGA, L. & McCONKEY, R. (1987) Home based learning programmes for mentally handicapped people in rural areas if Zimbabwe. *International Journal of Rehabilitation Research,* **10**, 175–183.

MASLOW, K. (1954) *Motivation and Personality.* London: Harper and Row.

MILES, C. (1986) *Special Education for Mentally Handicapped Pupils: A Teaching Manual based on Experience in North West Frontier Province, Pakistan.* Peshawar: Mental Health Centre.

MITTLER, P. (1984) *What is the International League of Societies for Persons with Mental Handicap.* Brussels: ILSMH.

——— (1992) Assessing people with mental retardation; an overview. In *Assessment of People with Mental Retardation.* Geneva: World Health Organization.

*——— & SERPELL, R. (1985) Services: an international perspective. In *Mental Deficiency: The Changing Outlook* (4th edn) (eds A. M. Clarke, A. D. B. Clarke & J. M. Berg), pp. 715–787. London: Methuen.

MDWG (Multi-Disciplinary Working Group) (1992) *Pre-natal Screening for Toxoplasmosis in the UK*. London: Royal College of Obstetricians and Gynaecologists.

NABUZOKA, D. (ed.) (1986) *Reaching Disabled Children in Zambia*. Lusaka: University of Zambia Institute of African Studies.

NARAYANAN, H. S. (1981) A study of prevalence of mental retardation in Southern India. *International Journal of Mental Health*. **10**, 28–36.

O'BRIEN, J. & TYNE, A. (1981) *The Principle of Normalisation; A Foundation for Effective Services*. London: Campaign for Persons with Mental Handicap.

ORLEY, J. H. (1970) *Culture and Mental Illness*. Kampala: Makerere Institute of Social Research.

O'TOOLE, B. (1987) Community-based rehabilitation (CBR): problems and possibilities. *European Journal of Special Needs Education*, **2**, 177–190.

PACKER, B. (1989) *A Manual of Appropriate Paper-based Technology*. Harare: IRED.

SAUNDERS, C. A. (1982) The epidemiology of handicap in the child population of Plateau State. In *The Developing Child; a Nigerian Perspective* (ed. V. Curran). London: Routledge.

SERPELL, R. (1986) Specialised centres and the local home community; children with disabilities need them both. *International Journal of Special Education*, **1**, 107–127.

——, MARIGA, L. & HARVEY, K. (1993) Mental retardation in African countries: conceptualisation, services and research. *International Review of Research in Mental Retardation*, **19**, 1–40.

STEIN, Z., DURKIN, M., DAVIDSON, L., *et al* (1992) Guidelines for identifying children with mental retardation in community settings. In *Assessment of People with Mental Retardation*. Geneva: World Health Organization.

TAO KUO-TAI (1988) Mentally retarded persons in The People's Republic of China: a review of epidemiological studies and services. *American Journal of Mental Retardation*, **93**, 193–199.

—— (1990) *Report of National Collaborative Study on The Prevention, of Mental Retardation in the People's Republic of China*. English version from Manila, Regional Office for the Western Pacific, WHO.

THORBURN, M. J. (1986) Early intervention for disabled children in the Caribbean. In *Childhood Disability in Developing Countries: Issues in Habilitation and Special Education* (eds K. Marfo, S. Walker & B. Charles). New York: Praeger.

TOWELL, D. (1988) *An Ordinary Life in Practice*. London: King's Fund.

WERNER, D. (1977) *Where There is no Doctor*. Palo Alto, Hesperian Foundation (TALC edition). London: Institute of Child Health.

—— & BOWER, B. (1982) *Helping Health Workers Learn*. Palo Alto, Hesperian Foundation (TALC edition). London: Institute of Child Health.

—— (1987) *Disabled Village Children*. Palo Alto, Hesparian Foundation (TALC edition). London: Institute of Child Health.

WHITE, M. & CAMERON, S. (eds) (1988) *Portage: Progress, Problems and Possibilities*. Windsor: NFER-Nelson.

WORLD HEALTH ORGANIZATION (1978) *Mental Disorders: Glossary and Guide to their Classification in Accordance with the Ninth Revision of the International Classification of Diseases*. Geneva: WHO.

—— (1980) *International Classification of Impairments, Disabilities and Handicaps*. Geneva: World Health Organization.

—— (1985) *Iodine-Deficiency Disorders in South-East Asia*. SEARO Regional Health Papers 10. New Delhi: WHO.

*—— (1986) *Mental Retardation: Meeting the Challenge*. Offset Report 86. Geneva: WHO.

—— (1987) *The Community Health Worker: Working Guide; Guidelines for Training; Guidelines for Adaptation*. Geneva: WHO.

—— (1992) *The Education of Mid-Level Rehabilitation Workers; Recommendations from Country Experiences*. Geneva: WHO.

YAMAGUCHI, K., SHIMIZU, N., DOBOSHI, T., *et al* (1990) *A Challenge to Potentiality: Vision of Early Intervention for Developmentally Delayed Children*. Proceedings of International Portage Conference. Tokyo, 1988. Tokyo: Japan Portage Society.

ZAMAN, S. S., KHAN, N. Z., ISLAM, S., *et al* (1990) Validity of the 'Ten Questions' for screening serious childhood disability; results from urban Bangladesh. *International Journal of Epidemiology*, **19**, 613–620.

*Denotes a general review of epidemiological literature, or a book containing a wide range of relevant material.

13 Anxiety and anxiety related disorders

R. GIEL

Anxiety is such a common emotional state or trait that its pathological manifestation has received less explicit attention in the epidemiological and transcultural psychiatric literature than, for example, the affective state of depression. DSM–III (American Psychiatric Association, 1981) has played a major role in recent attempts to research the field, because of its specification of diagnostic criteria. ICD–10 (World Health Organization, 1992) has also contributed for similar reasons of definition. In this chapter data regarding the prevalence of anxiety and related disorders will be presented, and the classification and transcultural manifestation of this group of disorders will be discussed.

Pathological anxiety does not differ in any essential way from ordinary anxiety. It tends to be more severe, more incapacitating, less easily put aside, and it is initially often experienced as life-threatening. In addition, if it is not free-floating and diffuse but instead associated with objects or situations, it tends to be disproportionate to that object or situation. A state of panic implies such acute and overwhelming anxiety that the victim can no longer contain him- or herself and has to do something to rid himself of the unpleasant emotional state and the concomitant physical arousal. Phobias involve fear of objects or situations that are commonly not fearsome, but nevertheless do not fail to frighten the person, leading to avoidance of the situation or object.

At this point it is important to note that anxiety is just as much a state of physical arousal, with all kinds of vegetative signs, as it is a frame of mind. Anxiety can also be considered a cognitive state, because the person first recognises and then is affected by his own state of bodily excitation. Culture and social environment are likely to influence perception of the meaning of what goes on inside the body. This aspect of anxiety will be discussed later on in this chapter.

Prevalence of anxiety

We have to look towards the Western world for more solid data on the prevalence of anxiety disorders. The results depend on which level in the pathway to care is studied:

a) The general population, nowadays, is examined with the help of a structured interview, such as the Diagnostic Interview Schedule (Robins & Regier, 1991).

291

b)   Primary care attenders, who are generally surveyed with a self-reporting questionnaire such as the General Health Questionnaire (Goldberg, 1972), followed by a structured interview such as the Diagnostic Interview Schedule or the Present State Examination (Wing *et al*, 1974).

c)   Mental health service attenders diagnosed by clinicians, in their traditionally unstructured way, or according to DSM–III or ICD–10 criteria.

The above methodological differences render comparison of prevalence rates at the successive levels somewhat hazardous. As far as they can be compared, we expect fewer and fewer cases per 1000 population filtering through to the higher levels in the pathway of care. Not everyone with anxiety in the population will attend a primary care provider, and not every case of anxiety will next be referred to a mental health service. Cultural norms and social environment are bound to influence the stresses causing anxiety, the patterns of illness behaviour, the diagnostic attitudes and decisions of the care providers, as well as the availability of primary care and specialist services.

Level I (population)

The Epidemiologic Catchment Area project in the USA rendered the following information (Robins & Regier, 1991):

● at any one time one in 12 people (8%) aged 18 years or more suffers from a DSM–III anxiety disorder;
● the lifetime prevalence is 20%; of the latter about half are simple phobias. Agoraphobia was found in 6% of the samples and panic disorder in 1.6%.

Apparently, anxiety disorder is a very common kind of human problem, because the point-prevalence of all psychological disorder at this level was 32%, and the lifetime prevalence was also 32%. The point- and lifetime prevalence rates of affective disorder were much lower (5% and 8%). Rates were quite similar in Germany (Wittchen, 1987) and New Zealand (Joyce *et al*, 1989). Panic, general anxiety and phobia were twice as common in women than in men.

Level II (primary care)

The following data summarise a number of studies (Hoeper *et al*, 1979; Schulberg *et al*, 1985; Goldberg *et al*, 1987; Grayson *et al*, 1987; Von Korff *et al*, 1987; Barrett *et al*, 1988; Ormel *et al*, 1990).

● One in three to four successive primary care attenders (25–32%) has a psychological disorder. If we assume that in the Western world the population visits primary care services on average at least once a year, then the annual prevalence of all psychological disorder at this level is about similar to that in the general population. This concerns morbidity not necessarily all recognised by the primary care provider.
● The prevalence of anxiety disorder varies greatly across studies, from 25–50% of all psychological disorder. One difficulty is the diagnostic distinction between anxiety and depression, because anxiety and depression do not exclude each other. In other words, the diagnostic criteria can force the direction.

TABLE 13.1
Rates of anxiety at level III

	Point-prevalence (n)	Incidence (n)	Annual prevalence (n)	Per 1000 population	% of annual prevalence
Anxiety	44	23	67	1.5	5.6%
Phobia	4	5	9	0.2	0.7%

● Phobia prevails in 2–8% of primary care attenders, panic disorder in 0.1–1.7% and general anxiety in 5–16%.

The above figures do not exclude the possibility that patients attend the primary care service for reasons other than that of anxiety.

Level III (mental health care)

The most complete data are collected in a case register covering all mental health service contacts from a circumscribed area. The data shown in Table 13.1 are extracted from a Dutch case register.

More anxiety occurs at this level than is indicated in Table 13.1, but then as part of other diagnostic categories. It is obvious, however, that few cases of anxiety in the general population or among primary care attenders filter through to the level of specialist care, as shown even in the Netherlands which is richly provided with specialist services. Therefore, observations concerning anxiety should take into consideration the level at which they are made, and the factors determining the filters between those levels. They include awareness and interpretation of anxiety, help-seeking behaviour, availability of the various health care providers and the policies of the latter.

For example, in the Netherlands Ormel *et al* (1990) found that recognition of anxiety by general practitioners is low compared to that of depression. One of the reasons may be that patients do not see their phobia as something worth mentioning to the general practitioner.

Again, it is the Epidemiologic Catchment Area project which gives us an indication of the fate of people suffering from anxiety (Shapiro *et al*, 1984; Boyd, 1986; Robins & Regier, 1991). Contacts of the respondents with the health care system during the six months preceding the survey were studied, and the results are shown in Table 13.2.

Table 13.2 reflects illness behaviour of the respondents and admission policy of the health agencies, indicating that anxiety disorder is more often interpreted as

TABLE 13.2
Patients with anxiety in contact with the health care system

	% of respondents in contact with the health care system			
	Somatic health care		Mental health care	
	Out-patient	In-patient	Out-patient	In-patient
Panic	86	34	51	17
Phobia	68	17	17	4
General anxiety	40	8	25	2

physical illness than as a mental health problem. A panicky person in particular suffers this fate. Phobia and general anxiety maintain a relatively low profile in mental health care.

As far as these figures represent attitudes in Western cultures, they seem to indicate a fairly strong physical orientation towards anxiety in societies said to favour introspection and psychologisation of experience.

Anxiety in non-Western cultures

Although the reported greater sensitivity of Japanese people to alcohol imposes caution, it seems that human physiology is less culture-bound than human psychology. If this applies to the physiology of anxious arousal, then cultural diversity in the perception of physical arousal becomes of particular interest to transcultural psychiatry. Kleinman (1981; Fig. 13.1) put it as follows: ". . . affects

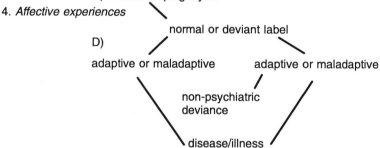

A) Cultural beliefs and values will in part determine if a stimulus is perceived as a stressor and how it is ranked in a hierarchy of potential stressors.
B) Cognitive processes through which an affect is perceived, labelled and valuated. Culture will exert an impact here via the cultural construction of affective structures and the ways in which such categories are applied and interpreted.
C) Culturally constituted cognitive coping mechanisms come into play to manage secondary affects, especially strong or dysphoric affects.
D) A, B and C give rise to affective experiences that are either socially sanctioned as normal or labelled as deviant. Either social category may include personally adaptive or maladaptive experiences. Maladaptive normal or deviant affective experiences may be further classified as disease/illness. Adaptive deviant experiences fall into a class of non-psychiatric deviance.

Fig. 13.1. Model of the cultural impact on affects and affective disorders (Kleinman, 1981).

occur as universal psychobiological states, but they are cognized before they take on the form of perceived, felt, labeled, and evaluated experiences recognized as emotions".

The model illustrated in Fig. 13.1 helps us disentangle the cultural component of otherwise universal psychopathology. Next, we will review some culture-bound syndromes involving anxiety as the basic emotional problem.

Culture-bound anxiety syndromes

Simons & Hughes (1985), while reviewing the literature, observed that "although the meanings assigned to unusual experiences and behaviours vary markedly from site to site, salient features of those experiences and behaviours are sometimes surprisingly similar in historically unrelated and culturally dissimilar times and places". It became increasingly apparent that many of the so-called culture-bound syndromes could be sorted readily into phenomenologically similar sets, of which he discerned seven taxa: 1) startle matching; 2) sleep paralysis; 3) genital retraction; 4) sudden mass assault; 5) running; 6) fright illness; and 7) cannibal compulsion. He believed that it is more useful to make a distinction between features which account for a syndrome's description and those which account for its being endemic to one site and absent from another. Factors which determine why a syndrome occurs in one place and not another are not necessarily the same as those which account for its descriptive features. This may affect the adequacy of explanatory considerations using factors which on closer scrutiny appear not present in all cultural settings.

Only in two of the taxa listed above did Simons & Hughes (1985) find indications for a DSM–III diagnosis of anxiety: sleep paralysis 300.01 (panic disorder); and genital retraction 300.01 (panic disorder).

Sleep paralysis is found among the Inuits of Alaska (Uqamairineq). It probably has a neurophysiological explanation, where it is related to spontaneous awakening during rapid eye movement sleep at a time at which the muscular relaxation typical of this stage in the sleep cycle is still in force. The point is that in the mind of the Inuits it represents the separation of body and soul occurring when a person dies. During sleep and particularly during dreaming the soul is supposed to start wandering. However, before waking up the soul finds the body again. Waking up in a paralysed state, therefore, must be a terrifying experience to the Inuit who will think that the merger has not taken place.

In Newfoundland (Ness, 1985), sleep paralysis is called 'old hag', carrying a less threatening meaning. It is supposed to be common when you are sleeping on your back or when you have done too much physical effort. It is not considered a symptom of illness but an unimportant circulatory problem.

Other and more frightening forms are the 'kokma' spirits in the Caribbean and the 'Zar' spirits in Ethiopia and Egypt, which may try to possess and smother you during the night. The Zar has a sexual connotation, and may cause infertility.

It is obviously the cultural meaning, perhaps combined with personal vulnerability, which turns a not uncommon experience into a panic, further paralysing the victim.

Koro (Hughes, 1985), which was first thought to be indigenous to South-East Asia, has since been reported to occur elsewhere, notably in Nigeria, Sudan, England and the United States. It is characterised typically by complaints of genital hyperinvolution and fear of impending death. The origin of the term is not altogether clear, whether stemming from Sulawesi or China. In any case, it is connected with fatal retraction of the genitals into the abdomen, even though there is no official medical record of fatal cases. Leng (1985), presupposes the following cycle: information about koro on hearsay plus some sexual fears and subjective sensations in the genitalia either of a normal nature such as associated with the sexual act, defaecation or micturition, or of an abnormal nature such as an insect bite plus fear lead to koro, which in turn causes more fear and heightened koro.

While anxiety concerning the genitalia and sexuality appear universal, it remains unexplained that koro is such a rare condition according to the literature. Sleep paralysis and koro are both examples of affective experiences which are primarily less culture-specific than was originally assumed, giving rise to culture-specific secondary affects because of their culturally determined meaning and stimulating culture-specific coping mechanisms, such as tying up the genitals to keep them from entering the body.

Culture-bound phobias

Taijin-kyofu-sho (TKS) has long been regarded as a common culture-bound syndrome in Japan, characterised by fear of hurting the feelings of others (or even causing physical damage) by certain imagined shortcomings within oneself (Si-Hyung, 1987; Kasahara, 1987; Prince, 1991). Offending others may occur in many ways: embarrassing others by blushing; making others uncomfortable by the nature or intensity of one's gaze, through one's facial expression, or through deformities, body odours or shakiness of the voice. Of late TKS has also been observed to be common in Korea.

This persistent and irrational fear is similar to that described under the label of social phobia in ICD–10, except that the patient is not afraid of his own exposure but of that of others.

Kasahara distinguishes four 'stages' of phobia: 1) a transient type; 2) a pure social phobia fitting the definition of ICD–10; 3) a social phobia that takes on the quality of a delusion of reference; and 4) social phobia arising as a prodrome of schizophrenia or as a post-psychotic symptom during remission. The question is whether these are separate disorders or constitute a sequence in one and the same disorder.

In Korea the concept of 'noonchi' appears central to the disorder, where it refers to non-verbal communication: in addition to the burden of being conscious of others, one has also to determine what is in another's mind through noonchi. Social phobic sufferers constantly question how others evaluate them, accept and like them. They have to answer the question through noonchi, i.e. the way others talk, their gestures and facial expression, and every single detail of non-verbal cues. This is to some extent Korean culture, where in order to live in harmony and peace under the crowded conditions of most Korean households, one must constantly scrutinise others' needs and feelings, and especially those of the household's seniors. One can be deceived by talk but not through noonchi. Noonchi, according to Si-Hyung and as described by Prince (1991), is a condition in which the ego boundary between self and other is fused and undifferentiated and loses objectivity. One moves into the other and measures how one is affecting the other by becoming the other's eyes and ears, and even the other's mind in order to read their mind. In Western culture, where clear-cut verbal communication is essential, no equivalent of noonchi appears to exist.

This irrational fear and distress in social situations and the resulting compelling desire to avoid them appear just as central features of the condition as in the ICD–10 definition of social phobia. Therefore, the only difference is in the direction of the embarrassment. Application of Kleinman's model suggests a cultural difference in the cognitive labelling of the primary affect of anxiety. A pertinent question here is whether the emphasis in ICD–10 on patients' personal humiliation rather than on that of the other should be considered a cognitive feature bound to Western culture. The perception that a Saudi man has of his social situation may represent the other extreme. Regarding the latter, Al-Sabaie (1989) reported social phobia as a common condition in Saudi males. Their presentation usually comprised complaints of shyness and fear accompanied by excessive avoidance of certain situations where the person felt under scrutiny. Overt criticism, limited privacy, the attribution of exaggerated importance to appearance and judgement on first impression are all highly characteristic social features of Saudi Arabian male culture. Deviation from rigid social codes and highly valued customs can be detrimental to vulnerable individuals.

Social phobia offers a good example of secondary transcultural differences in the meaning of affective experiences which are basically similar across cultures.

Clinical guidelines for the diagnosis of anxiety and phobia

There are a number of features of anxiety which we have to confirm before the condition is diagnosed. Is the experience unusual for the patient (state anxiety) or has he always been an anxious person (anxiety as a trait)? Is the anxiety out of the blue, or is it generated by a specific situation or object? And, if the latter is the case, is the anxiety or fear reasonable or unreasonable (phobia)? Finally, is the experience accompanied by physical phenomena: trembling, sweating, palpitations, dizziness, a choking feeling, the urge to urinate or defaecate or not?

As stated before, pathological anxiety is in essence no different from normal anxiety. It is, however, more severe and incapacitating, and more of an existential threat and less reasonable. A panic is a sudden and unanticipated attack of overwhelming anxiety, which the person has to overcome by taking some kind of action (leaving the house, calling one's partner or taking a bath). Next, fear for another attack can become just as incapacitating as the original anxiety, and behaviour avoiding all situations that provoke anxiety can begin to dominate daily life. Finally, it can assume a more generalised and lasting character.

A phobia is a disproportionate fear of an object or situation, which itself does not warrant such strong emotions. Nevertheless, the patient cannot retain his fear, and tries to avoid the object or situation at all cost, even the thought of it.

He knows his fear to be irrational, but cannot suppress the accompanying physical arousal.

A simple phobia concerns only a specific situation or object, e.g. fear of water. A social phobia keeps a person away from others for fear of, for example, blushing. In case of agoraphobia, there is fear of a breakdown or a panic attack in a public place, where there is no-one available to ask for help without causing embarrassment. In all cases autonomic arousal is an essential feature of the condition: trembling, palpitations, sweating, hyperventilation, or churning. The patient knows that he should not be so full of fear, but this does not give him any relief. If, on the contrary, he thinks that his fear is realistic, we have to consider a delusion.

Obsessive–compulsive disorder

Mr P. complains about having to think certain things, particularly when he feels stressed. These thoughts always concern people who have died, his father-in-law but also others. If he does not follow precisely the content of his thoughts, then he feels that he insults the deceased person. If at such a moment he does not stop combing his hair or brushing his teeth, then this is an insult to the one he mourns. He tries to avoid all that has to do with death, the cemetery, the chair of his father-in-law, for fear of insulting the latter. During the interview he interrupts himself to indicate that he has to say something in a special way, so as not to insult his father-in-law. He is aware that these thoughts are his own, but he considers them alien to his nature and unpleasant. At times, everything around him appears strange and distant. If he does not allow these thoughts to have their way, he starts to feel anxious and depressed. These thoughts date back to the shameful sexual fantasies he used to have as a schoolboy, about the girlfriend of one of his friends. Lately, he has been impotent with his wife and during occasional extramarital contacts.

These are clear examples of obsessional thoughts. Often unpleasant, aggressive, obscene and senseless, which arise against a person's will, but which are recognised as one's own. Compulsive acts have the same character, they are aimed at preventing unlikely events or disaster. Initially, the patient does his best to resist the ideas or acts, but ultimately his life is transformed by them.

Adjustment disorder

Obsessive–compulsive disorders are disorders in which anxiety, without realistic origin, is the central theme. The anxiety is experienced undisguised, or disguised as a phobia or an obsession as the result of neurotic coping strategies, fending off early unconscious conflicts. The adjustment disorders, however, result from recent drastic changes or life events, threatening continuity and self-respect and sometimes leading to more lasting difficult circumstances. The response is usually non-adaptive and counterproductive, impeding the fulfilment of social roles.

Acute stress reactions are transient responses to an overwhelming traumatic life experience: war, disaster, rape, an accident or other drastic change in a person's social position or network, for example, imprisonment or becoming a refugee. Although the trauma is generally very severe, not everyone will respond in the same manner. Therefore, individual vulnerability is supposed to play a role. First, the victim becomes dazed, his attention is restricted, and his comprehension and orientation are reduced. This can develop into a state of stupor or agitation and overactivity, accompanied by autonomic arousal. This response is almost immediate, and can last several hours or days, depending on whether the victim has the opportunity to leave the disaster area. Usually the symptoms diminish with time, even if the threatening situation persists. The victim can develop amnesia for the traumatic episode.

Post-traumatic stress disorder is a late development, following the same kind of trauma. Characteristic are 'flashbacks', vivid and unasked for recollections of what has happened, and nightmares. The person is either depressed, listless and apathetic; or jumpy and aroused, and particularly sensitive to situations reminding him of the trauma. The latter response usually appears after a period of latency, and does not persist for more than six months. However, it can become chronic, with signs of anxiety, depression and suicidal ideation or alcohol abuse.

In adjustment disorder the trauma is less overwhelming, while the role of individual vulnerability and coping is more prominent. Life events involving loss or threat provoke the reaction, in the form of anxiety and depression or of deviant behaviour: aggressive, histrionic or regressive behaviour. Again, the response follows within a matter of weeks, and rarely lasts more than half a year.

Somatisation

A history of many physical complaints without clear organic pathology is said to be common in non-Western cultures. 'Crawling under the skin' or 'heat in the body' are some of the typical worries patients present. Indicative are also the tenacity of the illness behaviour and the concern about what the complaints might ultimately lead to. Kirmayer (1984*a,b*), who reviewed the subject extensively, sees somatisation as a discrepancy between where the observer believes a problem, concern or event is located or how he expects it to be expressed and the patient's experience and expression of it in the body.

Various definitions of somatisation prevail: a) the presentation of physical symptoms in the absence of organic pathology, or the amplification of physical complaints accompanying organic disease beyond what can be accounted for by physiology; b) the presentation of somatic symptoms in place of personal or social problems; and c) a mechanism by which emotions can give rise to somatic signs and symptoms of illness. Adhering to one of these definitions, however, does not exclude the validity of the others. Culture features in all three definitions: in the preoccupation with certain parts of the body or in the prevailing organic pathology; in the transactions dictated by the preoccupations of the provider of health care; and in the culture-specific cognition of primary affects or in coping styles. Kirmayer considers the view of somatisation as a culture-bound anomaly hard to sustain in the face of its widespread prevalence: "Instead, it is the more exotic phenomenon of 'psychologisation', occurring among an educated Western urban minority, that may require special explanation" (Kirmayer, 1984*a,b*). Psychologisation, i.e. the tendency towards introspection and interpretation of distress in psychological terms, is probably related to decades of predominance of psychodynamic theory.

A culture-specific example of somatisation symptoms is 'brain fag' in students in Ethiopia and Nigeria, consisting of inability to concentrate and to retain learned material, a variety of paraesthesias, and blurred vision. They are associated with brainwork, such as studying. Nichter (1981) found somatisation a common way of expressing social distress among Brahmin women. A manifold of somatic complaints – poor appetite, general weakness, body pain, etc. – were often recognised by the traditional healer as related to psychosocial problems. Nichter even suggested that such symptoms are a means of social protest, among other idioms of distress including refusal to cook or to perform purification rights. Perhaps psychiatrists in Europe and the United States are more inclined to emphasise the depressive component in such syndromes.

As to the relationship between somatisation and psychologisation, Mechanic (1980) identified the following sources of association between physical and mental symptoms of illness or distress:

- some symptoms, like fatigue and loss of appetite are general symptoms that occur in many circumstances;
- psychological states may contribute to physical symptoms by a direct psychophysiological effect or by influencing habit patterns and lifestyle;
- psychological orientations may be associated with bodily arousal that can be appraised as symptoms by the individual;
- the psychological state may affect how persons monitor their bodies and their readiness to interpret bodily changes as illness;
- physical illness may induce such symptoms as anxiety and depression.

In other words, somatisation involves complex mechanisms that give rise to both somatic and emotional symptoms, cognitive attributional processes that characterise symptoms as belonging to body or mind, and social processes that encourage or sanction particular styles of illness behaviour.

Presentation of somatoform disorders

Most important is the act of complaining about bodily phenomena, also after physical examination has revealed nothing, or has produced findings which do not justify the complaints. Even if the complaints, as to their onset or persistence, are clearly related to difficulties in the life of the patient, the latter still denies this attribution. Apparently, secondary illness gain (i.e. the emotional and material advantages of the sick role) is too substantive to relinquish the act of complaining. The patient is often anxious and depressed.

In somatisation disorder proper, there are multiple, vague and continuously changing physical symptoms. The patient has consulted various specialists, almost never to his satisfaction. In the worst case multiple surgery and medication has been attempted. He lives a life dependent on medication and disturbed by illness behaviour. The problem of organic illness finally emerging in such a patient should not be overlooked.

In hypochondriasis the patient is continuously worried about a specific disease or the affliction of a particular bodily function or organ. The worries concern not so much what is, but into what it might develop. Physical examination briefly calms the patient, but soon his worries will return. Distinction from a hypochondriacal delusion can be difficult.

Somatoform autonomic dysfunction is a more specific disorder focusing on one of the bodily systems, e.g. cardiovascular or digestive. In other words, one of the systems, largely under autonomic control, is affected. The symptoms betray a state of arousal: palpitations, sweating, blushing, trembling, or increased bowel movements. In addition, there are subjective symptoms without accompanying physical phenomena. Again, a major concern of the patient is what they might lead to. The irritable bowel syndrome and cardiac neurosis are examples.

Psychogenic pain belongs to the same category of a physical sensation without an underlying organic substrate, although it may have had its origin there. Usually, it is closely related to an emotional conflict or psychosocial problem, and has firmly established itself in the patient's life pattern and his family. The secondary illness gain is often too great to permit disappearance of the pain.

Nowadays, conversions are dealt with under the heading of dissociation; in the case of a conversion, sensory experience is dissociated (cut off) from ordinary awareness. The image one has of oneself is affected. It is presumed that, in this manner, an anxiety provoking unconscious conflict is symbolically warded off. This is called the primary illness gain of the conversion, but in addition there is its secondary illness gain in the form of the emotional attention and consideration given by the environment. The conversion manifests itself in a physical dysfunction (paralysis, blindness) without organic substrate to explain it. Usually, the dysfunction does not check precisely with the (neuro)physiological systems and mechanisms that operate the function, but more with the image the patient has of his body. Unfortunately, the emotional conflict is often difficult to trace and identify. Of diagnostic importance are the emotional indifference towards the dysfunction and the denial of any emotional conflict.

Possession and psychiatry

Ritualised dissociation (possession): an example from Ghion, Ethiopia. Every morning at about 8 o'clock several hundred people crowd into the place of worship which is especially built for this purpose. Some of the Coptic priest's disciples direct the visitors to their seats. Men and women sit apart and people of importance occupy the front rows. Some of the more disturbed patients are led to the rear of the building.

Abandoned amulets, handcuffs discarded by those who were violent at one time, insects and other vermin vomited in the process of healing adorn the walls and attest to the cures that took place. In front of the pulpit is an open space where a simple chair awaits those who are to become possessed. Soon the priest starts his sermon. Prayer, readings from the Bible and the stories of the Saints enlighten those who can understand the Amharic language. Soon someone in the audience, often a woman, starts to groan. Attendants, four or five in number rush forward to support the swaying possessed, who is rarely violent at this stage, to the chair. Here the victim is held with arms and legs in a crosslike posture. The Coptic priest, interrupting his sermon, descends from his pulpit and quietly approaches his client. Putting his cross with some force against her forehead the priest starts to question the woman: *Who are you that has occupied this woman?*

Splashes of water and repetitions of this question direct the attention of the possessed, whose groaning stops and gives way to the voices of the spirits who make themselves known as seytan, buda or zar.
How many are you?
Again the spirits speak up and they state their numbers. From one up to more than a hundred are cited.
How many years is it that you have possessed her?
The spirits answer they have entered 1, 2 or even 50 years ago.

The spirits claim for example, that it happened during a wedding or near a forest. The questions are always the same and put in a domineering way, leaving little room for any variation of the answers. At this point the priest orders the spirits in a strong voice to go in the name of God, and then he retreats to his pulpit to continue the service. The attendants release the woman, who cries out with renewed force and goes into a violent and rhythmic sprawling or jumping phase. Gradually the violence subsides and finally she slumps to the floor to be picked up and led away by the attendants, in a somewhat dazed condition. Throughout, the priest remains in complete control of the situation. The state of possession lasts from 1 to 3 minutes, and the occasional spirit that lingers on is severely told to go and then does so.

At one point during a sermon a groaning man was taken to the chair, but had to be kept on the floor, because he was suffering from a severe grand mal seizure of considerable duration. We felt some anxiety about the treatment of this particular case. However after a glance, the priest calmly told his audience that he would not question the man because he would be unable to answer.

After the sermon is over the priest consecrates the water to be used in the proper healing session. A great many throng into the side-room to be baptised by the priest and to be showered abundantly with holy water while the priest touches the diseased parts of their body with his cross. Occasionally someone cries out and goes into trance. A record is kept of all those who become possessed. It is at this stage of the service that the disabled come forward. The full spectrum of diseases can be observed: hemiplegia, parkinsonism, mental deficiency, spastic children, severe oedema, leprosy, cutaneous leishmaniasis, deafness, mutism and blindness to mention only some of them.

The state of possession or trance in psychiatric terminology is sometimes equated with dissociative reaction, hysteria or hypnosis, and is essentially a state of altered consciousness. In order to understand the nature of this alteration we have first to define what is meant by consciousness. According to Kräupl-Taylor (1966) consciousness refers to the reactivity of psychoneural functions manifesting themselves not only in awareness of what we see, hear, think, remember or feel, but also in the awareness that we are seeing, hearing, thinking, remembering or feeling. The level of consciousness can be assessed objectively by evaluating a person's alertness and attentiveness. Any reduction or limitation in responsiveness is taken as a sign of altered consciousness. However, even a completely clear consciousness does not imply that we pay the same degree of attention to all of our experiences. Some are in the centre of attention, others are at the fringe. We can be partially absent-minded in that we can perform two mental activities simultaneously, one of which is automatic, like driving a car absent-mindedly along a familiar road and at the same time being preoccupied with a meeting we are going to attend. Only when we narrowly escape bumping into another car do we realise that we have been driving automatically, and that we have no reminiscence of the route we followed. When this state of absent-mindedness becomes complete we speak of 'trance'. According to Kräupl-Taylor all mental processes in a state of trance are vague and move only in a range that is narrowly associated with the motivation that dominates the fringe attention. Contact with the environment is precarious in such a state. In a deep trance, contact is almost completely lost and the person is entirely absorbed by some phenomena in his mind. In a more superficial trance there is some interaction with the environment, but in the same way as the absent-minded driver who is automatically keeping to his course. In such a state the interactions may be restricted to objects and events which are related to one's absent-minded motivations, like responding only to the standard questions of the priest and revealing the number and type of spirits to be expelled.

There are many factors facilitating the attainment of a trance. Sometimes it is the high prestige attached to it because of the supposed contact during a trance with supernatural powers, sought by man in his desire to control nature (Frazer, 1959). Or inductive stimuli are employed, like the rhythm of drums or dancing. Then there are the many examples of social indoctrination, by which whole populations are put into a trance, perhaps starting with those who are constitutionally more susceptible. Finally, there is the more scientific method of inducing a state of trance (hypnosis) by means of suggestive measures. In the latter it is of course important that people attend in the right frame of mind, expecting that something is going to happen.

Though absent-mindedness is very much a feature of normal life, the relation of total absent-mindedness or possession to mental illness is less clear. Viewpoints tend to differ, perhaps mainly with the background and the sphere of interest of those who discuss the phenomenon. The true anthropologist may consider possession a normal and important attribute of the leaders of a society: kings, chiefs, priests or priestesses.

Even under these circumstances, it is sometimes stressed (Radin, 1957) that some form of emotional instability is essential to acquire such an important role. Possession is then accepted as normal only in certain people taking up particular roles. Bateson & Mead (1942) described how young Balinese dancers have to go into a trance before they start their performance which is inspired by the deity. Occasionally spectators or assistants are induced to a state of possession by the preliminary proceedings. They are invariably taken away from the scene because their behaviour is considered as highly inappropriate. Another and extreme position is taken up mainly by psychiatrists who almost without exception link possession to hysteria, schizophrenia and other mental illnesses. Others, taking up an intermediate position, speak of all those being possessed as 'patients' (Messing, 1959) and of 'hysterical' possession (Loudon, 1965). At the same time, however, they state that 'frustrated status ambitions' (Loudon, 1965) can lead to the attainment of possession. Or that in some societies "the steps which are socially defined as those appropriate in cases of illness are often substantially the same as those considered appropriate in relation to other misfortunes" (Loudon, 1965).

Apparently possession can also be an attribute of the 'underdog', the loser in the struggle for power and prestige. Among the Tanala of Madagascar, the younger son, who will not inherit his father's wealth, tries to better his lot by means of possession (Kardiner, 1961). In this case possession may be a normal, culturally accepted tool to achieve one's goal, and not part of an illness; people relying on possession cannot be called 'patients' indiscriminately, even though mentally disturbed people will be especially attracted to its use.

When taken as a psychiatric symptom one tends to compare, or even equate possession with a dissociative reaction, as occurs in hysteria. A dissociative reaction is an episodic disturbance in the stream of consciousness in a case of overwhelming anxiety, when defence mechanisms (repression) govern consciousness, memory and temporarily even the total individual, with little or no participation of the normal personality. Anxiety provoking experiences are banned from consciousness before they can interfere with the normal peace of mind. The repression causes a selective inattention with the continuation of impulses at the unconscious level. In extreme cases aspects of the personality, normally altogether excluded from awareness, manifest themselves vigorously, and are often hallucinated as illusory personifications coming from outside.

The same defence mechanism of repression causes amnesia, which occurs after the event of a dissociative state. Anxiety apparently is the central issue in a dissociative reaction. To equate hysterical or psychotic dissociation with possession would imply that anxiety is also the main theme of possession. When considering the trance states at Ghion in the light of the above, it is important to note that possession is not a feature of mental illness only. The trance states we could observe (about 20), followed a standard pattern which was very much under the control of the priest. People came in a mood of expectancy, enforced perhaps by economic sacrifice, days of travelling and the obligation to accompany relatives. They saw possessions occur right before their eyes. Finally they were subordinate to the dominating personality of the priest and his standardised and suggestive questioning. His actions determined their behaviour and responses. They communicated with him only, when they were possessed. The stage of groaning lasted as long as it took him to direct his attention to them. When he had approached them the groaning stopped and some sort of conversation became possible. As such, this state of trance resembled very much the more superficial absent-mindedness which is described by Kräupl-Taylor.

We were able to examine two women right after they had been possessed. One of them was fully conscious when we interviewed her. She appeared to have no knowledge of what had occurred. This was in accordance with the information we obtained from other cases, stating that they did not remember at all what they had said when they were possessed. Their companions had informed them afterwards. The second woman who had thrown hysterical fits at home, behaved differently when we examined her. When we addressed her she seemed drowsy. However, when we talked to her husband she appeared to be fully aware of what was going on. She stated that she had a vague knowledge of communicating with the priest. Her spirits had refused to go. We thought that she might have had a hysterical dissociative reaction, as there was evidence of the neurotic anxiety, which is considered to be central in the mechanism of dissociation. In some of the other mentally normal people we had little proof for such neurotic anxiety.

The state of possession or trance appears not to be specifically related to mental illness, but to be learned absent-mindedness in the majority of cases, with many factors contributing to the process of learning, like the expectant mood in which people arrived, the daily example of trance states, and the definitely inductive actions of the priest.

In our opinion the state of possession has to be distinguished from a hysterical dissociative reaction resulting from strong repression in case of overwhelming anxiety, a condition which perhaps occurs in some of the cases.

Presentation of dissociation

A 12-year-old Ethiopian girl was so ashamed of her low marks at school, that she tampered with her semester results. She was found out in school, and was told to bring her father in. Thereupon she left school and started to roam, not knowing where she was heading. Several hours later she reappeared near her home, anxious, agitated and in a state of shock. Her parents invited a priest, who exorcised devils. This increased her anxiety, but soon she was so exhausted that she fell asleep. Next morning she woke up, refreshed and calm. However, she had regressed in time to three months earlier, as if still on holiday. She denied all knowledge of what had happened the day before, and of her problems at school. She had never had a similar experience before.

Commonly, we are able to give direction to our attention, while integrating our sense of the present and the past. Memories and present experience merge into a meaningful perception of ourselves and the environment. During a state of dissociation this capacity is lost, or unstable.

In the past, this was called hysterical dissociation. It was considered to have a psychogenic basis, originating in an unconscious conflict, which is reactivated by a recent stressful event. Usually, this connection is consciously denied. The dissociation begins suddenly, and tends to resolve in a matter of days or weeks.

It is a matter of choice whether to call depersonalisation and derealisation the result of partial dissociation of consciousness. In this case, patients experience themselves or their environment as if unreal and at a distance. Everything appears dead or artificial, an imitation of the real thing. The experience of 'as if' is important, because if the patient is convinced that he is dead or a robot, then this would be evidence of a delusion of depersonalisation.

Dissociative amnesia is a circumscribed, but often changing almost daily in extent, loss of memory. Frequently, the patient accepts the loss with indifference.

During a dissociative fugue or twilight state the patient is totally absent-minded but moves and acts in a purposeful manner. He takes care of himself, and maintains a normal appearance. This is different from a dissociative stupor, during which the patient remains immobile and unresponsive to outside stimuli. Muscle tone, posture, respiration and eye movements indicate that the patient is not asleep.

Finally, there is the state of meditation, which is an absent-mindedness which is sought on purpose. It is as if the meditating person tries to disconnect his focus of attention from the present central and shared world, while allowing access to stimuli from the fringe of his attention. Like possession, it is a state of mind which can be trained.

General observations on the management of patients

Language constitutes a barrier in transcultural psychiatry; much more so does the difference in the worlds of meaning in transcultural communication. Yet, the material presented so far does not suggest basic differences in pathology. We can assume that essential therapeutic strategies, such as drug treatment or the application of behavioural techniques, remain valid.

The differences are in the cultural varnish enveloping largely universal pathology, and in the illness behaviour of the patient to which the health professional has to respond. In addition, the professional's diagnostic and therapeutic behaviour is by no means culture-free.

In recent times, we have witnessed significant changes in professional behaviour, based on an increased awareness of factors other than physical pathology influencing illness behaviour of the patient. We have learned that psychosocial distress can overrule the expression of physical distress. The doctor is not only managing pathology but also a relationship. This is where the differences may emerge, according to the expectations of the patient. The latter may have anticipated authoritative directives and instructions, and not digressions into his inner world of emotions or into his social situation. He may, for example, be concerned about his sexual performance and be willing to discuss it, but not his sexual relationship.

Nowadays, it is customary in Western society to establish some sort of equality in the doctor–patient relationship, where the patient is requested to explore the nature of his problems and to take the initiative in seeking their solution. In other cultures this is the expected role of the healer, who is supposed to instruct his patient after due exploration of the problem. The terms under which the healing occurs may remain the secret of the healer.

Hall's (1959) discussion of the crossroads of transcultural communication helps to understand the difficulties that may arise. He poses that people learn and communicate at three levels. 'Formal' learning is by precept and admonition; it is implicit and occurs at an early age. The adult moulds the young according to patterns he himself has never questioned. Corrective communications imply that no other form of behaviour is conceivably acceptable, therefore the situation is charged with emotion. 'Informal' learning is chiefly by imitation. The message is: "Don't ask questions, look around and see what people do". It concerns behaviour that cannot be explained, other than by "this is what people usually do". There is some room and understanding for other patterns, such as how late one can be for an appointment and still be on time. 'Technical' learning is entirely explicit, all knowledge rests with the teacher. If the teacher is clear enough, she can put her message in writing. In transcultural communication in particular, the difficulty is that we are not mutually aware of the level at which we are communicating, and whether it is the same level for both participants.

In transcultural psychiatry we are trying to carry the burden of continuous awareness at all three levels. We have to be explicit about common matters that are largely implicit. This rule in the management of mental illness applies not only to the transactions between cultures, but also to those between social strata within one and the same culture.

In the following paragraph a more detailed management protocol will be described.

The management of somatising patients

Once anxiety, mostly disguised in physical symptoms, has been detected as the central problem of the patient, it has to be decided how far the health worker will go in its management. This depends not only on the problem of the patient, but also on the level of training of the health worker, and whether referral to a specialist is at all possible. The primary health worker in her health station or the medical assistant in a health centre at the next level of care may do little more than proceed with the first tentative steps in the total management of such cases. All medical staff will have the following spontaneous responses in common, which will tend to steer them towards a physical diagnosis:

1. Because of the symptoms of physical arousal or the physical focus of the complaint, they will experience the challenge to their medical responsibility not to miss a serious physical illness.
2. They will be under pressure of time in their busy out-patient clinic.
3. They may feel frustrated by their failure to come to grips with the symptoms indicative of somatisation.
4. They will, in such cases, tend to defer a decision by referring the patients for further examinations.
5. If they do suspect an emotional background for the symptoms, they may not dare to touch it, either because they consider a person's emotions his private property or because they are afraid to be confronted with socially unacceptable emotions.

If the health worker remains focused on a physical diagnosis, further escalation in that direction may result. Denial of the underlying anxiety or disqualification of the complaint as not indicative of any significant physical condition will force the patient to come forward with another symptom. Referral for specialist or laboratory examination will emphasise the seriousness, particularly of the physical side of the complaint, and lead to unjustified medical attention. The health worker's focus should shift towards the management of a patient's attitude towards his complaint, and the relationship between patient and health worker. A stepwise reinterpretation or reattribution from physical towards emotional experience is required:

Step 1: while taking the history of the patient, the health worker should be aware of the patient's behaviour and of her own attitude towards the complaint and the complainer. Recognition of their emotional aspects should follow only after all possible physical causes have been excluded.
Step 2: a physical examination, strictly within the limitations of the clinic and the capabilities of the health worker, should be made to show patients that any physical suffering is taken seriously.
Step 3: next, the patient should be confronted with the negative physical findings and comforted with regard to possible worries about physical illness. If examination reveals a physical condition, not coinciding or inadequately explaining their physical sensations, patients should be told of this discrepancy, while their physical condition is treated. Depending on the

training, time and interest of the health worker, management of the case can stop here, with an explanation that this is as far as they can go.

Step 4: health workers with more interest, time or training may, at this stage, explore the patient's life situation for a recent loss or threatening experience. They may also venture to suggest a solution or refer the patient to community agents for advice and assistance. If no such events can be traced and a neurotic conflict is suspected, the health worker may decide to close the case.

Step 5: this step brings the health worker, without undue effort and with a possibility of success, into the realm of psychiatry, because it involves giving the patient insight into the emotional side of his problems. Particularly in case of somatisation, the objective is to have the patient reattribute his worries and concerns. More difficult is to show patients how their illness behaviour and dependent attitude are influencing their relationships, and the extent to which they provide them with a self-defeating protection. Here the main problem for health workers is that, whatever they do, they will immediately be confirmed more strongly in the dependent relationship with the patient with the danger of an escalation of medicalisation on their part and of further somatisation on that of the patient. In this case, the health worker will have to focus on this relationship with the patient, striving for a less helpless attitude in the patient. It is essential at this stage for the health worker to set a limit on the number of contacts with the patient. This will prevent false expectations on both sides or the continuation of a relationship which no longer serves a useful purpose.

If the health worker remains unsuccessful, referral to a mental health service can be considered, but it should be noted that, in most 'neurotic' cases, the psychiatrist does little more than has been described under steps 4 and 5.

Medication can be introduced, in the form of benzodiazepines, at each step. But their prescription needs very careful consideration, because they may lead to dependency or become part of a process of escalation as prescription carries also a message to the patient. It is first necessary to enquire what drugs have already been used, for how long and in what dosage. The chances are that the patient has already exhausted the list, because they are among the most widely distributed drugs in the developing world. If medication is unavoidable, it should aim at a clearly indicated symptom or complex of symptoms, and the drug should be prescribed for a limited period of only two or three weeks. If the drugs do not help they should be discontinued with an explanation that they are obviously not the answer to the patient's problem.

Escalation of medication takes two forms. Either patients want endless continuation of a prescription because it worked and they fear recurrence of their anxiety, or they demand other and stronger prescriptions because the previous one was ineffective. Requests for medication can become instrumental in manipulating the doctor–patient relationship, with a tendency on the part of the health worker to yield too easily to compensate their sense of failure.

This discussion of the management of anxiety and its related phenomena shows that for most health workers it is more a matter of what not to do. There are, however, special techniques to overcome anxiety, e.g. relaxation, but they require special training.

References

AMERICAN PSYCHIATRIC ASSOCIATION (1980) *Diagnostic and Statistical Manual of Mental Disorders* (3rd edn) (DSM–III). Washington, DC: APA.

AL-SABAIE, A. (1989) Psychiatry in Saudi Arabia: Cultural perspectives. *Transcultural Psychiatric Research Review,* **26**, 245–262.

BARRETT, J. E., BARRETT, J. A., OXMAN, T., *et al* (1988) The prevalence of psychiatric disorders in primary care practice. *Archives of General Psychiatry,* **45**, 1100–1119.

BATESON, G. & MEAD, M. (1942) *Balinese Character. A Photographic Analysis.* New York: Academy of Sciences.

BOYD, J. H. (1986) Use of mental health services for panic disorder. *American Journal of Psychiatry,* **143**, 1569–1574.

FRAZER, J. G. (1959) *The Golden Bough.* New York: Criterion Books.

GOLDBERG, D. P. (1972) *The Detection of Psychiatric Illness by Questionnaire (GHQ).* Maudsley Monograph 21. London: Oxford University Press.

GOLDBERG, D. & BRIDGES, K. (1987) Dimensions of neurosis seen in primary-care settings. *Psychological Medicine,* **17**, 461–470.

GRAYSON, D. A. (1987) The relationship between symptoms and diagnoses of minor psychiatric disorder in general practice. *Psychological Medicine,* **17**, 933–942.

HALL, T. A. (1959) *The Silent Language.* Greenwich: Fawcett Publications.

HOEPER, E. W., NYCZ, G. R., CLEARY, P. D., *et al* (1979) Estimated prevalence of RDC mental disorder in primary medical care. *International Journal of Mental Health,* **8**, 6–15.

HUGHES, C. C. (1985) Culture-bound or construct-bound? The syndromes and DSM–III. In *The Culture-bound Syndromes* (eds R. C. Simons & C. C. Hughes). Dordrecht: Reidel.

JOYCE, P. R., *et al* (1989) The epidemiology of panic symptomatology and agoraphobic avoidance. *Comprehensive Psychiatry,* **30**, 303–312.

KARDINER, A. (1961) *The Individual and his Society.* New York: Columbia University Press.

KASAHARA, Y. (1988) Social Phobia in Japan (Abstract). *Transcultural Psychiatric Research Review,* **25**, 145–150.

KIRMAYER, L. J. (1984*a*) Culture, affect and somatization, I. *Transcultural Psychiatric Research Review,* **21**, 159–188.

———— (1984*b*) Culture, affect and somatization, II. *Transcultural Psychiatric Research Review,* **21**, 237–262.

KLEINMAN, A. (1981) *Patients and Healers in the Context of Culture.* Berkeley & Los Angeles: University of California Press.

KRÄUPL-TAYLOR, F. (1966) *Psychopathology, its Causes and Symptoms.* London: Butterworths.

SI-HYUNG, L. (1988) Social phobia in Korea (Abstract). *Transcultural Psychiatric Research Review,* **25**, 145–150.

LENG, G. A. (1985) Koro – A Cultural Disease. In *The Culture-bound Syndromes* (eds R. C. Simons & C. C. Hughes). Dordrecht: Reidel.

LOUDON, J. B. (1965) Social aspects of ideas about treatment. In *Transcultural Psychiatry* (ed. Ciba Foundation Symposium). London: Churchill.

MARKS, I. M. (1986) Epidemiology of anxiety. *Social Psychiatry,* **21**, 167–171.

MECHANIC, D. (1980) The experience and reporting of common physical problems. *Journal of Health and Social Behaviour,* **21**, 146–155.

MESSING, S. D. (1959) In *Culture and Mental Health* (ed. M. K. Opler). New York: Macmillan.

NESS, R. C. (1985) The Old Hag phenomenon as sleep paralysis: a biocultural interpretation. In *The Culture-bound Syndromes* (eds R. C. Simons & C. C. Hughes). Dordrecht: Reidel.

NICHTER, M. (1981) Idioms of distress: alternatives in the expression of psychosocial distress. A case study from India. *Culture, Medicine and Psychiatry,* **5**, 379–408.

ORMEL, J. & GIEL, R. (1990) Medical effects of nonrecognition of affective disorders in primary care. In *Psychological Disorders in General Medical Settings* (eds N. Sartorius, D. Goldberg, G. de Girolamo, *et al*). Toronto: Hogrefe & Huber.

PRINCE, R. (1991) Transcultural psychiatry's contribution to international classification systems: the example of social phobias. *Transcultural Psychiatric Research Review,* **28**, 124–132.

RADIN, P. (1957) *Primitive Religion*. New York: Dover Publications.

ROBINS, L. N. & REGIER, D. A. (1991) *Psychiatric Disorders in America. The Epidemiologic Catchment Area Study*. New York: Free Press.

SCHULBERG, H. C., SAUL, M., McCLELLAND, M., *et al* (1985) Assessing depression in primary medical and psychiatric practices. *Archives of General Psychiatry*, **42**, 1164–1170.

SHAPIRO, S., SKINNER, E. A., KESSLER, L. G., *et al* (1984) Utilization of health and mental health services. Three Epidemiologic Catchment sites. *Archives of General Psychiatry*, **41**, 971–978.

SI-HYUNG, LEE (1988) Social Phobia in Korea (Abstract). *Transcultural Psychiatric Research Review*, **25**, 145–150.

SIMONS, R. C. & HUGHES, C. C. (1985) *The Culture-Bound Syndromes*. Dordrecht: Reidel.

VON KORFF, M., SHAPIRO, S., BURKE, J., *et al* (1987) Anxiety and depression in a primary care clinic: comparison of DIS, GHQ and practitioner assessments. *Archives of General Psychiatry*, **44**, 152–156.

WING, J. K., COOPER, J. E. & SARTORIUS, N. (1974) *Measurement and Classification of Psychiatric Symptoms: an Instruction Manual for the PSE and Catego Program*. Cambridge University Press.

WITTCHEN, H. U. (1986) Epidemiology of panic attacks and panic disorders. In *Panic and Phobias: Empirical Evidence of Theoretical Models and Longterm Effects of Behavioral Treatments* (eds I. Hand & H. U. Wittchen). Berlin: Springer Verlag.

WORLD HEALTH ORGANIZATION (1992) *The Tenth Revision of the International Classification of Diseases and Related Health Problems* (ICD–10). Geneva: WHO.

14 Psychiatric disorders of children and young adults

MORUF L. ADELEKAN

This chapter will address different aspects of psychiatric disorders occurring in childhood and adolescence in developing countries.

By definition, developing countries are less industrialised than developed countries and have limited resources for service development. Their populations are relatively young and predominantly rural. They also have established traditional cultures which are now at different stages of transition due to economic, political and educational influences (Nikapota, 1991).

Development of psychiatric services for children and young adults recorded a significant growth in developing countries only within the past three decades despite the fact that children under the age of 15 years constitute 40–50% of the population (Asuni, 1970; Basheer & Ibrahim, 1976; Minde, 1976; Olatawura, 1978). This lack of priority is largely due to the lack of lobbying power children have upon the deployment of scarce medical resources in these countries (Olatawura, 1978). The lack of specialised manpower has also contributed significantly to the slow development of services. Even where such services are available, the local beliefs and attitudes of the people as to what constitutes psychiatric disorders in their children and the treatment deemed necessary sometimes prevent a full utilisation of the services. The resultant effect is that many of these disorders either go undetected or are poorly reported to orthodox psychiatric centres. Most of the patients are treated within the setting of adult psychiatric units; separate child/adolescent units are hard to come by, even in university teaching and specialist hospitals. Consequently, there is a dearth of literature on childhood psychiatric disorders in the developing world, and hardly any written specifically on the adolescent age group. There is no journal in the developing world which deals specifically with the emotional needs of children, although progress is now being made in some Asian and African countries (Minde, 1976).

Epidemiology

Epidemiological data on childhood and adolescent psychiatric disorders in the developing world are derived from sources such as community surveys involving households or primary health care centres, school-based surveys and data derived from out-patient clinics and other hospital facilities.

311

Community household surveys

Community household surveys are a reliable means of gathering comprehensive epidemiological data on children and young adults. Several such surveys have been conducted in developed countries (Miller *et al*, 1974; Rutter *et al*, 1974, 1976; Richman *et al*, 1975; Kruprinski *et al*, 1976; Graham & Rutter, 1977). They are labour and capital intensive but additional problems are involved in conducting them in developing countries, including poor financial, personnel and material resources. Standardising questionnaires developed in industrialised countries and translating them into several languages also presents problems, as does poor numbering of houses and the fact that such enquiries are usually viewed with extreme suspicion (Narayanan, 1981). There are also special difficulties involved in carrying out clinical, biochemical and psychometric evaluations in the field. Despite these enormous difficulties, some successful household surveys have been carried out in some developing countries within the past two to three decades.

Cederblad (1968) focused on specific psychological symptoms in children. In 1965 she screened all 1716 children aged 3–15 years who lived in three adjacent Sudanese villages with a total population of about 5000, with respect to stuttering, sleep walking, enuresis, encopresis and sleep disturbances. Children showing more than one of the above symptoms and a Swedish control group were then studied in more detail. Cederblad found the Sudanese children to have a generally lower rate of severe symptoms than those of the Swedish sample (8% versus 25%). The Sudanese, however, showed a higher incidence of aggression and nocturnal enuresis than their Swedish controls. One of the limitations of this report is that medical students who were engaged in interviewing the families involved in the study had little experience in psychiatric phenomenology and interview techniques (Minde, 1975).

In 1979/80 Rahim & Cederblad (1984) did a follow-up study on the effects of rapid urbanisation on child behaviour and health in Hag Yousif, a newly urbanised part of Khartoum and one of the villages used in the 1965 study. The procedures used in the two studies were similar, although additional sociological–anthropological investigations were included in 1979/80 to enable a meaningful interpretation of the results. Some of the symptoms found in both studies were fear of darkness, psychogenic headache, nocturnal enuresis, aggressive behaviour and psychomotor hyperactivity. Rare presentations included daytime enuresis, encopresis, depression and conduct disorders. Behaviour symptoms were found to be higher in boys than in girls, and more prevalent in older than in younger children, probably in proportion to the extent of their exposure to new external influences. Some of the favourable aspects of community life in the study area included extended family relations, durable marital commitments with very low divorce rates, mutually supportive communal interdependence and traditions of social control present in the form of a deep-rooted Islamic religion.

Cederblad (1988) also carried out a cross-cultural review of the pattern of childhood psychiatric disorders in three countries (Sudan, Nigeria and Sweden) using data derived from household surveys in which she was involved either directly (Sudan, Sweden) or indirectly (Nigeria). A two-stage technique was used in the three studies. Children's mothers were interviewed by social workers and psychologists in the first stage, and psychiatrists made a global assessment on a sample of possible cases and some non-cases during the second stage. All the Swedish and Sudanese children were aged 3–15 years and the Nigerian children 5–15 years. Urban and rural areas of the countries were selected for study. The prevalence rates of psychiatric morbidity in the urban areas were: Sudan 13%, Nigeria 18%, and Sweden 19%. The corresponding figures for the rural areas were 8%, 11% and 15%. Differences in symptom profile were observed. For example, sleeping problems, eating problems, tics and anxiety were common in the Swedish sample, while nocturnal enuresis was more frequent in the Nigerian and Sudanese eight-year-olds.

Several important findings emerged from this cross-cultural review. For instance, the rate of disturbance tended to increase with age among boys, especially in the Swedish group. Background factors known to covary with behavioural problems in children of developed countries showed similar connections in developing countries. Thus behavioural problems were common in children of low status fathers in urban Sudan as well as in Sweden. Psychiatric problems in parents or a negative emotional climate in the home were associated with greater behavioural problems in all children. Poor physical health, severe punishment, or corporal punishment were all associated with increased rates of behavioural problems in Nigeria and Sudan. In Sweden, living with a single mother, being born to a mother under the age of 20 at delivery, having more than two siblings and living in a large apartment house increased the rate of behaviour problems. There was also a much higher rate of divorce and alcoholism among Swedish parents. Although the African samples suffered from a lot of health and educational hardships, they seemed to enjoy a lot of protective factors as earlier highlighted (Cederblad, 1988).

As part of a general psychiatric community survey of two Ethiopian villages, Giel *et al* (1969) found that 3–4% of all children under the age of nine and 10% of those ten years and older showed psychological abnormalities. No detailed breakdown of symptomatology was given.

Surveys based at primary health care centres

Diop *et al* (1980) found in a primary health care centre in Senegal that 17% of 545 children aged 5–15 years were suffering from some form of emotional problem, behaviour disturbance or neuropsychiatric disorder.

A more extensive World Health Organization-sponsored survey (Giel *et al*, 1981) involved children aged 5–15 years attending primary health care (PHC) centres in four developing countries: Sudan, Philippines, India and Colombia. The first stage of screening involved a series of ten questions called the Reporting Questionnaire for Children (RQC) which were directed at an accompanying adult. The second stage involved an independent assessment of the child by a child psychiatrist using a semi-structured approach. The primary health worker was also expected to provide an overview of the child's problems. The study reported a 12–29% psychiatric morbidity in the study countries. No specific diagnoses were made, although attempts were made to use the 5-axis diagnostic instrument by Rutter (1975). Frequent symptoms found on the RQC include headaches, sleep disturbance and speech disturbance. On the other hand, 'running away from home' and 'stealing from home' were infrequently found. The authors noted that people who accompany children to PHC centres do recognise mental health problems, particularly when carefully interviewed. They also observed that PHC workers in the areas studied picked up only 10–20% of these problems. The results of the study were used to design appropriate training programmes for PHC workers.

School-based surveys

Well-designed surveys have been conducted on primary school-aged children in Uganda (Minde, 1975), China (Yu-Feng *et al*, 1989) and Hong Kong (Wong, 1990). The three-stage procedure used was quite similar to those described in Western studies (Rutter *et al*, 1976; Graham & Rutter, 1977; Kolvin *et al*, 1981). The first stage required teachers of all the children in the sampling to complete a primary screening questionnaire such as the Children's Behaviour Questionnaire (Rutter, 1967) or a multiple criteria screening procedure (Kolvin *et al*, 1977). In the second stage, a sample of the children who scored above the cut-off point ('problem children') and a sample of controls were further interviewed by a child psychiatrist who was blind to the scores of the first stage screening. The third stage involved an interview of the parents of both the problem children and control samples interviewed in stage two by either medical students or social workers, to find out more on the children's developmental and psychosocial history. The authors of each of the three studies confirmed the high reliability of the screening instruments, although these were developed primarily for British children, and arrived at definite psychiatric diagnosis. The prevalence rates of definite psychiatric disorders were found to be 18% (Uganda), 8.3% (China) and 16.3% (Hong Kong). These figures are comparable to those reported from the Western world (Miller *et al*, 1974; Rutter *et al*, 1976; Graham & Rutter, 1977). Some common covarying factors emerged such as broken or disharmonious home, lesser involvement of parents in their children's education and poor academic performance.

Data collected from health institutions

The majority of the available reports on childhood and adolescent psychiatric disorders in developing countries are gathered from the records of patients seen in child guidance clinics, psychiatric units of teaching and specialist hospitals and general out-patient departments. A major limitation is that they only reflect patients considered ill enough to be brought to see a physician. There is also the problem of evaluating these data as most of the authors give only a very general description. Some do not cite age and gender of the patients described. In the majority, the diagnosis was not based on any stated criteria and no definite classificatory scheme was used. This leads to a tremendous variation in the clinical material presented and also to problems in comparisons. Some recent authors (e.g. Malhotra & Chatuverdi, 1984; Wong, 1990) have used the ICD–9 (WHO, 1978) to classify their patients.

A high percentage of clinic attenders presented with evidence of brain damage in the form of mental retardation, epilepsy, and other organic brain conditions usually complicated with behavioural problems: 36–44% of all clinic patients in Sudan (Basheer & Ibrahim, 1976; Rahim, 1976), 50% in

Nigeria (Izuora, 1976; Olatawura & Odejide, 1976), 50% in India (Malhotra & Chatuverdi, 1984), 64% in Sri Lanka (Nikapota, 1983), and 55%–67% in Uganda (Minde, 1974a; Muhangi & German, 1975). About 50% of these brain damaged cases have been attributed to prenatal and postnatal causes (Tao, 1988) compared to 25% from same causes reported from Western countries (Hagberg, 1978). (Other factors associated with mental retardation are discussed in chapter 12.) There are proportionately few children brought to clinics because of conduct disorders. No mention was made of this condition by Muhangi & German (1975) and the figures quoted in other studies were generally low and ranged between 3% (Basheer & Ibrahim, 1976; Rahim, 1976) to 10–15% (Izuora, 1976; Olatawura & Obejide, 1976; Wong, 1990) and 27% (Nikapota, 1983).

Although there are hardly any in-patient psychiatric admission facilities for children and adolescents in developing countries, some severely disturbed children are admitted to adult psychiatric wards. Oyewunmi (1989) reported on the socio-demographic and clinical characteristics of 84 adolescents aged 12–20 years (mean=17 years) admitted to a teaching hospital in Nigeria within a two-year period. The pattern of psychiatric disorders reflected that found in the adult population. Major psychoses comprising schizophrenia (44%), organic brain syndrome (23%), and affective disorders (16%) predominated. There were also cases of psychosis associated with infections (14%) (typhoid, pneumonia, meningitis) and use of cannabis (5%). Two cases of attempted suicide by ingestion of poison were also reported. Parry-Jones (1986) also reported that most children admitted to in-patient facilities in China appeared to be suffering mainly from schizophrenia, affective psychosis, and epilepsy, with a small number manifesting hysterical and other neurotic symptoms. Gilles de la Tourette syndrome was reported to be unexpectedly common and infantile autism and anorexia nervosa are rare. Neurotic symptoms may be commoner in out-patients.

Mbatia (1979) described 219 patients aged 18 years and below who were managed as in- and out-patients at the psychiatric unit of Muhimbili Hospital, Dar-es-Salaam, Tanzania within a two-year period. The male–female ratio was 2:1. The majority (66%) were adolescents, while 17% were less than seven years old. The diagnostic categories were organic brain syndrome (including seizures) (42%), neurotic disorders (38%), functional psychosis (11%), personality disorders (5%) and mental retardation (4%). The classification used was amorphous and followed no standard scheme. Thus neurotic disorders included, among others, behavioural disorders, crisis of identity, social problems relating to overprotection and so on.

Classification

In ICD–10 (WHO, 1992), WHO has harmonised the merits of both the ICD–9 and DSM–III (American Psychiatric Association, 1980). Disorders which are specific to childhood and adolescence are covered under Sections F80–89 'disorders of psychological development', and F90–98 'behavioural and emotional disorders with onset usually occurring in childhood and adolescence'.

Some examples of the syndromes listed under Section F80–89 are:

F80   Specific developmental disorders of speech and language, e.g. specific speech articulation disorders (F80.0).
F81   Specific developmental disorders of scholastic skills, e.g. specific reading disorder.
F82   Specific developmental disorder of motor function.
F84   Pervasive developmental disorders, e.g. childhood autism, other forms of disintegrative disorders, Rett's syndrome, and Asperger syndrome.

The following major sub-sections are contained under Section F90–98:

F90   Hyperkinetic disorders.
F91   Conduct disorders.
F92   Mixed disorders of conduct and emotions.
F93   Emotional disorders with onset specific to children.
F94   Disorders of social functioning with onset specific to childhood and adolescence.
F95   Tic disorders.
F98   Other behavioural and emotional disorders with onset usually in childhood and adolescence.

Problems of classification in developing countries

As noted under the section on epidemiology, most of the earlier clinical reports from developing countries used diagnostic sub-groups that do not follow any internationally accepted classificatory schemes. A possible reason may be related to the poor level of the development of childhood and adolescent psychiatric services in general in these countries. Even in most established service centres, there is no classificatory scheme built into the record-keeping system. There are a few centres, however, where such schemes are used and computerised (Wong, 1990). In order that developing countries might be able to exchange their scientific findings with the rest of the world, it appears essential that the use of a standard classificatory scheme should be built into the already existing ones. Computerisation of such records should be a feasible and desirable long-term goal.

Clinical sub-syndromes

General considerations

This section will deal mainly with sub-syndromes that have been commonly reported in developing countries. Epilepsy, mental retardation, and drug abuse are considered in separate chapters.

The diagnostic criteria of childhood psychiatric disorders in developing countries are similar to those used in most Western countries where most of the practitioners had their medical training. The criteria for emotional and conduct disorders are more difficult to apply than those for psychosis or retardation. This is because presenting complaints may be couched in simple concrete terms relating to physical disabilities, for example 'fever', 'abdominal pain stopping the child from speaking' or 'worms stopping the child from growing or walking' (Mughangi & German, 1975). There is also the problem of apparent scarcity of words or phrases in local dialects to describe relevant psychiatric symptoms and issues. At other times, the accompanying adult may demonstrate a lack of awareness that emotional issues are important in illness and that doctors are interested in this.

Assessment and management of patients is usually limited by available personnel and facilities. In most developing countries, there is a gross inadequacy and/or maldistribution of both. The present emphasis on primary health care is aimed at correcting some of this imbalance. The thrust of the discussion on management will therefore be on what is achievable at the primary care level. Where relevant, a distinction will be made between short-term and long-term goals of management. Facilities for assessment will also need to take due cognisance of cultural factors, accessibility and affordability.

Emotional disorders

These are found in about 2.5% of pre-adolescent children. They are equally distributed between the sexes in early childhood but as childhood progresses, become more common among girls (Rutter *et al*, 1976). The disorders are characterised by anxiety, shyness, tearfulness, self-depreciation and sadness. The clinical picture is more undifferentiated and less disabling than adult neurosis and because of this, Rutter (1972) thought a more appropriate term was 'emotional disorder specific to childhood and adolescence'. A small percentage of affected children however, display incapacitating symptoms which do not improve with time and qualify to be diagnosed as neurotic. Emotional problems can manifest as anxiety, depression, and phobia of all types. Hysterical reactions, hypochondriasis, obsessive–compulsive states and school-refusal are among others.

In most reports from developing countries, emotional disorders were not broken down into sub-groups. They were sometimes referred to as 'neuroticism' (Izuora, 1972), considered together with behavioural disorders as 'neurotic and behavioural disorders' (Basheer & Ibrahim, 1976) or simply referred to as 'psychoneurosis' (Rahim, 1976). Epidemiological studies focus mainly on 'symptoms' and not 'syndromes' and no attempts were made to formulate diagnoses from the former. Some of the symptoms, however, suggest emotional problems. For example, Rahim & Cederblad (1984) described the following symptoms in their epidemiological study: fear of darkness in 26.1% of their sample, psychogenic headache in 16.6%, conversion hysteria in 4.5%, anxiety in 3.1%, sleep disturbance in 2.3% and depression in 0.9%. Rates varying from 18–30% were reported for emotional disorders in out-patient clinic reports (Mughangi & German, 1975; Nikapota, 1983; Malhotra & Chatuverdi, 1984; Wong, 1990). Prevalence tends to increase with age. Thus, Nikapota (1983) reported a rate of 30% in the 11–16-year-old group in his clinic population compared to 7% in those who were ten years or younger.

Rahim (1976) described the symptoms of emotional disorders as diverse, ranging from definitive symptoms like headaches of varying severity, sensation of fear, nightmares, poor sleep, poor appetite and palpitation to vague and indefinite symptoms.

The 'brain-fag syndrome' is the name given to a neurotic condition associated with studying among African students (see page 296). First described by Prince (1960), other authors (Minde, 1974*b*; Morakinyo, 1980) have commented further on this condition. The affected student usually complains of a variety of symptoms associated with muscle tension such as headaches, pain in the eyes, chest or abdomen. Morakinyo (1980) reported an association with nervous predisposition, sleep deprivation and psychostimulant abuse, the latter two being self-imposed to ensure successful outcome in examinations. Some authors (e.g. Minde, 1976) have however questioned the need for a different terminology for this condition which seems to share many symptoms in common with anxiety neurosis.

A brief description of clinical features and management of the different sub-groups is now given.

Separation and social anxiety of childhood

Here, behaviour may be clinging, dependent and infantile. Patients often experience disturbed sleep with frequent nightmares. Concentration may be poor, leading to poor school performance. Physiological disturbances associated with autonomic over-activity, such as frequency of micturition (sometimes bed wetting), diarrhoea, nausea, vomiting and sleep disturbance are all common and may be the reason for bringing the child to attention. Appetite may either be increased or decreased. Irritability is common with inappropriate displays of aggression. The cause may be a short-lived frightening experience, such as admission to hospital, or a prolonged stress, for example frequent rows between parents. It may be associated with parental anxiety or a reflection of an anxiety-prone temperament in the child.

In management, account should be taken of aetiological factors or ongoing life stresses such as academic pressure, a specific learning problem, parent marital disharmony and so on. The clinician should offer advice to significant others on how to reduce the stresses. Sometimes, parents too may need help in their own right. If a child is old and verbal enough, he should be helped to talk over his worries. This may be a difficult but still essential task in most developing countries where the culture does not usually allow children to verbalise their feelings. With a bit of tact on the part of the physician, a lot can still be achieved. Anxiety-reducing activities (e.g. relaxation techniques, occupational therapy) can help but only culture-modified variants of these may be available in most developing countries. Anxiolytic drugs should be avoided except for temporary relief of extreme anxiety.

School refusal

School refusal refers to a situation where there is extreme reluctance to attend or to remain at school (Berg & Nursten, 1995). A child may not be at school for various reasons, physical illness being the commonest. A small number are deliberately kept at home by parents to help with domestic work or for company. Some are truants who could go to school but choose not to, often as a form of rebellion.

Some anxiously avoid school because of victimisation there. The typical school refuser stays away from school without there being any justification for the fear experienced. School refusers have been described as having above average intelligence and possessing a dependent, inhibited or timid personality. They also tend to come from families characterised by overprotection and a history of neurotic disorders (Hersov, 1960).

Cases of school refusal are reportedly common among out-patient clinic attendees in developed countries although reports from developing countries do not suggest that it is a big problem (Rahim & Cederblad, 1984).

The clinical picture may take the form of a child who suddenly and completely refuses to attend school. More often, there is an increasing reluctance to set out with signs of unhappiness and anxiety when it is time to go. In some, somatic symptoms of anxiety such as headache, abdominal pain, diarrhoea or vague complaints of being ill are predominant. Some leave home but get increasingly distressed as they get nearer school.

The main aetiological factor in younger children is separation anxiety. In older ones, there may be a true school phobia, that is a fear of certain aspects of school life or fears of failure and rejection, often associated with depression.

Management involves making arrangements for an early return to school. This may involve working closely with social workers and school teachers. In a few cases, a graded behavioural plan may be necessary. It is important to treat underlying causes (e.g. severe anxiety and depression). The child should be encouraged to talk about his feelings, while support and reassurance should be given to parents.

Phobic anxiety disorder

A phobia is an intense fear of an object or situation, recognised as irrational by the sufferer who is nonetheless incapable of overcoming it. Minor phobic symptoms are common in childhood. They usually concern animals, insects, the dark, school and death. Phobias may occur as part of a generalised anxiety state, but sometimes may be monosymptomatic.

Most childhood phobias improve without specific treatment. Some children do not improve and in such cases, simple behavioural treatment can be combined with reassurance and support. The essential ingredient in the behavioural therapy is encouraging the child to confront the feared object in circumstances which enable her or him to experience a diminution of the anxiety.

Dissociative (conversion) disorders

The term 'hysteria' is often used loosely and in a derogatory way to describe dramatic behaviour, or behaviour which others feel forces them into a caring role. Its psychiatric use should be restricted to disorders involving the dissociation or loss of a mental ('dissociation disorder') or physical function ('conversion disorder') in the absence of a structured abnormality. Hysteria is known to occur more commonly in adolescence than in childhood. Conversion disorders (e.g. paralyses, abnormalities of gait, inability to see or hear normally) are known to be commoner in children than dissociative form disorders (e.g. trance or fugue states). As in adults, however, conversion symptoms can occur in the course of organic illness as well as in the primary syndrome of hysteria. Physical symptoms may be misdiagnosed as hysteria. It is therefore advised that the diagnosis of hysteria should be made only after the most careful search for organic disease.

Although hysterical reactions are described as rare in children in Western countries, 90% of all children diagnosed as 'neurotic' in an Indian child guidance clinic presented with hysterical symptoms (Malhotra & Chatuverdi, 1984). The authors explained that conversion of emotional feeling to bodily symptoms is the only way out for the child as the society is authoritarian and does not allow free verbal expression in children. Reports also exist on the epidemic form of hysteria (see Basheer & Ibrahim, 1976).

Dissociation or conversion should be treated as promptly as possible as delay may allow for an entrenchment of symptoms due to the appearance of social or psychological advantages of being ill (secondary gain). Conversion symptoms can usually be removed by suggestion, demonstrating to the child that he can use the affected part normally. Subsequently, the child should be encouraged to talk about his problems while the clinician explores other ways of helping to reduce stressful events.

Obsessive–compulsive disorder

Recurrent thoughts which provoke anxiety out of all proportion to their content ('obsession'), which might seem to the patient silly or far-fetched, and urges to master anxiety by ritual actions to counter anxiety ('compulsion') are rare in childhood. Mild compulsive behaviour is however common in the form of adherence to ritual (e.g. touching lamp posts). Severe and persistent obsessional thoughts or compulsive symptoms occurring in childhood are usually secondary to an anxiety state. Primary obsessive–compulsive neurosis is less common. When it occurs symptoms may appear as early as six years of age but seldom appear in full form before late childhood. These children often involve their parents in their rituals or ask that they should be given repeated reassurance about their obsessional thoughts. Most obsessional children are known to come from compulsive, perfectionistic families. Ritualistic behaviour is common among autistic children.

In management, the parents should be advised to accept the rituals without comment since appeals to the child to control them may result in anxiety which serves to intensify the behaviour. Possible underlying causes of the behaviour should be sought and treated along the lines for anxiety neurosis.

Depression

Some depressive symptoms (sad mood, tearfulness, etc.) are common in emotionally disturbed children but the full syndrome of depression is rare before puberty, although it probably occurs more often than it is diagnosed. Children may appear miserable in unhappy circumstances, such as the serious illness of a parent, the death of a family member or parental disharmony. They may be tearful and lose interest and concentration. They may eat and sleep badly. These symptoms may co-occur with anxiety symptoms or conduct disorder. Some psychiatrists (e.g. Cytryn & McKnew, 1972) have argued that 'masked' depression is present in most cases of conduct disorders, but most psychiatrists restrict the diagnosis of depression to a syndrome including depressed mood which is abnormally persistent and out of proportion to precipitating factors.

Depressive symptoms in childhood are treated by reducing unhappy circumstances and helping the child to talk about his feelings. Children with manifest depressive disorder respond to tricyclic antidepressants, though by no means constantly or predictably. In general, these drugs should be reserved for older children with definite symptoms of a severe depressive disorder.

Conduct disorders and mixed disorders of conduct and emotions

Conduct disorders are characterised by severe and persistent antisocial behaviour. In the United Kingdom, they form the largest single group of disorders in older children and adolescents (Rutter *et al*, 1976). In developing countries, however, conduct disorder symptoms rank very low in epidemiological studies (Giel *et al*, 1981; Rahim & Cederblad, 1984; Cederblad, 1988). They also constitute a low percentage of out-patient clinic attendance (Basheer & Ibrahim, 1976; Rahim, 1976; Wong, 1990). Conduct disorders in children are a more significant problem in developing countries than these figures would suggest. Many parents perceive difficult behaviours in children as issues to be solved through advice or harsh discipline given by either the parents themselves, elders or even community leaders, not health services. Others take their children to traditional or religious healers for treatment while some children end up in probation services, juvenile courts, special schools or remand homes. A large number may form peer groups or gangs who engage in minor criminal activities (stealing, burglary, drug abuse) and may escape arrest by law enforcement agencies for a long time.

The clinical features of conduct disorders take the form of a persistent abnormal conduct more serious than ordinary childish mischief. The initial symptoms may comprise stealing, lying, disobedience together with verbal or physical aggression first noticed at home. Later the behaviour becomes evident outside the home as well, especially at school as truanting, delinquency, vandalism, poor school work, as well as reckless behaviour or alcohol and drug abuse. The conduct disordered child presents with a superficial toughness, hiding low self-esteem and a feeling that he has been unfairly treated. He blames others for his difficulties, is egocentric, reckless and impulsive. His frustration makes for frequent displays of temper.

'Juvenile delinquency' represents a more serious form of conduct disorder where the individual comes into contact with the law or has the potential for being charged for an offence. It represents a serious financial problem to society involving as it does aggressive behaviour towards others and their property. Vandalism, fire-setting, stealing and truancy are some of the manifestations. Alcohol and substance abuse are common among older children and sexual promiscuity or prostitution may enter the picture. Delinquency rates rise with industrialisation and urbanisation and are higher in low-income, culturally deprived families.

In the assessment of the conduct-disordered child, a thorough clinical history should be taken to rule out any evidence of other psychiatric disorder, such as emotional disorder which may co-occur with conduct disorder. There should also be a full psychological work-up including an assessment of the intelligence and educational attainment. A social worker or mental health worker may be able to provide valuable information on the home background.

Conduct disorders usually run a prolonged course in childhood and may persist into adulthood. If the disorder is assessed as mild, the treatment may involve only simple advice to parents as well as the patient. In severe cases, the treatment should be directed at the family. The aim should be to help the delinquent child build up a stable and secure interpersonal relationship and a feeling of responsibility for himself and toward society. A simple form of operant behaviour therapy is sometimes used in treatment. In this, desirable behaviour is rewarded while reinforcement is withheld from undesirable behaviour. Group therapy, utilising peer pressures, may be beneficial. Remedial teaching may help where there are associated reading difficulties. Medication is of little value. It is important to maintain treatment on an out-patient basis as much as possible. Residential treatment may evoke a further feeling of rejection in the child which in turn may lead to an increase in anger and aggression. Where residential treatment is considered absolutely necessary, it is essential to involve parents fully in the management plans drawn up at the institution and the treatment should be for a defined period.

Hyperkinetic disorder

This disorder manifests in early childhood, and affects boys more than girls. It is diagnosed in about 1.5% of children referred to psychiatric hospitals in the Western world. In developing countries, higher figures of between 5–10% have been reported (Malhotra & Chatuverdi, 1984; Wong, 1990). This difference may be connected to the strong association between hyperkinetic syndrome and brain damage, since the latter has been reported to be more prevalent in developing countries.

The main clinical features include extreme motor restlessness, impulsiveness, uncontrolled activity and poor concentration which are noticed by parents in children usually at around the age of 3–4 years when normal children begin to acquire impulse control. Learning difficulties may occur, due in part to impaired attention, and they affect both school work and the acquisition of social skills and standards. Minor forms of antisocial behaviour are common, particularly disobedience and aggression. Temper tantrums are also common and signs of depression may also be evident.

As a baby, the hyperkinetic child may have been noticed to be overactive. More often, however, the significant problems begin when the child starts to walk. Hyperactive children show bursts of activity which may lead to compulsive or dangerous actions, constant restless movement, or upset in the home. Sleep may be disturbed. At school the child may be disruptive in the classroom and fail to attend to lessons.

Parents need to be given support from the start of the treatment because of the physical as well as emotional exhaustion they experience due to the hyperactivity of the child. Teachers also need advice and remedial teaching may be required. Some form of behaviour modification schedules may be worked out to reduce overactivity. When attention deficits are severe, stimulant drugs, in particular the stimulant methylphenidate, may be tried. Care must be taken in the use of stimulants because of the significant side-effects of appetite suppression, mood disturbance and, in high doses, growth retardation. Phenobarbitone and benzodiazepines are to be avoided because they can have the paradoxical effect of increasing overactivity.

Pervasive developmental disorders

This is used as a collective term for several serious disorders which always begin in childhood. They include childhood autism, autistic spectrum disorders including Asperger syndrome, disintegrative psychosis and other rare deteriorating disorders such as Rett syndrome. In addition, adult psychoses are seen occasionally in older children, namely schizophrenia and manic–depressive disorder.

Estimates of the prevalence of pervasive developmental psychoses in the general population vary according to the diagnostic criteria used. Conservative estimates put the prevalence at about 40 per 100 000 children, probably half of this being cases of infantile autism. Childhood psychosis occurs twice as commonly in boys as girls. From developing countries, Wong (1990) reported that 9.1% cases referred to a child psychiatric clinic in Hong Kong had infantile autism while Izuora's (1976) figure for a Nigerian clinic was 3%. Longe (1972) described in detail four autistic children seen in her clinic in Lagos, Nigeria. She found family characteristics in her sample which were very similar to those described in Western literature. Other authors merely report on 'psychoses' without further differentiating them and figures here range from 2% (Malhotra & Chatuverdi, 1984) to 16% (Olatawura & Odejide, 1976) and 23% (Basheer & Ibrahim, 1976). The diagnosis of schizophrenia mostly occurring in older children was however made in some reports: 2% in Sri Lanka (Nikapota, 1983) and 24% in Sudan (Rahim, 1976).

Infantile autism will be considered in more detail below while the other forms of psychoses will be reviewed only briefly.

Childhood autism

The condition was first described in 1943 by Leo Kanner who identified four main features which are still used to make the diagnosis. These are a characteristic type of abnormal functioning in social interaction, communication, and behaviour which is restricted and repetitive; abnormal or impaired development is also apparent before the age of three.

The prognosis may be poor. Only about one in six have a reasonably satisfactory work and social adjustment in adolescence, but about 60% have a poor outcome and often need long-term hospital or other care. In the differential diagnosis, it is important to rule out other causes of childhood psychoses arising after the age of 30 months. The clinician should also aim to differentiate the condition from pure deafness, developmental language disorder and mental handicap.

Behavioural methods using contingency management (i.e. positive reinforcement of desired behaviour) may control some of the abnormal behaviour. In developing countries, the psychiatrist or psychologist may design this together with the PHC worker who can supervise parents who would carry it out at home. Special schooling with an emphasis on active and consistent teaching, much of it on a one-to-one basis between the teacher and the child, may be beneficial. If the condition is severe, residential accommodation (or admission to long-stay hospitals in developing countries) may be necessary. Parents require long-term support in understanding and caring for the child and coming to terms with the condition.

Childhood disintegrative disorder

Childhood disintegrative disorder is a pervasive developmental disorder in which there is a period of normal development followed by a definite loss of previously acquired skills in several areas and abnormal development of social interaction, communication and behaviour. This loss usually occurs over a few months. There may be restlessness and intellectual impairment. Clinical reports on this condition are few, even from developed countries. Ogunlesi (1987) described the syndrome in a nine-year-old Nigerian child who grew up normally until he was about five years of age and then gradually but steadily manifested all the classical symptoms of the disorder over a four-year period. No organic basis was found in this patient even after extensive investigations. The disorder is however known to be strongly associated with some organic conditions, for example encephalitis, lipoidosis, and leucodystrophy.

Schizophrenia

This condition usually starts around puberty. It rarely occurs in younger children and is almost unknown before the age of seven years. The whole range of clinical features that characterise schizophrenia in adults can also be found here. About 80% of those affected are reported to be odd, timid or sensitive as children. History of delayed speech development is not uncommon. The presence of these non-specific symptoms may make diagnosis difficult in the early stages.

Manic–depressive psychosis

This is typically a disturbance of adult life and it is characterised by periodic and profound alterations in mood (depression and mania), but it is rare in childhood. Isolated reports of mania have however been made.

Specific developmental disorders

These are circumscribed developmental delays which cannot be accounted for by another disorder. They are put on a separate axis from that used to code psychiatric disorders in the WHO (1992) multi-axial system but not in DSM–IV (APA, 1994) where they are considered as Axis I disorders. Examples include specific reading retardation, developmental speech and language disorder, specific motor retardation, specific arithmetic retardation and so on. When present in a child, they may lead to poor performance in school with possibly accompanying psychological problems of low self-esteem, anxiety, depression or conduct disorders. Some of these conditions are now briefly reviewed.

Specific reading disorder

Reading disorder is a serious handicap in childhood. It is sometimes defined by a reading age for ten-year-olds of 28 months or more below the level expected from the child's age and overall ability. It was present in 4% of 10–11-year-olds in the Isle of Wight (Rutter *et al*, 1976). The condition is 3–4 times as common in boys as in girls. The child presents with a history of serious delay in learning to read, sometimes preceded by delayed acquisition of speech and language. Writing and spelling are also impaired but these children are good at other school skills, for example mathematics.

The aetiology of this condition is thought to be multifactorial. Factors include possibly a sex-linked genetic predisposition to developmental disorders (all much commoner in boys than girls); a poor pre-school language environment such as exists in culturally deprived and large families; poor teaching in schools with rapid turnover of children and staff, and minor neurological abnormalities in a minority. A strong association was found between this condition and conduct disorders in the Isle of Wight study (Rutter *et al*, 1976). About one-third of children with conduct disorders were reading-retarded compared with 4% of the general population.

Specific development disorders of speech and language

These are conditions in which, in spite of normal intelligence and adequate language stimulation in the home background, the child is slow to develop language, and when speech is acquired it is commonly marked by defective articulation. Usually there is also an undue persistence of infantile pronunciation, especially of consonants (dyslalia), but in most of these mild cases language comprehension is unimpaired. Educational handicaps become apparent as these children grow older, when they may manifest problems with reading and writing. These children have lower scores on 'verbal' than 'performance' items in standard intelligence tests, show difficulties in left–right orientation and in verbal (rote) learning.

Specific developmental disorder of motor function

Some children display clumsiness in school work or play as a result of delayed motor development. These children can carry out all normal movements but they have poor coordination. The clumsiness may affect such skills as dressing, walking and feeding. They tend to break things and are poor in handicrafts and organised games. They may have problems with writing, copying and drawing. They usually score better on verbal than performance sub-tests in intelligence tests.

Assessment of specific developmental disorders

It is essential to carry out a full psychometric assessment, including intelligence testing, using a test such as the Wechsler Intelligence Scale for Children (Wechsler, 1974) which gives separate scores for different abilities, as well as tests of attainment in reading, spelling and arithmetic. There is also the need to conduct a careful appraisal of the child and his background, if possible by a social worker. Assessment should also cover other possible causes of school backwardness, for example intellectual handicap, physical defects (visual, hearing, etc.), attention deficit and emotional problems.

Management

The emphasis in management is remedial education tailored to the need of the child. These children need to go at a slower pace than their peers. They may need to be in 'special' schools where classes are small and the child receives individual help. Support should be given to parents and due cognisance taken of possible emotional effects of the developmental delay on the child.

The situation in developing countries

Very little mention has been made of specific learning problems by workers from developing countries. Izoura (1976) reported 2.5% of his out-patient clinic population as having 'dyslexia'; Olatawura & Odejide (1976) found 'developmental disorder' in 8% of their own clinic population. The questionnaires used in epidemiological studies in these countries hardly contained any items aimed at identifying specific developmental delays. This dearth of information does not however imply total absence or rarity of the conditions: first, teachers may not be sensitised enough to identify them; second, there are few specialised services set up specifically to help children with learning problems. Also, as parents may not perceive learning problems as having any relevance to psychiatric disorders, they are likely to seek non-orthodox methods of treatment. Mental health workers in developing countries therefore have a great responsibility to alert other professional groups, parents as well as policy makers on the special needs of children with specific developmental delays.

Enuresis

Functional nocturnal enuresis is the repeated involuntary voiding of urine during sleep occurring after an age at which continence is usual, in the absence of any identified physical disorder. It is important to differentiate nocturnal enuresis (bed wetting) from the diurnal type which occurs during waking hours. Most children achieve day and night time continence by three or four years of age. A child without learning disability or urinary abnormality who wets clothing or bed-linen after five years of age may require attention. Nocturnal enuresis is very common from clinical as well as epidemiological reports from both developed and developing countries (Rutter *et al*, 1976; Giel *et al*, 1981; Cederblad, 1984; Rahim & Cederblad, 1984). It is a symptom that can cause great unhappiness and distress, particularly to the child but sometimes to the whole family. Some parents may tolerate the problem up to a time at home but they become embarrassed and anxious when the affected child has to go to a boarding school or stay with other families or friends for a fairly long period.

The aetiology of functional nocturnal enuresis is uncertain. In the primary type, where the child has never been dry, a developmental delay affecting the neuromuscular control of the bladder could be the cause. There is some evidence from general population and twin studies for a genetic basis. Also, early life stresses have been shown to predispose to enuresis. Rarely, congenital abnormalities of the urinary tract or spina bifida of sufficient degree to produce other neurological abnormalities may be associated with it. Several studies have shown an association between enuresis and urinary tract infection, particularly among girls, although the cause and effect are not clear. It has been suggested that children with nocturnal enuresis have abnormally deep sleep and their bladder capacity is smaller than usual, although both claims have not gained universal acceptance.

Secondary enuresis which occurs after the child has become dry is practically always associated with emotional disturbance, and some children wet when tension rises at home. It is necessary to rule out other causes of bed wetting such as a degenerative disease of the nervous system, polyuria associated with diabetes or incontinence produced by epileptic fits.

In assessing the enuretic child, it is important to be sure that the bed wetting is of a functional type and not due to the other physical disorders previously mentioned. An assessment should also be made for other psychiatric disorders, of the extent of distress caused to the child, and the attitude of the parents and siblings. A physical examination and urinalysis (microscopy and culture) are essential.

The management of the patient requires an energetic and interested approach on the part of the mental health worker. She should try and diffuse family tension through counselling of parents and the child, and should also advise parents against using punitive measures, which are very common in developing countries. There is a need to build confidence in the child and to reassure him that the problem can be solved. The patient should be actively involved in the treatment by compiling a star chart, with stars (and possibly other records) being awarded every dry night. The parents should also be encouraged to take part in the treatment, for example by waking the child up two or three times during the night to void. Severe restriction of fluid intake at bedtime is not advised.

If symptoms persist after carrying out the above, the 'pad and buzzer' apparatus may be used with the patient. Problems of accessibility and cost may however limit the use of this apparatus in most developing countries. Drug treatment with imipramine is often effective, but the relapse rate after drug discontinuation is high.

Child abuse

Wilson-Oyelaran (1989) includes the following under this heading: (i) neglect of the child's survival and developmental needs; (ii) physical or emotional injury or harassment; (iii) subjecting a child to measures, situations and experiences which interfere with a child's healthy development towards adulthood (e.g. labour which overworks the child or interferes with the child's participation in formal education).

This encompassing description incorporates a wide variety of mistreatments, such as physical abuse, physical neglect, sexual abuse, abandonment, or educational neglect. Each type of mistreatment may have a different aetiology and a different set of psychosocial dynamics and consequences.

There is a lack of systematic research on child abuse in developing countries today, and the available anecdotal as well as scientific data would suggest that the problem is by no means negligible. Deliberate neglect of unwanted children because of illegitimacy or severe disability is well known. Sexual abuse may take different forms, for example, arranged marriages of under-age girls, or abuse of housemaids by their masters. It may also involve the abuse of very young school girls by wealthy or influential people in the society. Incest is known to occur in many communities, but because it is often a taboo, it is very seldom reported. Sexual defilement of boys is rarely reported although anecdotal reports exist of such practices in popular tourist cities.

Exploitative child labour is common in developing countries. Some children can be found working in both the formal and informal sectors. They work as beggars' assistants, street hawkers, load carriers, housemaids, hotel workers, apprentice mechanics, factory labourers, or commercial agricultural labourers. For the most part, the conditions are characterised by long working hours, hazardous environments, exposure to crime, harassment and meagre remuneration.

The 'battered child syndrome' is a form of physical abuse that has received some attention (Nwako, 1979; Lieh-Mak *et al*, 1983). The syndrome should be suspected when there are multiple contusions, unusual or unexplained fractures, particularly of the limbs, subdural haematomata, or head injury. Some of the characteristics of the parents of victims include poor living circumstances or the presence of a psychiatric illness. They may be undergoing severe stress at the time of their action or may be addicted to alcohol and drugs. They are also likely to have been victims of battering themselves or to have had unhappy childhoods (Lieh-Mak *et al*, 1983). Unwanted or illegitimate children, children with chronic illnesses or disabilities, or difficult to manage children are more likely to be victims.

A form of physical abuse that is common in many developing countries is severe corporal punishment administered with the hand or with the aid of sticks or whips, which sometimes results in bodily harm to the child. The action is acceptable in many cultures and seen as a way of instilling discipline in the 'difficult' child.

Street children constitute another high-risk group for psychiatric morbidity (some of these children are the victims of discrimination on religious or traditional grounds). Children can also be the victims of the violence or armed conflicts which are rampant in developing countries. The conflicts usually result in the displacement of the families with the attendant problems of poverty, mulnutrition, poor education and disruption of normal living.

The management of child abuse in whatever form should be based on detailed assessment of the situation. This should involve the multidisciplinary medical team approach. PHC workers together with social welfare officers should play a leading role in the identification of cases and education of the community. Appropriate governmental and non-governmental bodies as well as the whole community should be mobilised in the rehabilitation of victims. The legal provisions that protect the child against any form of exploitation should be strictly enforced. General measures aimed at raising the living standard of individual countries may reduce the incidence of exploitative child labour.

Anorexia nervosa

This is an extremely rare clinical condition in developing countries compared to developed countries where reported rates range between 0.37–1.6 per 100 000 population per year (Kendell *et al*, 1973). Most patients are young women, for whom the condition usually begins in adolescence, most often between the ages of 16 and 17. In males, the peak onset is earlier, about the age of 12. A disproportionately large percentage of patients come from upper-class backgrounds.

The main clinical features are a body weight less than 75% of average weight matched for age and gender; fear of fatness; revulsion for food, self-induced vomiting, a denial of thinness despite pronounced weight loss and emaciation which may lead to death. There could be episodes of binge-eating (bulimia) usually followed by self-induced vomiting. Amenorrhoea occurs early in the development of the condition in women and in about a fifth of cases, it precedes obvious weight loss.

The rarity of this condition in developing countries has led to its being termed a culture-bound syndrome. Crisp (1980) described it in some Arab patients while Buchan & Gregory (1984) described what is probably only the third case in a black African recorded in the literature. In Malaysia, Buhrich (1981) collected information from 17 psychiatrists on 30 patients suffering from anorexia nervosa seen in their practice over an average period of nine years. The prevalence was very low compared with Western figures, although the study confirmed a preponderance of the female gender (14 to 1) and upper social class (5 in 6).

Why is anorexia nervosa very rare in developing countries? The real reasons are unknown although some have been suggested. Affluence appears to be a strong predisposing factor (Crisp, 1980) and this is a rare commodity in most developing countries. There are however 'affluent' people, albeit in tiny proportions in developing countries whose children are most likely to have had intense exposure to Western values and cultures. Could it be then that the condition is under-diagnosed particularly in these groups? There is a need to intensify research efforts in this direction.

Another possible reason for the rarity has to do with the attitude of many cultures in developing countries towards food and stature. Many traditional cultures consider being 'plump and robust' as a visible sign of success, affluence and sometimes nobility. The opposite is the situation in many Western countries where women are under immense pressures to become slim through advertisements in the mass media and role modelling by 'stars'.

Whether or not other suspected aetiological factors such as inheritance, hypothalamic dysfunction, family factors, and influences and personality of the patient contribute to the difference in prevalence rates can only be elucidated through cross-cultural researches.

Drug and alcohol abuse

Since this is the main subject of another chapter of this book, this short review will only highlight the current trend observed in substance use and abuse among youths in the developing world.

According to Basheer (1989), technological advances, rapid transportation, increasing urbanisation and other aspects of socio-cultural changes have produced drastic changes for the worse in the pattern of alcohol and drug abuse in developing countries within the past 2–3 decades. Adolescents have been particularly affected in this regard. Apart from lacking the skills and/or support to cope with the above stated changes, many of them are subjected to other effects like peer pressure, curiosity and experimentation, unstable homes, or adolescent crises. Increased availability of the substance is another important factor as many of the developing countries in Africa, South-East Asia, or South America are popular production and trafficking centres of substances such as cannabis, opium, heroin, cocaine, methaqualone, amphetamines and morphine (Tongue, 1988).

Most epidemiological and clinical reports on substance use and abuse among children and adolescents in developing countries utilised different research methodology and the available data are thus not strictly comparable. Wide variations in rates do occur in different countries and even in different locations within the same country. Broad generalisations will therefore be difficult to make and only specific examples will be possible here.

In Nigeria, substances most commonly used by young people are the socially acceptable and widely available ones such as alcohol, cigarettes, or stimulants, (Adelekan, 1989). There are however several clinical reports of a high percentage of young people being treated for psychiatric disturbances temporally related to cannabis and amphetamine abuse (Oviasu 1976*a,b*). Hard drug abuse (mainly cocaine and heroin) is also becoming a big problem among young people, particularly those from a middle-class background who live in the cities. More men than women misuse drugs although the preponderance of men is falling.

Khat (*Catha edulis*) is a psychostimulant with the active ingredients cathine and cathinone which produce pleasurable euphoric effects. Students are known to chew this plant in order to improve their academic performance. Khat abuse is reported to be common in Ethiopia, Kenya, Somalia, Tanzania, Madagascar and the south-west of the Arabian peninsula.

Vapour inhalation is associated with social deviancy and delinquency. Petrol (gasoline) (Ibrahim, 1974) 'thinner', plastic cements, cements for bicycles, shoe dyes and industrial glues (de la Fuente, 1980) are all inhaled. Vapour inhalation has been reported from Sudan, Mexico, Kenya, Somalia, Swaziland and Zambia. Habitual inhalation causes severe damage to the central nervous system, liver, kidney and bone marrow.

The abuse of hard drugs (heroin, cocaine) is also reported in Kenya, Liberia and Mauritius while cannabis abuse remains generally popular among young people in many developing countries. More extensive epidemiological and clinical research using internationally standardised instruments are needed to better define the extent, pattern and psychosocial correlates of substance abuse among youths in developing countries.

Aetiological factors

Most of the aetiological factors associated with childhood psychiatric disorders in developing countries have been discussed in the sections on epidemiology and clinical sub-syndromes. This section will therefore only briefly underscore some of these biological and socio-cultural factors.

Biological factors

Biological factors are regarded as the main aetiological factors in the severe forms of mental retardation globally. Thus, in those developing countries where facilities for extensive investigations exist, factors such as inborn errors of metabolism or chromosomal abnormalities have been isolated. For example, in a review of 36 severely mentally retarded people in the Karnataka State of southern India, Narayanan (1981) identified such aetiological factors as phenylketonuria and Tay–Sach's disease, true microcephaly, harelip and polydactylism, birth injury, low birth weight, and Down's syndrome. In the mild form of mental retardation (familial–cultural form) however, environmental factors such as poverty, malnutrition and infection are considered to be contributory.

Malnutrition is particularly damaging to the foetus and the child under the age of two years. This period is characterised by prodigious neuronal multiplication, brain growth and myelination of nerve fibres. Associations have been found between severe malnutrition and intellectual impairment (Stoch *et al*, 1982; Galler, 1983). Thus, the malnourished child in the developing country may present with intellectual impairment and poor school record.

Socio-cultural factors

Social factors in the aetiology of child psychiatric disorders in the developing world are similar to those in the Western world. Thus, studies from both regions show that conduct disorders are commoner in boys and emotional disorders are commoner in girls; the incidence of both disorders increases with age (Rutter *et al*, 1976; Rahim & Cederblad, 1984). There is also agreement that urbanisation tends to increase the vulnerability of children despite possible advantages of easier access to health care and educational facilities (Minde, 1975; Rutter *et al*, 1976; Cederblad, 1984). Multiparity, broken homes or marital disharmony, poverty, school underachievement, are other associated factors, as are parental unemployment, alcoholism or psychiatric disorder (Sartorius & Graham, 1984).

Some child rearing practices in developing countries have been found to be associated with an increased risk. Most of these have been considered under child abuse (e.g. physical abuse, physical neglect, child labour). Some of these conditions might be resistant to change as they are deeply entrenched in and sanctioned by the culture. The role of highly restrictive cultures in the development of psychosomatic and hysterical disorders in children in developing countries has been noted (Goodall, 1972; Mughangi & German, 1975; Malhotra & Chatuverdi, 1984). Superstitious beliefs and taboos abound in developing countries and these can constitute the basis of severe anxiety symptoms in children and adolescents (Rahim, 1976; Nikapota, 1983).

Other factors have been identified which may have a protective effect on children in developing countries. Mention has been made of the close physical contact between the child and mother in the first few weeks of life (Cederblad, 1988); the support derived from the extended family system (Sartorius & Graham, 1984; Cederblad, 1988; Yu-Feng *et al*, 1989); durable marital commitments with low divorce rates, extensive mutual community support and a strong adherence to religion and traditional values as sources of social control (Rahim & Cederblad, 1984). Most of these factors need to be further studied for their significance in the face of rapid socio-cultural changes.

Preventative aspects

Primary prevention of mental ill-health in children can be achieved by the amelioration of harmful influences likely to produce mental ill-health by the provision of good obstetric care, for example. In secondary prevention, the aim is to reduce prevalence through early detection and prompt treatment. Tertiary prevention deals with how to minimise the effects of residual disabilities and take advantage of remaining assets after mental disorder has been recognised and treated.

Primary and secondary prevention are particularly important in developing countries. The majority of child mental health problems identified in these countries are due to preventable causes, for example poor obstetric care leading to brain trauma, severe malnutrition, infections, ignorance as to what constitutes ill-health and the appropriate treatment necessary. Moreover, separate and comprehensive child mental health services as they exist in developed countries are rare in most developing countries. The human and material resources needed for such services are also limited or sometimes non-existent.

Mental health prevention services for children in developing countries should be prioritised based on the prevalence of disorders, perceived community needs, available resources and expected outcome of intervention. Prevention should be a routine part of general medical care and should be integrated with the PHC system. Aspects of child mental health should be incorporated into the curricula of the PHC workers. Training packages such as those produced by the World Health Organization (WHO, 1982, 1987) could be found useful for such an exposure. Procedures for liaison with secondary and tertiary levels of care should be clearly laid out for the PHC workers.

The school system should be involved. Generic teachers as well as those who specialise in guidance and counselling should be taught about mental health matters. They can assist in early detection of cases and also in giving guidance in the school setting. This has worked successfully in India (Kapur *et al*, 1980). Schools can also encourage the formation of groups such as the Boy Scouts, Girl Guides and so on which can provide social experience for the isolated youngsters.

There is a need to mobilise and utilise all available resources within and outside the traditional health services. The mental health team will therefore need to work with teachers, community leaders, law-enforcement agencies, governmental and non-governmental child welfare associations, and parents' associations.

There should also be liaison with the community physician, the midwife, the traditional birth attendant, the obstetrician and the paediatrician. Adequate attention should be paid to the physical and psychological aspects of pregnancy. The mother should be immunised against diseases that can be transmitted to the child, for example rubella. The mother should receive education on the need for adequate nutrition during pregnancy and on the possible effects of drugs, alcohol and nicotine on the foetus.

Delivery should be carefully monitored and instrumentation, if necessary at all, should be handled by an expert. Immediate referral for treatment of treatable postnatal conditions, for example haemolytic jaundice, and care of the premature are also important preventative measures. *In utero* screening for detection of abnormalities or screening of infants for signs of handicap (e.g. phenylketonuria) may only be possible in a few specialised centres.

Public education, given through the print and electronic media, should be targeted at teachers, parents and the community as a whole. It should aim at educating the public about psychological disorders in children, on where help can be sought, and on child abuse and how it can be prevented.

In order to mitigate the serious physical and psychological problems that beset the child from an impoverished background, governments should, as a matter of policy, make special welfare provisions such as free health care, free education, and subsidised feeding to affected children. As earlier suggested by Sartorius & Graham (1984), child mental health needs should be taken into account in the formulation of national health and social development policies.

Service issues

The inadequacy of available services for managing mental health disorders of children in developing countries has been mentioned in other sections of this chapter. The aim of this section is to briefly highlight the existing services and offer possible suggestions towards improving services.

Existing services

Out-patient facilities. Children are normally seen in general out-patient psychiatric clinics alongside adult patients. There are a few dedicated child guidance clinics in the developing world, as shown by studies in Sri Lanka (Nikapota, 1983), India (Malhotra & Chatuverdi, 1984), Nigeria (Asuni, 1970; Izuora, 1976), Malaysia (Krahl *et al*, 1981), and Hong Kong (Wong, 1990) among others. Most of these clinics have been described as grossly inadequate in terms of their number and the services they can offer to clients.

In-patient facilities. In-patient facilities in the form of either a unit or ward in a psychiatric or paediatric hospital are rare. Children who need admission because of the severity of their illness get admitted to adult psychiatric wards. Although far from ideal, this arrangement can be made workable (see for example Wong, 1990).

Special services for 'difficult' children. In some countries, voluntary charitable organisations such as churches, the Red Cross, or the Rotary, have founded remand homes and homes for motherless infants and children in need. Remand homes are used for children beyond parental control or those who run away from home because of various stresses. The few approved special schools are overcrowded, resulting in children roaming the streets or being detained in police custody (Olatawura, 1978).

Primary health care services. A WHO survey (1984) found that child psychiatric cases were seen in health centres in China, Brazil, Chile, Honduras and India.

Other services. Some parents utilise the services of traditional or faith healers for the treatment of disturbed behaviour in their children. This could be a reflection of the parents' perceived causation of the illness or of an awareness of the inadequacy or absence of orthodox facilities.

Suggestions for improving services

Child mental health services should be incorporated into the primary health care system with an emphasis on primary and secondary preventative services. Details of this have been outlined in the section on 'Preventative aspects'.

The child psychiatrist in a developing country will need to play the role of a planner, teacher, researcher and not simply that of a clinician (Nikapota, 1991). She would need to spend substantial time designing training and intervention programmes for other categories of workers (e.g. PHC workers, teachers, or general practitioners) who would be working directly with children. She should also play a leading role in influencing governments' policy decisions on issues relating to mental health needs of children.

Centres of excellence should be established to provide specialised care. Here, there should be separate out-patient and in-patient psychiatric facilities for children and a full complement of specialists (i.e. child psychiatrists, psychologists, psychotherapists, educational psychologists, and social workers). More remand homes and special schools for educationally backward children will be needed for special care.

Training and research needs

Training needs

As earlier noted, the child psychiatrist in the developing world will be involved in the training of the different cadres of primary and secondary health care staff. The exposure should cover the essentials of child mental health as well as psychopathology. The training should also be extended to those who are likely to be dealing significantly with mental disorders and with tasks that could promote the mental health of children (Sartorius & Graham, 1984). Examples of the latter include teachers, members of the paediatric health team, non-governmental voluntary organisations, youth organisations and other volunteer groups in the community.

The psychiatric curriculum for undergraduate medical students should contain some basic elements of child psychiatry. At the postgraduate level, there is a need for resident doctors in general psychiatry, general practice and paediatrics as well as trainee psychologists and trainee guidance counsellors to have some exposure to the theory and practice of child psychiatry. Their training should prepare them to disseminate knowledge and impart skill to workers at the primary and secondary levels of care.

The training of the child psychiatrist in a developing country constitutes a problem as courses are available only in the Western world. The cost of such training is high and many developing countries may not be able to sponsor candidates. It has been suggested (see Nikapota, 1991) that some form of input from specialised centres in the Western world could be arranged into such training courses based in individual developing countries or regional blocks. This could be a useful form of collaboration between developed and developing countries.

Research needs

There is a place for intensive research in developing countries in the following areas:

(i) Epidemiological studies on the extent and pattern of child psychiatric disorders. At the moment, these are few and scattered. Longitudinal studies should provide useful answers to pressing questions on aetiology, correlates and prognosis. Such data will also be useful in programme and policy formulation.
(ii) Improvement of mental health assessment procedures with the aim of developing culture-appropriate instruments.
(iii) Services and their evaluation, including the determination of the effectiveness of health-promoting interventions.
(iv) Systematic evaluation of treatment approaches feasible for use in centres with limited resources.
(v) Child-rearing methods and their impact on the development of the child.
(vi) Development of culture-appropriate indicators for development.

Concluding comments

Available epidemiological and clinical data on psychiatric disorders of children in the developing world have revealed prevalence rates quite comparable to those obtained in the Western world. The fact that children constitute a sizeable proportion of the population in developing countries further stresses the necessity for giving them priority in health resource allocation. However, the present situation is far from ideal. The human and material resources needed to provide child psychiatric services are extremely limited. The other limiting factors to provision of adequate services have been highlighted in the different sections of this chapter. On the whole, there is a need for a total overhaul of the system that provides for the mental health needs of children in the developing world. It has been proposed in this chapter that the cornerstone of the services should be the PHC system with active liaison with the secondary and tertiary levels of care. Emphasis should be on primary and secondary preventative strategies and the whole community should be mobilised to achieve this. The role of the child psychiatrist in a developing country is multi-dimensional and this has been fully addressed. There is a strong place for international collaboration in the training of personnel, conduct of cross-cultural researches and the dissemination of knowledge relating to different aspects of child psychiatry.

References

ADELEKAN, M. L. (1989) Self-reported drug use among secondary school students in the Nigerian State of Ogun. *Bulletin on Narcotics (United Nations Publication)*, **41**, 109–116.

AMERICAN PSYCHIATRIC ASSOCIATION (1980) *Diagnostic and Statistical Manual of Mental Disorders, 3rd edn* (DSM–III). Washington: American Psychiatric Association.

——— (1994) *Diagnostic and Statistical Manual of Mental Disorders*, 4th edn (DSM–IV). Washington, DC: APA.

ASUNI, T. (1970) Problems of child guidance of the Nigerian school child. *West African Journal of Education*, **14**, 49–55.

BASHEER, T. (1989) Drug and alcohol problems and the developing world. *International Review of Psychiatry*, **1**, 13–16.

——— & IBRAHIM, H. A. (1976) Childhood psychiatric disorders in the Sudan. *African Journal of Psychiatry*, **1**, 67–68.

BERG, I. & NURSTEN, J. (eds) (1995) *Unwillingly to School* (4th edn). London: Gaskell.

BUCHAN, T. & GREGORY, L. D. (1984) Anorexia nervosa in a Black Zimbabwean. *British Journal of Psychiatry*, **145**, 326–330.

BUHRICH, N. (1981) Frequency of presentation of anorexia nervosa in Malaysia. *Australian and New Zealand Journal of Psychiatry*, **15**, 153–155.

CEDERBLAD, M. (1968) A child psychiatry study on Sudanese Arab children. *Acta Psychiatrica Scandinavica*, Suppl. 200.

——— (1988) Behaviour disorders in children from different cultures. *Acta Psychiatrica Scandinavica*, **78** (Suppl. 344), 85–93.

CRISP, A. H. (1980) *Anorexia Nervosa: Let Me Be*. London: Academic Press.

CYTRYN, L. & MCNEW, D. J. (1972) Proposed classification of childhood depression. *American Journal of Psychiatry*, **137**, 22–25.

DE LA FUENTE, R. (1980) Mexico: young inhalant abusers. In *Drug Problems in the Socio-cultural Context* (eds G. Edwards & A. Arif). Geneva: WHO.

DIOP, B., COLLINGNON, R., GUEYE, M., *et al* (1980) Psychiatric symptomatology and diagnosis in a rural area of Senegal. *Psychopathologie Africaine*, **16**, 5–20.

GALLER, J. R. (1983) The influence of early malnutrition on subsequent behavioural development 2. Classroom behaviour. *Journal of American Academy of Psychiatry*, **22**, 16–22.

GIEL, R., BISHAW, M. & VAN LUIJK, J. N. (1969) Behavioural disorders in Ethiopian children. *Folia psychiatrica, Neurologica Neurochirugica Nurlandica*, **72**, 395–400.

———, DE ARANGO, M. V., CLIMENT, C. E., *et al* (1981) Childhood mental disorders in primary health care: results of observations in four developing countries. *Paediatrics*, **68**, 677–683.

GOODALL, J. (1972) Emotionally induced illness in East African children. *East African Medical Journal*, **49**, 407–418.

GRAHAM, P. & RUTTER, M. (1977) Adolescent disorders. In *Child Psychiatry Modern Approaches* (eds M. Rutter & L. Hersov). Melbourne: Blackwell Scientific Publications.

HAGBERG, B. (1978) Severe mental retardation in Swedish children born 1959–1970: epidemiological panorama and causative factors. In *Methods and Costs of Prevention*. Holland: Elsevier.

HERSOV, L. A. (1960) Refusal to go to school. *Journal of Child Psychology and Psychiatry*, **1**, 130–136.

IBRAHIM, H. H. (1974) Benzine inhalation and dependence among Sudanese children. In *Proceedings of the Workshop in Alcoholism and Drug Addiction*, pp. 30–33. Kenya, Nairobi. Lausanne: ICAA.

IZUORA, G. E. A. (1976) The Enugu Child Guidance Clinic: its organization and growth tendency. *African Journal of Psychiatry*, **1**, 131–135.

KAPUR, M., CARIAPA, I. & PARTHASARATHY, R. (1980) Evaluation of orientation course for teachers on emotional problems amongst school children. *Indian Journal of Clinical Psychology*, **7**, 103–107.

KENDELL, R. E., HALL, D. J., HAILEY, A., *et al* (1973) The epidemiology of anorexia nervosa. *Psychological Medicine*, **3**, 200–203.

KRAHL, W., QUEK, S. L. & RAMAN, N. (1981) A community child and adolescent clinic in Malaysia. *Medical Journal of Malaysia*, **36**, 171–173.

KOLVIN, I., GARSIDE, R. F., NICOL, A. R., *et al* (1977) Screening school children for high risk of emotional and educational disorder. *British Journal of Psychiatry*, **131**, 192–206.

———, ———, ———, *et al* (1981) *Help Starts Here: The Maladjusted Child in the Ordinary School*. London: Tavistock.

KRUPRINSKI, J., BAIKE, A. G., STOLLER, A., *et al* (1976) A community mental health survey of Heyfield Victoria. *Medical Journal of Australia*, **1**, 1204–1211.

LIEH-MAK, F., CHUNG, S. Y. & LIU, Y. W. (1983) Characteristics of child battering in Hong Kong: a controlled study. *British Journal of Psychiatry*, **142**, 89–94.

LONGE, C. I. (1972) *Four Cases of Infantile Autism in Nigerian Children*. Paper presented at the 3rd Pan African Psychiatric Congress, Khartoum, November.

MALHOTRA, S. & CHATUVERDI, S. K. (1984) Patterns of childhood psychiatric disorders in India. *Indian Journal of Paediatrics*, **51**, 235–240.

MBATIA, K. J. (1979) The nature of psychiatric morbidity in patients under 18 years at Muhimbili hospital, Dar-es-Salaam. *East African Medical Journal*, **59**, 30–34.

MILLER, F., COX, S., KNOX, E., *et al* (1974) *The School Years in Newcastle-upon-Tyne*. Oxford: Oxford University Press.

MINDE, K. (1974a) The first 100 cases of a child psychiatric clinic in Uganda. *East African Journal of Medical Research*, **1**, 95–106.

——— (1974b) Study problems in Ugandan secondary school students: A controlled evaluation. *British Journal of Psychiatry*, **125**, 131–137.

——— (1975) Psychological problems in Ugandan school children: a controlled evaluation. *Journal of Child Psychology and Psychiatry*, **16**, 45–59.

——— (1976) Child psychiatry in developing countries. *Journal of Child Psychology and Psychiatry*, **17**, 79–83.

MORAKINYO, O. (1980) A psychophysiological theory of a psychiatric illness (Brain Fag syndrome) associated with study among Africans. *Journal of Nervous and Mental Diseases*, **168**, 84–89.

MUGHANGI, J. & GERMAN, G. A. (1975) Patterns of child psychiatric illness in Uganda: a study of a clinic and its patients. *East African Medical Journal*, **52**, 455–461.

NARAYANAN, H. S. (1981) A study of the prevalence of mental retardation in Southern India. *International Journal of Mental Health*, **10**, 128–136.

NIKAPOTA, A. D. (1983) Development of a child mental health service in Sri Lanka. *Journal of Tropical Paediatrics*, **29**, 302–305.

——— (1991) Child psychiatry in developing countries. *British Journal of Psychiatry*, **158**, 743–751.

NWAKO, F. A. (1979) Child abuse syndrome in Nigeria. *Medicine, Science and Law*, **48**, 56–61.

OGUNLESI, A. O. (1987) Possible Heller's syndrome in a Nigerian child. *West African Journal of Medicine*, **6**, 73–77.

OLATAWURA, M. O. (1978) Mental health services for children in the African region. *International Journal of Mental Health*, **7**, 34–38.

——— & ODEJIDE, A. O. (1976) Child psychiatric disorders in Ibadan. *Nigerian Journal of Paediatrics*, **3**, 9–14.

OVIASU, V. O. (1976a) The abuse of cannabis in Nigeria. *Nigerian Medical Journal*, **6**, 359–365.

——— (1976b) Abuse of stimulant drugs in Nigeria: a review of 491 cases. *British Journal of Addiction*, **71**, 51–63.

OYEWUNMI, L. K. (1989) Inpatient adolescent psychiatry in a teaching hospital in Nigeria. *Acta Psychiatrica Scandinavica*, **80**, 639–643.

PARRY-JONES, W. L. (1986) Psychiatry in the People's Republic of China. *British Journal of Psychiatry*, **148**, 632–641.

PRINCE, R. (1960) The "brain-fag" syndrome in Nigerian students. *Journal of Mental Science*, **106**, 559–570.

RAHIM, T. H. (1976) Psychiatric disorders in the Red Sea children. *African Journal of Psychiatry*, **2**, 115–117.

——— & CEDERBLAD, M. (1984) Effects of rapid urbanization on child behaviour and health in a part of Khartoum, Sudan. *Journal of Child Psychology and Psychiatry*, **25**, 629–641.

RESNICK, C. A., DHADFHALE, M. & LUKWAGE, M. G. (1988) Socio-demographic background of children referred to psychological assessment clinic. *East African Medical Journal*, **65**, 658–660.

RICHMAN, N., STEVENSON, J. E. & GRAHAM, P. J. (1975) Prevalence of behaviour problems in 3-year-old children: an epidemiological study in a London Borough. *Journal of Clinical Psychology and Psychiatry*, **16**, 272–287.

RUTTER, M. (1967) A children's Behaviour Questionnaire for completion by teacher: preliminary findings. *Journal of Child Psychology and Psychiatry*, **8**, 1–11.

——— (1972) Relationships between adult and child psychiatric disorder. *Acta Psychiatrica Scandinavica*, **48**, 3–21.

——— (1975) *A Multi-axial Classification of Child Psychiatric Disorders*. Geneva: WHO.

———, YULE, W., BERG, M., *et al* (1974) Children of West Indian immigrants. *Journal of Child Psychology and Psychiatry*, **15**, 241–262.

——, ——, GRAHAM, P., *et al* (1976) The Isle of Wight studies, 1964–1974. *Psychological Medicine,* **6,** 313–332.

SARTORIUS, N. & GRAHAM, P. (1984) Child mental health: experience of eight countries. *WHO Chronicle,* **38,** 208–211.

STOCH, B., SMYTHE, P. M., MOODIE, A. D., *et al* (1982) Psychosocial outcome and CT findings after gross undernourishment during infancy: a 20 year developmental study. *Developmental Medical and Child Neurology,* **24,** 419–436.

TAO, K. T. (1988) Mentally retarded persons in the People's Republic of China: a review of epidemiological studies and services. *American Journal of Mental Retardation,* **93,** 193–199.

TONGUE, E. (1988) International overview of drug abuse problems. In *Handbook of the African Training Courses on Drug Dependence* (eds J. C. Ebie & E. J. Tongue). Lausanne: ICAA/CIPAT.

WECHSLER, D. (1974) *Wechsler Intelligence Scale for Children – Revised.* New York: Psychological Corporation.

WILSON-OYELARAN, E. B. (1989) The ecological model and the study of child abuse in Nigeria. *Child Abuse and Neglect,* **13,** 379–389.

WONG, C. K. (1990) Child psychiatry in Hong Kong: an overview. *Australian and New Zealand Journal of Psychiatry,* **24,** 331–338.

WORLD HEALTH ORGANIZATION (1978) *Mental Disorders: Glossary and Guide to their Classification in Accordance with the Ninth Revision of the International Classification of Diseases* (ICD–9). Geneva: WHO.

—— (1982) *A Manual on Child Health and Development.* Parts I–IV. New Delhi: WHO.

—— (1984) Mental health care in developing countries: a critical appraisal of research findings. *Technical Report Series,* 698.

—— (1987) *Recognition and Management of Children with Functional Complaints. A Training Package for the PHC Physician.* WHO/SEA/MENT/93. New Delhi: WHO.

—— (1992) *Tenth Revision of the International Classification of Diseases and Related Health Problems* (ICD–10). Geneva: WHO.

YU-FENG, W., YUCUN, S., BO-MEI, G., *et al* (1989) An epidemiological study of behaviour problems in school children of Beijing. *Journal of Child Psychology and Psychiatry,* **30,** 907–912.

Section IV. Training and research

15 Training for mental health

JOHN ORLEY and GIOVANNI DE GIROLAMO

Developing countries, where the majority of the world population lives, have large and unmet mental health needs. Even in 1975 the World Health Organization (WHO) noted that "The most important constraint in meeting mental health needs in the developing countries is the extreme scarcity of mental health professionals. This situation is unlikely to improve within the next decades, because of the small numbers at present being trained in mental health care, and the migration of those who have completed their training to developed nations" (WHO, 1975).

This chapter will discuss problems and perspectives related to the training of psychiatrists and the training of general health personnel in matters of mental health.

Training of psychiatrists

In 1984 a survey carried out by the World Psychiatric Association found that there were some 12 000 psychiatrists in developing countries (Lenz, 1984). Their distribution over the continents was, however, very unequal: in Latin America there was an average of two psychiatrists per 100 000 inhabitants, whereas in African countries the average was about one per million and in Asian countries about two per million inhabitants. The same survey found that many of the psychiatrists from developing countries were trained in developed countries: about 90% of psychiatrists from sub-Saharan African countries, about 50% of those from Middle Eastern countries and about 25% of those from Latin American countries. This is largely due to a shortage of training institutions in the psychiatric trainees' homelands. For instance, a survey carried out in 1977 in 15 African countries showed that complete specialist training was available only in four of the countries while another five countries provided up to one year's training (Harding et al, 1977). The situation in the region has improved since then but is still poor.

Overseas psychiatric training in Europe and North America has been decreasing over recent years. In particular the number of government-sponsored students (generally long-stay) from Africa and the Middle East has been declining (Appleby & Araya, 1990). This is partly because it has become so expensive. Increasingly, collaboration is now taking place between the developing countries. In a recent estimate, there were close to 300 psychiatric trainees in Latin America and perhaps half that number in the training centres of Asia and Africa. The projections for the developing world as a whole for the year 2000 suggests a very approximate total of 1500 potential psychiatric trainees per year looking for training in their country of origin, plus another 450 travelling abroad in search of training. Among others, one of the main distortions created by overseas training has been the way in which it encourages the 'brain drain'. As an example, it is possible to consider the case of Pakistan where there are fewer than 100 trained psychiatrists. The number of Pakistani psychiatrists in the UK and USA however exceeds 700 (Gonzalez & de Alarcon, 1989). It is therefore clear that new policies and programmes are needed to address the specific needs of psychiatric trainees in or from developing countries; the main points to be considered are discussed below.

Role of psychiatrists in developing countries

The role of psychiatrists in developing countries encompasses specific features which need to be considered in training. The treatment of mental disorders is still an important aspect of a psychiatrist's work; nevertheless, especially in the developing countries, a broader concern for mental health is required of psychiatrists and their role is very different from that of psychiatrists in Western countries. Psychiatric needs among the majority of the world's population, especially in the developing world, can only begin to be met adequately by interventions at the primary health care level. The major role for any psychiatrist in a developing country is therefore mainly educational, supervisory, and consultative. Psychiatrists in these countries have therefore to be competent in setting up, supervising and administering treatment services and related teaching programmes at many levels. They also need the skills to organise financial support for these services and to improve their cost-effectiveness. Part of their job is also likely to be advising government agencies regarding services and public health measures, with an awareness of socio-political change in their countries. The accomplishment of these tasks demands the development of some very special skills which are not commonly taught in training programmes for psychiatrists. These skills include the ability to motivate, teach, lead, supervise, and encourage the primary health worker and other health personnel.

Postgraduate training

Postgraduate training in psychiatry should, wherever possible, be given in the trainee's own country or region. This ideal is still not fully attainable but is the goal toward which all countries should strive. Only through training in the indigenous setting are the young professionals likely to learn to appreciate the realities of the cultural, social and economic conditions in which they are going to work.

When overseas training is needed, several psychiatrists with extensive experience of work in developing countries suggest that the psychiatric trainees should have at least a minimum of one year's exposure to psychiatric practice in their own country *before* they embark on training abroad (Ndetei, 1984). This helps them to put what they learn into a context relevant to their future work and to plan for what they might do on their return. One particular training scheme in Manchester (UK), organised by the University Department of Psychiatry (a WHO Collaborating Centre for Research and Training in Mental Health) takes psychiatric trainees from developing countries, primarily from Africa, with at least one year of psychiatric work in their own country, for a period of two years. These trainees are employed within the UK National Health Service and work as junior doctors/residents. As such they join the regular training scheme for all psychiatric residents in the area, but additional sessions are provided dealing with issues more specific to their home countries. The Manchester area (fortunately for this scheme) has more established posts in the National Health Scheme for psychiatric residents than can be filled by local medical graduates. Because of the links existing within the British Commonwealth, it is relatively easy for medical graduates from many of the other countries within the Commonwealth to practise, at least as trainees, in paid posts in Britain (Tantam & Goldberg, 1988).

Sub-speciality training

For the foreseeable future a need will continue for sub-speciality training which can be offered to psychiatrists in centres in countries foreign to the trainee. Since children under the age of 15 years constitute up to one half of the population in developing countries, training in child and adolescent psychiatry should represent a priority. Another area mentioned in this context is forensic psychiatry.

Although not needing 'sub-speciality training', organic conditions presenting with psychiatric symptoms and signs (including neuropsychiatric disorders related to AIDS) are particularly common in developing countries, substantially more common than in developed countries, and should therefore receive adequate space in training programmes.

Training settings

Psychiatric training should be 'service-led'. Training should as far as possible be in services which are of a type similar to those in which the trainee will have to work in the future. Thus university clinics and hospitals may not be the appropriate places for the majority of trainees to learn most of their psychiatry. On the other hand, some state institutions do not provide the necessary facilities nor the variety of treatment options which are necessary for good training. Under these circumstances it is important that the trainee is provided with a number of different training settings, not just to get experience of different treatment techniques, but also to get experience of different forms of service delivery such as security settings, community psychiatric services or vocational rehabilitation.

Keeping up to date

Training should not be restricted to any one type of arrangement and encouragement should be given to innovation. Psychiatry is at different stages of evolution in different parts of the world, and training needs must be seen as continuously evolving rather than static. A high degree of flexibility is therefore necessary together with the ability to rethink and recast training in the light of changing requirements. In addition, transcultural training should achieve a balance between universality and cultural sensitivity.

Research training

Research training should receive proper attention. Psychiatrists from developing countries require research training. Above all, they need to be trained for 'action-orientated research'. Epidemiological research and methods bearing on service evaluation are likely to be particularly appropriate. Emphasis should therefore be given to the development of a psychiatric database for that country, with the encouragement of epidemiological studies, the evaluation of psychiatric programmes, the evaluation of training activities and problem-orientated research in that locality.

The importance of research is by no means a universally held ideal, either among individuals or training centres. The number of psychiatrists who continue research after qualifying is small, even in the developed countries (10% in the USA and 5% in the UK), however those who believe in the need for the teaching of research have argued that it is an essential component of education. The contribution of research may not appear to be so significant in providing students with knowledge or skills for their future role as clinicians, but it is vital in fostering an attitude of scientific curiosity and critical observation which is so essential for a medical specialist. For this reason it is important that the learning of research should be fully integrated with all aspects of training as an essential component in teaching scientific objectivity. Finally, the problems of developing countries are very complex and varied. Often the solutions evolved in industrialised countries are not applicable or relevant. By developing a scientific attitude, health professionals will be more able to modify existing technology for local needs.

The learning of research techniques by 'hands-on' experience is by far the best method and wherever possible, learning should be made into a problem solving exercise. Divorced from practical research, the methodology and statistics can appear pointless and boring, but learned directly for the purpose of carrying out a small piece of research, it becomes interesting and can even develop into a passion. This type of experience can be gained by undertaking a modest research project in an informal manner, or can be formalised into the requirement of preparing a practical or theoretical thesis.

Administrative skills

The training in administrative skills should be adequately covered. Although the majority of psychiatrists would regard themselves as clinicians, nevertheless they become increasingly involved in administration as their careers progress. However, while psychiatrists in the developed countries are 'protected' from some of this burden by various levels of professional administrators who have been trained to deal with the financial and administrative aspects of health care, the psychiatrist in a developing country is likely to carry the whole burden.

In developing countries there is an increasing need for better planning, programming and organisation of services, and a growing demand for good team work. With these changes goes the requirement for better training in relevant areas of administration, especially:

- managerial processes in the planning and development of psychiatric care, including leadership of the primary health care team;
- setting of priorities;
- monitoring and evaluating planned activities;
- skills of communication;
- promotion of knowledge and skills in understanding the structure and function of complex organisations;
- understanding and making effective use of group dynamics;
- the production of public information and encouragement of community participation and mobilisation of resources;
- organisation of teaching;
- mobilisation of international support and contact with international organisations.

In many of the models for psychiatric care, the importance of the psychiatrists' role in administration is highlighted by their executive role at the top of a wide pyramid of health care workers.

The problem of providing adequate training in administration for psychiatric trainees who may be visitors from other countries may be complicated by their training in centres where their role is essentially supernumerary. Even in centres where the trainees are in established posts, they usually have little exposure to real administration and hence the importance of providing appropriate teaching of administration as part of a course in psychiatry.

If these points are carefully considered in the planning and implementation of training programmes for psychiatric trainees from developing countries, it is likely that they will be better able to fill the existing gaps in the mental health field in those countries.

The training of general health workers

The primary health care setting represents the main area for mental health interventions. Several well-conducted studies have demonstrated that a significant proportion of primary care attenders show different types and degrees of psychological disorders, from a low of 11% to a high of 46% with a median prevalence value of 25% (de Girolamo, 1990).

Unfortunately, several surveys have shown that the mental health knowledge of primary care personnel, including medical doctors, is poor. In general, between one to two-thirds of all primary health care attenders with psychological disorders go unrecognised by the general practitioner or the primary health care worker (Harding *et al*, 1980; Shulberg & Burns, 1987). The common somatic presentation of minor psychiatric morbidity is one of the reasons for it not being detected in primary and general health care. This makes the need for an appropriate training in the area of mental health for primary health care personnel an unavoidable priority.

Training in disease-related skills

Hitherto, only mental health specialists have acquired the skills to diagnose, assess and manage mental illness and psychological disorder. The concept of integrating mental health care into primary health care now requires that all general health personnel be equipped with at least some of these skills. Over the past 20 years, much has been done to define the mental health skills required by general health workers, to determine how much they are capable of learning and doing, and to produce appropriate training manuals (WHO, 1990). In fact, the easiest conditions to detect – and, in many cases, to manage – are those manifested by the greatest behavioural disturbances, such as the psychoses, epilepsy, and acute states of severe emotional disorder; referral to specialised facilities is, in many cases, unnecessary, provided that the primary health care personnel have been adequately trained. However, satisfactory mental health care by non-specialised personnel needs good supervision from specialist staff working at secondary and tertiary levels of the health system.

Psychosocial skills

The development of psychosocial skills and sensitivity to the emotional and psychological problems of patients is an important need. Patients presenting with physical symptoms may be unaware of underlying psychological causes, or may be trying 'silently' to communicate deeper emotional problems. Diagnosis of the true nature of such complaints and the provision of appropriate treatment or management may be difficult, and health workers must learn to interview skill-fully and listen carefully.

The need for training in this area has often been overlooked in the past, psychosocial skills having been regarded as somehow inherent in all health workers. However, the lack of such skills, and of sensitivity and understanding, is more often a cause of dissatisfaction and complaint among patients than is lack of technical expertise. The acquisition of these skills and sensitivity is probably a more time-consuming and subtle process than that of learning how to treat mental illness, and relies heavily on the development of appropriate attitudes. These attitudes must be instilled early and reinforced throughout training. It is as important to allow trainees to learn from example, by observing the behaviour of senior personnel, as it is to present them with factual information.

Emphasis should therefore be placed on the development of interpersonal skills, including simple counselling techniques, empathic listening skills, and the capacity for guidance and persuasion, taking account of local community beliefs, values and cultural attitudes.

Training experiences in developing countries: some results

There have been a number of effective mental health training programmes for general health workers carried out in developing countries. One of the most relevant was realised in the context of a WHO Collaborative Study in six developing countries. An objective of this study was to train general health personnel and evaluate the effectiveness of the various, locally adapted training programmes. In some sites simple research screening questionnaires (the Self-Reporting Questionnaire and the Reporting Questionnaire for Children) were employed as training tools (Ignacio *et al*, 1983). The design of the instruments, with short, easily understandable questions to which a 'yes' or 'no' answer can be given, proved to be very useful for training purposes and clinical work. At an 18-month follow-up it was found that the improvement of general health workers in knowledge, skills and ability to provide mental health care was still demonstrable and was of equal magnitude in all the countries (Ignacio *et al*, 1989). At the follow-up assessment, when compared with a baseline evaluation, more workers maintained spontaneously the link between somatic symptoms and mental disorders; recognised that mental health care should be an integral part of their daily work; and were able to describe the correct use of psychotropic drugs available in the health centre. In one site within this collaborative study, specific flow charts and management outlines were developed (Srinivasa Murthy & Wig, 1983).

Flow charts have been used as teaching aids for simple methods of diagnosis, assessment, management and referral. One set has been developed for the more serious mental disorders and requires only minor modification to give it local relevance (Essex & Gosling, 1982). With this set of flow charts, most patients with a disturbed mental state or behaviour can be classified into one of the following eight categories: (1) violence to others; (2) violence to self; (3) delusions and hallucinations; (4) withdrawal; (5) abnormal speech; (6) abnormal behaviour; (7) anxiousness; and (8) depression. These flow charts can be adapted to meet with local needs. One such adaptation was developed in Lesotho and general nurses without previous training in psychiatry were instructed, over a period of 13 hours, in the use of the charts for the identification and management of mental health problems (Meursing & Wankiiri, 1988). They then prepared management plans, with the aid of the charts, for 105 patients with suspected mental health problems attending three primary care clinics. The same patients were also seen separately by trained mental health workers who made a diagnosis and wrote up a management plan, without any knowledge of the plan prepared by the general nurses. The two sets of management plans were subsequently compared. Seventy-eight of the 105 patients (74%) were identified and treated correctly by the nurses. Certain problems in the charts were found, which if corrected would have improved their capacity to indicate a correct management plan.

Other programmes have been addressed to primary care doctors. In south India, 78 medical officers who underwent two weeks training in mental health care were assessed using a standardised multiple choice questionnaire before and after the sessions (Sriram *et al*, 1990). The doctors demonstrated a significant gain in knowledge; with younger doctors scoring significantly higher after the training and older doctors showing less gain.

Though limited in number, these examples clearly show the feasibility and effectiveness of specific training programmes targeted to general health care personnel.

Conclusions

In the larger part of the developing world, mental health services are inadequate, and in some places even non-existent. It is toward the amelioration of that entirely unacceptable situation that collaborative training efforts must now be directed. If efficient use is to be made of the scarce resources which are available to support such training and manpower development, these efforts will have to be planned, monitored and reviewed. WHO is in a position to help in these efforts, strengthening international collaboration, facilitating the exchange of information and experiences and fostering the national capabilities in order to achieve the goal of 'Health for All in the Year 2000'.

References

APPLEBY, L. & ARAYA, R. (1990) Postgraduate training in psychiatry 1977–87: disturbing trends in the pattern of international collaboration. *Medical Education*, **24**, 290–297.

DE GIROLAMO, G. (1990) Epidemiology of mental disorders in health care facilities. In *Psychiatry: A World Perspective. Volume 4: Social Psychiatry; Ethics and Law; History of Psychiatry; Psychiatric Education.* Proceedings of the VIII World Congress of Psychiatry, Athens, 12–19 October 1989 (eds C. N. Stefanis, C. R. Soldatos & A. D. Rabavilas), pp. 96–102. Amsterdam: Excerpta Medica.

ESSEX, B. & GOSLING, H. (1982) *Programme for Identification and Management of Mental Health Problems.* Harlow: Churchill Livingstone (Tropical Health Series).

GONZALEZ, R. & DE ALARCON, R. (1989) Psychiatry in the developing world: difficulties but no grounds for despair. In *Postgraduate Training in Psychiatry: Options for International Collaboration* (eds N. Holden & G. Edwards), pp. 9–12. Geneva: WHO (WHO/MNH/MEP/88.7).

HARDING, T., MOSER, J. & RAMAN, A. (1977) Mental health training in Africa: analysis of information from 23 countries. *African Journal of Psychiatry*, **12**, 17–30.

————, DE ARANGO, M. V., BALTAZAR, J., *et al* (1980) Mental disorders in primary health care: a study of their frequency and diagnosis in four developing countries. *Psychological Medicine*, **10**, 231–241.

IGNACIO, L. L., CLIMENT, C. E., DE ARANGO, M. V., *et al* (1983) Research screening instruments as tools in training health workers for mental health care. *Tropical and Geographical Medicine*, **35**, 1–7.

————, DE ARANGO, M. V., BALTAZAR, J., *et al* (1989) Knowledge and attitudes of primary health care personnel concerning mental health problems in developing countries: a follow-up study. *International Journal of Epidemiology*, **18**, 669–673.

LENZ, G. (1984) Postgraduate training in psychiatry in developing countries. In *Training and Education in Psychiatry* (eds J. J. Lopez Ibor Alino & G. Lenz), pp. 284–306. Vienna: Facultas.

MEURSING, K. & WANKIIRI, V. (1988) Use of flow-charts by nurses dealing with mental patients: an evaluation in Lesotho. *Bulletin of the World Health Organization*, **66**, 507–514.

NDETEI, D. M. (1984) The training needs of psychiatrists intending to work in developing countries – with specific reference to Africa. In *Training and Education in Psychiatry* (eds J. J. Lopez Ibor Alino & G. Lenz), pp. 348–357. Vienna: Facultas.

SHULBERG, H. C. & BURNS, B. J. (1988) Mental disorders in primary care: epidemiologic, diagnostic, and treatment research directions. *General Hospital Psychiatry*, **10**, 79–87.

SRINIVASA MURTHY, R. & WIG, N. N. (1983) The WHO collaborative study on strategies for extending mental health care, IV: a training approach to enhancing the availability of mental health manpower in a developing country. *American Journal of Psychiatry*, **140**, 1486–1490.

SRIRAM, T. G., CHANDRASHEDKAR, C. R., ISAAC, M. K., *et al* (1990) Training primary care medical officers in mental health care: an evaluation using a multiple-choice questionnaire. *Acta Psychiatrica Scandinavica*, **81**, 414–417.

TANTAM, D. & GOLDBERG, D. (1988) The Manchester scheme for training overseas psychiatrists. *Psychiatric Bulletin of the Royal College of Psychiatrists*, **12**, 444–446.

WORLD HEALTH ORGANIZATION (1975) Organization of mental health services in developing countries. *Technical Report Series*, **564**.

—— (1989) *Postgraduate Training in Psychiatry: Options for International Collaboration* (eds N. Holden & G. Edwards). Geneva: World Health Organization (WHO/MNH/MEP/88.7).

—— (1990) *Annotated Directory of Mental Health Training Manuals*. Geneva: World Health Organization (WHO/MNH/MND/90.6).

16 Conducting research

DAVID GOLDBERG and KENNEDY CRUICKSHANK

Research in developed countries is facilitated by ready access to well-stocked libraries, the possibility of asking for help from medical statisticians as need arises, and access to computers which perform elaborate statistical procedures. However, much useful research can be done with relatively simple designs that do not really need help from a statistician or a computer; and although access to journals is undoubtedly helpful both in suggesting ideas and in indicating which questions have already been answered, research can still be done even with limited access to a wide range of journals.

Thinking of an idea

What are the questions that need answering? Worthwhile research projects are those which question received wisdom, or those which establish the value of a particular procedure. An example of the former would be Gureje's (1988) demonstration that electroconvulsive therapy did not relate to either clinical features or cognitive decline in a population of schizophrenic patients in Nigeria; while an example of the latter would be the demonstration by Premalatha Chinnaya *et al* (1990) that a training course in India for paramedical staff produced appreciable changes in attitudes towards mental disorder. If an opportunity occurs of collaborating with an international collaborative study take it, since this will provide an experience with the latest research interviews, enable contact with researchers in other countries and perhaps even provide an opportunity to acquire some equipment. Sartorius (1988) has carefully defined the ten requirements that must be satisfied for such collaborative ventures to be worthwhile.

Keeping up with the literature

It is valuable to keep up with research in at least one journal, and ask whether the findings in the developed world really seem to apply to people with similar problems in your own culture. If they do, it is much less valuable to repeat the research than if they do not! It is unsatisfactory merely to repeat a study in order to show the same thing, since this only celebrates the message that we are all the same underneath our skins: but it is of great interest to shed light on the way in which symptoms and distress are to be best understood in the local own setting.

So, if you think that the clinical phenomena which surround you in your professional life are not perfectly well accounted for by the theories that you read about, ask yourself what explanations there may be for any differences, and how the variables that might account for the differences that might be present could be measured. It might then be worth repeating the study in the local setting, by including the additional variables in the new study.

Brody (1973) studied 254 first admissions to a mental hospital in Brazil using both a sociocultural questionnaire and one measuring psychopathology which included references to primitive beliefs and those derived from folklore. He noted that patients frequently mentioned belief in magic or spirits, but that there was no difference between patients who had attended African 'spiritist sessions' and those who had not. He noted the spiritist and cult-related beliefs were only rarely incorporated into delusional beliefs, although they were often used by patients to explain depression, weakness or anxiety.

Majodina & AttayahJohnson (1983) used WHO's Standardised Assessment for Depressive Disorders (SADD) interview in Ghana, and confirmed that the 'core' depressive phenomena described in the multinational study of depression occurred locally: however, they had recorded the religion of their patients, and they observed that the majority of patients with guilt and self-reproach were Christians.

Most clinical research projects will arise from daily work, but it is also valuable to develop tools that can be used for future projects locally. Such research usually takes the form of validating an existing screening procedure or case-finding interview in the local culture. An exception to the undesirability of replicating results elsewhere is when there may be an educational value for local colleagues: for example, if you wish that physicians in your local hospital were more aware of depressive illnesses among their patients it is no good telling them about how many cases are missed by physicians in London or Boston; they must be shown how many cases are missed in the best local clinics.

Finally, if services are to develop in your country it will be necessary to set up training courses for health workers, and such courses must be evaluated. Educational research has two main uses: it enables future courses to be improved by showing what has still not been achieved, and it can be used with administrators to justify resources for future courses. It may be necessary to consider leaving clinical settings altogether and carrying out survey work in the community. Surveys are used to plan services, and in particular to assess unmet needs for health care in a particular country. Each of these types of research – clinical, instrument development, educational and epidemiological – is discussed in more detail below, together with illustrative examples.

Clinical research

Although full-time research may not be possible, routine clinical work may provide access to clinical material which can be used to good effect. Occasionally one has the good fortune to make observations during everyday work which have important implications both for clinical colleagues and for our own view of a disease:

Muhangi (1972) described four cases of typhoid fever that presented psychologically in Uganda. He showed that they did not present with traditional organic signs such as confusion or impaired consciousness, but as catatonic schizophrenia, depression, hypomania and hysteria.

Alternatively, it may be possible to exploit unusual opportunities:

Dhadphale & Shaikh (1983) were asked to help sort out multiple cases of 'mysterious madness' in a Zambian school that had been reported in the local press. They arrived on the second day of the outbreak. A witch-finder's suggestion that poisoned food was responsible had led to rioting among the students. They found that the first girl to be affected had been anxious, and had felt controlled by spirits, and that the next cases were in her close knit group. Later cases demonstrated uncontrolled laughter, body twitching and aimless running. The authors diagnosed epidemic hysteria and found that a new administration in the school had imposed rigid sexual segregation, which had led to increased tension. They explained the nature of the malady and closed the school for two weeks. All went well thereafter.

Life is not always so dramatic. However, it can be of interest to document the effects of some change in the way that clinical services are being organised in your hospital:

Rwegellera & Mambwe (1977) began to insist that a diagnosis be made before treatment was instituted in the mental hospital in which they worked in Zambia. They wondered whether this would have an effect upon diagnostic practices. They therefore reviewed the diagnoses they had assigned to all new female indigenous patients admitted over the course of one year, and compared them with those admitted in a previous year. They found that schizophrenia had indeed become a less common diagnosis, and affective illnesses were diagnosed more frequently.

Sometimes it makes sense to graft a survey onto one's everyday work, so that interesting findings can be made provided that some additional observations are made:

Gureje (1989a) surveyed all chronic schizophrenic patients under his care in a large mental hospital to which he was attached in Nigeria. He surveyed each patient using a number of standardised clinical tests, and confirming diagnoses using research diagnostic criteria. He found that prominent negative syndromes were associated with poorer premorbid cognitive achievement, longer duration in hospital, cognitive impairment, behavioural deterioration and left eye dominance; while the positive syndrome had no such associations.

Instrument development

An instrument that works in one culture will not necessarily work in the same way in another, and one needs to find the best cutting threshold to discriminate between probable cases and probable non-cases for any screening test which is to be used in research. Thus, Shamasundar *et al* (1986) investigated the characteristics of the General Health Questionnaire (GHQ) in Bangalore, while Gureje & Obikoya (1990) did the same in Nigeria. Chan (1985) had shown that the

GHQ was influenced by the language in which it was presented: his subjects gave higher scores in English than they did in Chinese. Sriram *et al* (1989*a*) repeated Chan's observations in India, only this time they compared English with the local language, which was Kannada.

There is clearly no upper limit to research of this sort, although its interest is in direct proportion to the willingness of the investigators to examine local differences in responses carefully, and to offer possible explanations for them. Sometimes existing opportunities seem not to have been exploited: it would be of great interest to examine the effectiveness of Essex & Gosling's (1983) diagnostic algorithms, and perhaps to develop them further.

It is sometimes worthwhile to produce a local version of an established questionnaire if by doing so one obtains a better instrument for local use. Examples would be Cheng & Williams' (1986) Chinese Health Questionnaire (derived from the GHQ) for use in Taiwan, or Verma's (1975) psychiatric screening questionnaire for use in India.

Educational research

The World Health Organization's strategy for extending mental health care to general medical settings has generated a widespread need to develop and evaluate training courses, both for medical officers and for multipurpose care workers. The aims of such courses are to be found in a paper by Isaac *et al* (1982). It is vitally important that such training courses are intensively evaluated, since this will be the main vehicle for showing up shortcomings of the courses, and thus improving them:

> Sriram *et al* (1989*b*, 1990*a*) report the development and standardisation of MCQ material for use on such courses, and clinical case vignettes as a method for evaluating training in mental disorders provided for medical officers (Sriram, 1990*b*). Premalatha Chinnaya *et al* (1990) report the use of an attitude scale towards mental disorders used in the evaluation of training courses provided to paramedical staff, and show significant changes produced by attendance at the training course. They draw attention to 15 items where their teaching produced no change in attitudes, and show that attitudes before training were not related to age, gender, educational level or to length of service.

Epidemiological surveys in the community

Epidemiological surveys are expensive, and most of those carried out in developing countries have therefore relied upon funding provided nationally, for example Verghese *et al*'s (1973) study of morbidity near Vellore, or the four centre study of severe morbidity in India described by Isaac *et al* (1987). However, those with access to medical students can carry out modest surveys without external financial support:

> Otieno *et al* (1979) carried out the first ever epidemiological study of alcoholism in Kenya using an interview and questionnaire administered by 35 students supported by six members of staff. They visited 200 homes, and interviewed 200 people. One hundred and forty had drunk alcohol and of these no fewer than 50 were 'alcoholics'. Alcoholism was estimated to affect 24% of the female, and 27% of the male population. The authors draw attention to absence of treatment facilities. They point out

that their findings contrast sharply with those of Odejide & Olatawura (1977) in Nigeria, who found that only men were affected.

Choosing a method

If the purpose of a study is to evaluate unmet need in the community, factors that are associated with disease, or the need for medical services, then it will be necessary to carry out a prevalence survey. This may lead to problems in finding the resources, and deciding how to draw a representative sample of the population which is of interest.

However, most clinical investigations will not be prevalence surveys in the community but will use one of four basic designs: one-stage designs, two-stage screening surveys, case-control surveys, and cohort studies. Remember that use of these designs may allow risk factors to be studied in an interesting way, and we will therefore describe three measures of risk in detail.

The distinction between a one- and a two-stage design is that in the former all patients (or a random sample of patients) are included in the study, while in the latter a screening test is used to select patients of particular interest.

One-stage designs

It may be helpful for the psychiatrist to make independent assessments of patients seen by other physicians since this may lead to a greater understanding of psychological factors in disease by colleagues in other specialities.

> Bhatia *et al* (1989) examined 1000 female patients attending a surgical clinic in India. All were examined both by the surgeon and the psychiatrist. An added refinement of this study was that those with high scores on a screening questionnaire were examined by other psychiatrists. The investigators used a rather conservative view of what constitutes a psychological disorder, since they say that 'physical illness was ruled out in all psychiatric cases'. The psychiatrists found that 17.8% of the patients satisfied such criteria, while the surgeon only recognised 6%. Half of the psychiatric diagnoses were neuroses, and 20% of the remainder were physiological disorders arising from mental disorder.

Somehow or other the labour must be found to carry out a survey. It can be helpful to use medical students to make some of the assessments for you:

> Holmes & Speight (1975) used medical students to carry out initial assessments in 170 patients attending a general medical clinic in Tanzania. The two psychiatrists expanded the history obtained by the medical students where necessary, and carried out a physical examination. They found no structural disease present and a positive evidence of psychosocial disturbance in about half of the patients, while the remainder had some evidence of organic disease with, in some cases, coexistent psychological disorder. They then contrasted the psychological disorders seen in those with, and those without, evidence of physical disease. Depression was commonest in the former, while anxiety states were commonest in the latter. They identified the 'top 5' symptoms in the non-organic group as abdominal pain,

palpitations, chest pain, body weakness and genital complaints. Ninety-five per cent of those with chest pain, 75% of those with abdominal pain, and 70% of those with palpitations had no demonstrable physical disease. Abnormal sensations and headache were also very unlikely to be organically determined.

Two-stage designs

The idea of a two-stage design is to enable a population that may contain only a low proportion of cases to be screened using some inexpensive test, so that probable cases can be interviewed in depth by clinicians or researchers using standardised research interviews. To the extent that non-cases turn out to have low scores, the screening test has high specificity (and is therefore efficient in terms of the researcher's time), while to the extent that cases have high scores means that test has high sensitivity (and is losing very few cases). The problem is that if the threshold score is raised so that specificity is as high as possible this will be at the expense of sensitivity, while if the threshold score is lowered sensitivity will be improved at the expense of specificity.

If you want to miss as few cases as possible and do not mind wasting the researchers' time you will lower the threshold score, while if the most important thing is to select patients that are likely to be cases – and you do not mind if you miss some – you will raise it.

Validating a screening test

If it is decided to use a screening test that has been used before with similar patients, and the sensitivity, specificity and best cutting threshold are known – then the test can be used without further work. However, if the test has not been used before with similar patients in a particular country it will be necessary to find the best threshold for discriminating between cases and non-cases. This will involve making blind research assessments of high scorers and low scorers on the test. Provided that the prevalence of illness is reasonably high, there is much to be said for taking a random sample of patients if the sole aim of the study is to validate the test and determine the best threshold. This is because: (a) you will not have to weight the sample back to the score distributions in the original population before you calculate your validity coefficients; (b) your estimates of these coefficients will be more accurate; and (c) it will be easy for you to calculate a Receiver Operating Characteristic (ROC) curve (Goldberg & Williams, 1988).

The importance of weighting back your data in a two-stage screening survey can be illustrated from the original validity study of the General Health Questionnaire (GHQ; Goldberg, 1978) (Table 16.1).

Of the 107 non-cases at interview, 94 were low scorers – so if unweighted data were used, specificity would be reported as 94/107, or 87.8%. Similarly,

TABLE 16.1
Number of patients screened with the General Health Questionnaire and number subsequently interviewed with the Clinical Interview Schedule in a two-stage validity study

	Total number	Selected for	Non-cases	Cases
High scorers	178	102	13	89
Low scorers	375	98	94	4

TABLE 16.2
Weighted data prepared from Table 16.1

	Non-cases	Cases
High scorers	22.69	155.3
Low scorers	359.70	15.3
Total	382.39	170.6

unweighted sensitivity would be 89/93, or 95.7%. However, in the original sample there were unequal numbers of high and low scorers – and therefore we have to weight the sample back to represent the original score distributions. We can do this by multiplying the high scorers by 178/102, or 1.745; and the low scorers by 375/98, or 3.826. This produces the results shown in Table 16.2.

The figures shown in Table 16.2 have the great merit that they represent what would have been found if all 553 patients in the original sample had somehow been interviewed. We can therefore say that the true specificity is 359.7/382.39, or 94.07%; and the true sensitivity is 155.3/170.6, or 91.02%. We also notice that the 170.6 cases that would have been seen among the original 553 respondents would represent a prevalence of 30.8%. Note that had we used unweighted data we would have underestimated the specificity and overestimated the sensitivity of the screening test, and we could not have estimated the true prevalence without the use of some algebra.

It is permissible to use thresholds and validity coefficients from another study providing that it was done with comparable patients. Validity coefficients calculated for consulting populations cannot be extrapolated to community settings for any screening test.

Two stage designs are commonly used to document the kinds of psychological disorder that are encountered in general medical settings (for reviews, see Goldberg, 1989; Burvill, 1990; Lobo, 1990). A multinational study in four developing countries (Colombia, India, Sudan and the Philippines) was reported by Harding *et al* (1980), and single country studies have been reported in Kenya (Dhadphale *et al*, 1983) and India (Deshpande *et al*, 1989). These studies have by and large confirmed the findings in the developed world: between one-quarter and one-third of patients seen in general medical settings have mental disorders, most of these present with somatic symptoms, and only a minority are recognised to have a mental disorder by the doctor in charge of the case.

Case-control studies

This is perhaps the most widely used design to test aetiological hypotheses. Essentially one compares a group with an illness with a group without that illness who come from the same population and are matched for factors that are considered important, but about which one requires no further information. For example, if one matched the index and the controls for social class, one could never tell whether or not social class had any aetiological relevance for the disorder in which you were interested.

Otsyula & Rees (1972) wished to shed light on the aetiology of the 'East African tumbo syndrome': patients in general medical clinics with polymorphous symptoms including abdominal pain, but without physical findings. In the course of normal out-patient work one doctor selected 60 such patients from 200 new cases in the clinic, and another doctor confirmed his assessments independently. They selected a group of organic patients from the same population (few details are given in the paper, but they should have matched each case of 'tumbo' with a comparable organic control). Compared with the organic controls, patients with 'tumbo' were found to have symptoms in multiple bodily systems, to have had their symptoms longer and to overstate them, to have seen a larger number of doctors, and to improve little with symptomatic remedies. Detailed histories revealed domestic and professional difficulties in their lives.

Cohort studies

If you wish to study the natural history of a disorder, or if you wish to discover factors that predict the future course of an illness, it is necessary to select a representative group of patients – a 'cohort' – and follow them up, studying them initially and at one or more future time points. Jablensky (1989) describes the outcome of cohorts of schizophrenic patients seen in the International Pilot Study of Schizophrenia (IPSS) in both developing and developed countries, and shows that a much greater proportion had a favourable outcome in the former.

Dube *et al* (1984) carried out a 14-year follow-up study of the cohort of patients seen on the IPSS in Agra, India. Cases were followed by mail and personal interview, but contact was lost with 14%. The outcome of the schizophrenic patients and the manic depressive patients was similar, and both illnesses were found to lose their intensity over the years. Mortality in the schizophrenic group was shown to be higher than in the general population.

Other examples of longitudinal studies in developing countries are given below (Miller *et al*, 1988, 1990; Taylor *et al*, 1991).

Measuring risk

Perhaps because epidemiology is not included in the training of most psychiatrists from developing countries, measures of risk seem to have been largely neglected in the research carried out to date. This is a pity, since risk measures are important tools in understanding the aetiology of disease, or in deciding on the probability of a particular outcome – such as dying, or becoming depressed. We will consider three measures of risk: attributable risk, relative risk and odds ratios. The first two are used in analysing data from population surveys, while the latter is similar to relative risk, but can be used even in quite small projects.

Attributable risk

This is a measure of how much of an outcome can be attributed to a particular variable: for example, how much medical consultation is due to psychological disorder? It is defined as the rate of a disease in exposed individuals that can be attributed to that exposure. It is important in public health, since it measures the additional risk of a disease in a population exposed to a variable over a population that has not been exposed, and therefore allows us to estimate how much a disease would be reduced if a particular variable could be prevented. The measure is derived from subtracting the rate of an outcome among the unexposed from the rate among the exposed. In terms of our example, how much less would people consult doctors if they were not psychologically unwell?

> Williams *et al* (1986) divided subjects seen in a community survey into cases and non-cases, and found how many of each had consulted their doctor. Of the cases, let us say that 'a' had consulted, and 'c' had not; while of the non-cases, let us say 'b' had and 'd' had not.
>   The size of the consulting population is therefore [a+b], and we want to know what proportion of that was due to psychological disorder.
>   We know that 'a' psychological cases had consulted – but some of these would have consulted even if they had not been mentally unwell. That is not really difficult, since we know the probability of consulting among the non-cases [b/b+d], and we can easily multiply this by the total cases: [a+c]. So, $\{(a+c) \times (b/b+d)\}$ is the number of cases that would have consulted anyway.
>   The excess consultations by the cases are obtained by subtracting $\{(a+c) \times (b/b+d)\}$ from 'a'; and this must be expressed as a proportion of [a+b]. The attributable risk is therefore:
>
> $$\frac{a - \{(a+c) \times (b/b+d)\}}{(a+b)}, \text{ and this turns out to be } 0.20$$

Thus, 20% of all medical consultations can be attributed to psychological disorder.
  Miller *et al* (1988) used a related measure, 'population attributable risk', to study the explanation for the high death rates seen in those of Indian descent in Trinidad. This measure is similar to 'attributable risk', but takes age-adjusted prevalence of disease into account. They were interested in seeing how much of the excessive mortality in this group could be attributed to diabetes on the one hand, and hypertension on the other. Table 16.3 shows how much of the mortality from all causes can be attributed to diabetes and hypertension in people of four different ethnic groups.

Relative risk

The relative risk of any risk factor is given by comparing the incidence of disorder in those with the factor with the incidence in those without it – it is therefore a ratio, obtained by division. (An incidence rate is the number of new cases of a disorder per unit time.) The relative risk estimates the strength of a potential cause of a disease or outcome, and tends to be used for rare conditions like

TABLE 16.3
Population attributable risk of death (as percentages of all causes of mortality)

Cause	Subjects			
	African	*Indian*	*Mixed*	*European*
Blood sugar < 4.7 mmol/l	10.4	19.8	7.5	6.9
Blood pressure > 130 mm	20.8	17.4	16.4	17.9

schizophrenia. (If in doubt about whether a condition is rare, use the odds ratio described in the next section.)

In the following example the 'factor' is unemployment, and we are interested in finding the extent to which being unemployed increases the risk of parasuicide:

> Kreitman (1990) showed that the parasuicide rate for the unemployed in Scotland was 1345/100 000; while that among the employed was only 114/100 000. The relative risk of parasuicide in the unemployed was therefore 11.8. Put another way, parasuicide was nearly 12 times as likely in those without jobs.

Here is an example from a developing country, where the factor is drinking alcohol, and we are interested in finding what effect that has on dying from coronary heart disease (CHD):

> Miller *et al* (1990) carried out a prospective study of 1341 men in Trinidad between 1977 and 1986 in which they studied weekly alcohol consumption and scores on the CAGE questionnaire for alcohol dependence, as well as morbidity due to CHD. They counted the deaths in four groups: the abstinent, ex-drinkers, social drinkers and alcoholics. Compared to the abstinent, the relative risk of dying for a social drinker was 0.66, for an ex-drinker was 1.1, and for an alcoholic was 1.38. These figures suggested that social drinking conferred an advantage in terms of mortality, and the investigators showed that this was due to reduced deaths from CHD.

Odds ratios

If relative risks cannot be calculated because we do not know the incidence rates, we can still calculate a broadly similar measure of risk called the odds ratio. This measures how much more likely an event is to occur if a particular factor is present. It is the probability of the event occurring with the factor present divided by the probability of it occurring without it. It is rather like the odds you would use if you were placing a bet.

> Giel *et al* (1990) studied whether patients were referred by the general practitioners (GPs) to mental illness services in Holland. Of the patients with high neuroticism scores, seven were referred and 26 were not (a ratio of 1:3.71) and of the patients with low neuroticism eight were referred and 50 were not (a ratio of 1:6.25). The odds ratio (OR) just divides one ratio by the other, and is therefore 1.68. It means that if you are neurotic, you have a 1.68 times greater chance of being sent to a psychiatrist than if you are not. It is readily calculated by $[ad/bc]$ – since this is identical with the more cumbersome $\{a/c\}/\{b/d\}$. You should note that if a factor has no effect upon an outcome the OR will be 1. For example, being a single person had an OR of 1 in this study, showing that being unmarried has no effect whatever upon being referred, while being widowed had an OR of 4.25, meaning that widowed people were more than four times as likely to be referred.

Odds ratios are attractive to clinical researchers, since they do not depend upon large samples, and can be used with data from case-control studies:

Taylor *et al* (1991) were interested in whether poor vision was responsible for increased mortality in villagers living in Tanzania. They had previously studied a prevalence survey of 2510 inhabitants of three villages, and for the purposes of this study decided to carry out a case-control study among those in the age range 40–79. They identified 47 such people with poor vision at the time of their original survey, and chose two controls with normal vision for each index case with poor vision. They were able to gather information on 87% of the index cases and 82% of the controls 3.5 years later. Of the usually impaired subjects 40 had died while 37 were still alive; of those subjects with normal vision, seven had died and 70 were still alive.

The chance of death is thus 10/37 for the visually impaired, to be compared with 7/70 for those with normal sight – an OR of 2.72. This means that those with poor vision are almost three times as likely to die in the course of three years as those with normal vision.

The confidence limits of an OR are easy to calculate, and are given by:

$$(\log_e OR) \pm [1.96 \times (\text{standard error})]$$

for a 95% confidence limit. Substitute 2.58 for 1.96 for a 99% confidence limit. By looking up the natural logarithm of the OR in tables, one can readily calculate the standard error:

$$SE = (1/a + 1/b + 1/c + 1/d)^{1/2}$$

that is, the square root of the sum of the four reciprocals (Kahn & Simpson, 1989).

Putting idea and method together

Once an idea has been thought of, it must be committed to paper at once. This is usually done by writing a research protocol.

The research protocol

This can be quite short, provided it addresses four basic questions: (1) what are the aims of the research? (2) what methods will be used? (3) what measuring instruments will be used? and (4) what numerical calculations should be performed in order to achieve the aims?

Aim

The aim is usually the most difficult part of the exercise. Ideally, it should be in the form of a hypothesis. It may need to be revised several times, sharpening it up each time. You might start by wondering whether there was a link between depression and malnutrition. The first revision might be to ask whether depressed patients attending the clinic were any less well nourished than patients with psychotic illness. The final hypothesis might read that 50 consecutive out-patients satisfying ICD-10 (WHO, 1992) criteria for a major depressive episode will have lower body weights and lower levels of haemoglobin than 50 consecutive patients with psychotic illness. (This will be investigated by seeing whether the null hypothesis can be disproved, this being that there will be no difference between the two groups either in terms of body weight or circulating haemoglobin.)

Method

The method also needs careful thought. Where will the patients be found, how will inclusion criteria be decided, how will patients be sampled, and how big a sample should be taken? The availability of research criteria means that these will usually be used in order to define inclusion criteria – be sure that up-to-date information is available about the latest set of criteria! Sampling can be tricky: in survey designs, be sure that the sample studied is representative of the parent population. The size of the sample will be limited by how much work it is feasible for you and your colleagues to carry out – the only way to decide whether the sample is big enough is by carrying out a power calculation, which is described in the next section.

Measures

The measures should be those that are best at carrying out the job in hand: this is where your reading in the library, and discussions with more experienced colleagues should be helpful. Excellent advice may be found in *Measuring Health* by McDowell & Newell (1987), a book that gives full information on 68 current scales, and has the good sense to include the name and address of the person who developed each test. Don't be reluctant to write to such people if there is something that you do not understand about their test.

The statistical treatment of the results is dealt with in the next section.

The project log

Once you have your protocol, lose no time in producing a project log: an old exercise book is fine. The time budget is on the first page, and starts with today's date, and has the date on which you hope to finish writing the project up at the bottom of the page. Starting at the bottom and working up, allow at least three months for preparation of the manuscript; allow time for doing the calculations, depending upon how complicated they are likely to be – say two months; time for the main study – determined by how quickly you are likely to be able to work, or the supply of suitable patients; time for a pilot study if you need one; and time for training in any standardised procedures that you intend to use. If there is some time to spare, so much the better, you will probably need it.

In the remainder of your log you write down things as they happen, always putting in appropriate dates. When you come to write the project up, your log will be invaluable.

The pilot study

This tests the acceptability and practicality of your proposed procedures for both patients and other staff who may be involved. It familiarises others with your procedures, and allows you to make adjustments to your method in the light of experience. You may also decide to modify any research interviews you have designed specially for the study, and you can use the results of a pilot study to decide how large a group you are going to need, by measuring the variances in your main measures. (The variance is the square of the standard deviation: it is easy to see that the more variable the measure, the larger the sample that will be needed.) The main study is deemed to have begun only when you decide to make no further alterations either in your procedures or in your test measures.

Doing the calculations

Most one-man research projects can be done with a pocket calculator and really quite simple statistical procedures (chi squares, *t*-tests, analyses of variance). The beginner would be well advised to get hold of a copy of Siegel (1956), since a familiarity with non-parametric procedures will stand him or her in good stead. Do not rush to do the statistical tests: if possible, plot out the data yourself on a large sheet of paper. Gloat over it a bit: plot out things on squared paper, draw histograms, try out cross tabulations. If you are fortunate in having a computer with software to do all this for you, all well and good, but all the necessary procedures can be done perfectly well for a small data set without a computer. You will learn far more about your data by handling it yourself than the colleague who is squinting at the screen of his computer.

Power calculations

Two kinds of error can be made in scientific research: the claim that there is a relationship when in fact none exists, and observations made due to chance (a type 1 error); or fail to demonstrate a relationship that does in fact exist (a type 2 error). You can think of type 1 as a 'false positive error', and type 2 as a 'false negative error'. Scientists naturally dislike the first type of error even more than the second, since they do not like to make bogus claims.

The power of a test is the ability of the test to show that a relationship exists, when it really does exist: it measures how good the test is at avoiding a type 2 error. The power will increase as the sample size increases. In routine clinical research, one often sets the power at 0.80, that is, we like to have an 80% chance of showing that there is a relationship if one actually exists.

The significance of a test, on the other hand, is the probability that we shall make a false claim, and thus commit a type 1 error. In most routine clinical research we set the significance of our test at 0.05, that is, we only wish to have a 5% chance of claiming a relationship exists when it actually does not – that is to say, our positive result was due to chance. Once more, the bigger the sample the better.

Our task is to decide on a sample size necessary to give us sufficient power to demonstrate something positive, and sufficient significance to prevent us making a fool of ourselves. However, it is important to grasp that one can decide what significance level one wishes to use after the fieldwork is completed, but if a type 2 error is to be avoided one must choose a group of sufficient size at the design stage. Different statistical procedures are associated with different values of power and significance for a given sample size.

In order to decide how large a sample we need we must decide how small a difference between two groups we wish our procedure to detect. If we only want to detect really big differences we can get by with fewer subjects than if we wish to detect small differences. For most statistical tests, tables are available that show the required sample size to achieve selected power for specified differences and values of significance (Lachin, 1981; Machin & Campbell, 1987). For example, with power set at 0.80 and significance at 0.05, we would need 95 subjects to pick up a 30% difference, 160 for a 15% difference, and no fewer than 360 for a 10% difference. It can be seen that the small numbers chosen by many well-meaning clinical investigators would only pick up really big differences between the groups! More details on choosing the size of your sample can be found in Altman (1980, 1991); the text includes a nomogram which enables you to calculate the size of the sample you require without access to specialised tables.

Sophisticated statistical treatments

The ready availability of computers has meant that complex statistical treatments can now be carried out on data sets without the necessity for laborious calculations. When Binitie (1975) carried out a comparison between the structure of depressive symptoms in Africans and Europeans, it was necessary for him to come to London in order to use the BMD computer package. However, advances in computer technology now mean that elaborate calculations can be carried out by anyone with a desk computer and an appropriate software package.

> Gureje (1989*b*) examined 147 patients resident in the wards of a Nigerian mental hospital in order to investigate the prevalence of tardive dyskinesia (TD) and its relationship to other variables. He found no difference in prevalence between patients with schizophrenia and those with affective psychoses. Variables which discriminated between those with, and those without TD were identified using two sample *t*-tests. Two different syndromes of TD were discerned, and then separate stepwise multiple regression analyses were computed. It was shown that cumulative length of exposure to neuroleptics predicts appendicular TD, while length of hospitalisation predicts orofacial TD.

A simple but clear account of how computers work is to be found in Carey (1979), and a more ambitious but straightforward series of articles from the *British Medical Journal* has been published by Asbury (1983). Freeman (1991) discusses the use of computers in psychiatric research.

Writing up

It is still true that published research work is the most important single yardstick by which a future academic psychiatrist is judged. If you have had the good sense to plan your project so that it is not a mere replication of someone else's results, and if you remembered to try to address an interesting question in the first place, you should have no problems. Choose a journal that publishes similar research to your own, and write your study up using its house style. Read their 'instructions

TABLE 16.4
Step by step procedure to design a good research project

1. Look about you: what opportunities does your clinical work provide you with, and what help is available to you from colleagues or medical students?
2. Read the literature about your chosen topic as far as you are able to do so. Do the findings reported elsewhere seem to apply to your own setting? If you have a hunch concerning the factors that may account for any difference you expect, be sure to include those factors in your survey instruments. (A replication of a finding elsewhere is only worthwhile if it is likely to have an educational value for local colleagues.)
3. Do any new measuring instruments need validating in your setting?
4. What about setting up a training course, and evaluating it properly?
5. Is enough known about the longitudinal course of disease, and the factors that may affect it? Think of a cohort study.
6. If you are interested in the aetiology of a particular condition a case-control is the only design for studies by small groups of investigators.
7. Remember that either cohort or case-control studies lend themselves to the measurement of risk factors. It is highly likely that very little is known about these in your country!
8. Always ask for help from colleagues who are more experienced; from designers of any tests you decide to use; and from any statistical advisers who are available. Do a pilot study.

to authors' and do exactly what is asked. It is better to aim your work carefully, as it is counter-productive and exhausting to have your papers do the rounds of various journals – sooner or later your paper comes up against the same assessor for the second time! Try to be concise, and do not succumb to the temptation of slicing your project up into too many papers. Better one good paper that gets published, than several thin ones that do not. Avoid too many tables, and make your paper concise and to the point. Table 16.4 provides a useful summary of the steps to follow to produce a good research paper.

References

ALTMAN, D. G. (1980) Statistics and ethics in medical research: III – How big a sample? *British Medical Journal*, **281**, 1337–1340.
——— (1991) *Practical Statistics for Medical Research*. London: Chapman & Hall.
ASBURY, A. J. (1983) *ABC of Computing*. London: British Medical Association.
BECKLES, G. L., MILLER, G. J., KIRKWOOD, B. R., *et al* (1986) High total and cardiovascular disease mortality in adults of Indian descent in Trinidad, unexplained by coronary risk factors. *Lancet*, *i*, 1298–1300.
BHATIA, M. S., AGRAWAL, P., RASTOGI, V., *et al* (1989) Psychiatric morbidity in patients attending surgery OPD. *Annals of the National Academy of Medical Sciences (India)*, **25**, 331–336.
BINITIE, A. (1975) A factor analytic study of depression across cultures (African and European). *British Journal of Psychiatry*, **127**, 559–563.
BRODY, E. (1973) *The Lost Ones: Social Forces and Mental Illness in Rio de Janeiro*. New York: International University Press.
BURVILL, P. (1990) The epidemiology of psychological disorders in general medical settings. In *Psychological Disorders in General Medical Settings* (eds N. Sartorius, D. Goldberg, G. de Girolamo, *et al*). Bern: Hogrefe & Huber.
CAREY, D. (1979) *The Computer – How it Works*. London: Ladybird.
CHAN, D. W. (1985) The Chinese version of the GHQ– does language make a difference? *Psychological Medicine*, **15**, 147–155.
CHENG, T.-A. & WILLIAMS, P. (1986) The design and development of a screening questionnaire (GHQ) for use in community studies of mental disorders in Taiwan. *Psychological Medicine*, **16**, 415–422.

DHADPHALE, M. & SHAIKH, S. P. (1983) Epidemic hysteria in a Zambian School. *British Journal of Psychiatry*, **142**, 85–88.

———, ELLISON, R. H. & GRIFFIN, L. (1983) The frequency of psychiatric disorders among patients attending semi-urban and rural out-patient clinics in Kenya. *British Journal of Psychiatry*, **142**, 379–383.

DESHPANDE, S. N., SUNDARAM, K. R. & WIG, N. N. (1989) Psychiatric disorders among medical in-patients in an Indian hospital. *British Journal of Psychiatry*, **154**, 504–509.

DUBE, K. C., KUMAR, N. & DUBE, S. (1984) Long-term course and outcome of the Agra cases in the IPSS. *Acta Psychiatrica Scandinavica*, **70**, 170–179.

ESSEX, B. & GOSLING, H. (1983) An algorithmic method for management of mental health problems in developing countries. *British Journal of Psychiatry*, **143**, 451–459.

FREEMAN, H. & TYRER, P. (1991) *Research Methods in Psychiatry.* London: Gaskell.

GIEL, R., KOETER, M. W. & ORMEL, H. (1990) Detection and referral of primary care patients. In *The Public Health Impact of Mental Disorder* (eds D. Goldberg & D. Tantam), pp. 25–34. Bern: Hogrefe & Huber.

GOLDBERG, D. (1978) *The Manual of the General Health Questionnaire.* Windsor: National Foundation for Educational Research.

——— (1989) Mental health aspects of general health care. In *Health and Behaviour* (eds D. Hamburg & N. Sartorius), pp. 162–177. Cambridge: Cambridge University Press.

——— & WILLIAMS, P. (1988) *The User's Guide to the GHQ.* Windsor: National Foundation for Educational Research.

GUREJE, O. (1988) Schizophrenic patients treated with ECT: demographic, clinical and cognitive features. *East African Medical Journal*, **65**, 379–385.

——— (1989*a*) Correlates of positive and negative schizophrenic syndromes in Nigerian patients. *British Journal of Psychiatry*, **155**, 628–632.

——— (1989*b*) The significance of subtyping tardive dyskinesia: a study of prevalence and associated factors. *Psychological Medicine*, **19**, 121–128.

———, OSUNTOKUN, B. O. & MAKANJUOLA, J. D. A. (1989) Neuropsychiatric disorders in Nigerians: 1914 consecutive new patients seen in one year. *African Journal of Medical Science*, **18**, 203–209.

——— (1991) Gender & schizophrenia. *Acta Psychiatrica Scandinavica*, **83**, 402–405.

——— & OBIKOYA, B. (1990) The GHQ-12 as a screening tool in primary care. *Social Psychiatry and Psychiatric Epidemiology*, **25**, 276–280.

HARDING, T. W., DE ARANGO, M. V., BALTAZAR, J., *et al* (1980) Mental disorders in primary care – a study of their frequency and diagnosis in four developing countries. *Psychological Medicine*, **10**, 231–241.

HOLMES, J. A. & SPEIGHT, A. N. (1975) The problem of non-organic illness in Tanzanian urban medical practice. *East African Medical Journal*, **52**, 225–236.

ISAAC, M. K., KAPUR, R. L., CHANDRESHEKAR, C. R., *et al* (1982) Mental health delivery through rural primary care – development and evaluation of a pilot training programme. *Indian Journal of Psychiatry*, **24**, 131–138.

———, ———, KHORANA, A. B., *et al* (1987) *Collaborative Study of Severe Mental Morbidity.* New Delhi: Indian Council of Medical Research.

JABLENSKY, A. (1989) WHO studies in schizophrenia. In *The Scope of Epidemiological Psychiatry* (eds P. Williams, G. Wilkinson & K. Rawnsley). London: Tavistock.

KAHN, H. A. & SIMPSON, C. T. (1989) *Statistical Methods on Epidemiology.* London: McGraw Hill.

KREITMAN, N. (1990) Epidemiological and public health aspects of suicide. In *The Public Health Impact of Mental Disorder* (eds D. Goldberg & D. Tantam). Bern: Hogrefe & Huber.

LACHIN, J. M. (1981) Introduction to power analysis and sample size determination for clinical trials. *Controlled Clinical Trials*, **2**, 93–113.

LOBO, A. (1990) Mental Health in General Medical Settings. In *Public Health Impact of Mental Disorder* (eds D. Goldberg & D. Tantam). Bern: Hogrefe & Huber.

MACHIN, D. & CAMPBELL, M. J. (1987) *Statistical Tables for the Design of Clinical Trials.* Oxford: Blackwell.

MAJODINA, M. Z. & ATTAYAH JOHNSON, F. Y. (1983) Standardised assessment of depressive disorders in Ghana. *British Journal of Psychiatry*, **143**, 443–446.

MCDOWELL, I. & NEWELL, C. (1987) *Measuring Health.* Oxford: Oxford University Press.

MILLER, G., KIRKWOOD, B. R., BECKLES, B. L., *et al* (1988) Adult male all-cause, cardiovascular mortality in relation to ethnic group, systolic blood pressure and blood glucose in Trinidad, West Indies. *International Journal of Epidemiology*, **17**, 62–69.

———, BECKLES, G. L., MAUDE, G. H., *et al* (1990) Alcohol consumption: protection against coronary heart disease and risks to health. *International Journal of Epidemiology*, **19**, 923–930.

MUHANGI, J. R. (1972) Functional or organic psychosis. *African Journal of Medical Science*, **3**, 319–326.

ODEJIDE, A. O. & OLATAWURA, M. O. (1977) Alcohol use in a Nigerian rural community. *African Journal of Psychiatry*, **3**, 69–74.

OTIENO, B., OWOLA, J. A. & ODUOR, P. (1979) A study of alcoholism in a rural setting in Kenya. *East African Medical Journal*, **56**, 665–670.

OTSYULA W. & REES, P. H. (1972) The occurrence and recognition of minor psychiatric illness among out-patients at Kenyatta Hospital, Nairobi. *East African Medical Journal*, **49**, 825–829.

PREMALATHA CHINNAYYA, H., CHANDRASHEKAR, C. R., MOILY, S., *et al* (1990) Training primary care health workers in mental health care: evaluation of attitudes towards mental illness before and after training. *International Journal of Social Psychiatry*, **36**, 300–307.

RWEGELLERA, G. G. & MAMBWE, C. C. (1977) Diagnostic classification of first ever admissions to Chainama Hills Hospital, Lusaka, Zambia. *British Journal of Psychiatry*, **130**, 573–580.

SARTORIUS, N. (1988) Experience from the mental health programme of the World Health Organization. *Acta Psychiatrica Scandinavica*, **78**, 71–74.

SHAMASUNDAR, C., MURTHY, R. S., PRAKASH, O. M., *et al* (1986) Psychiatric morbidity in a general practice in an Indian city. *British Medical Journal*, **292**, 1713–1715.

SIEGEL, S. (1956) *Non-Parametric Statistics for the Behavioural Sciences*. Tokyo: McGraw Hill Kogakusha.

SRIRAM, T. G., CHANDRASHEKAR, C. R., ISAAC, M. K., *et al* (1989a) The General Health Questionnaire (GHQ). Comparison of the English version and a translated Indian version. *Social Psychiatry and Psychiatric Epidemiology*, **24**, 317–320.

——, ——, MOILY, S., *et al* (1989b) Standardisation of MCQ for evaluating medical officers. *Social Psychiatry and Psychiatric Epidemiology*, **24**, 327–331.

——, ——, ISAAC, M., *et al* (1990a) Training primary care medical officers in mental health care: an evaluation of an MCQ. *Acta Psychiatrica Scandinavica*, **81**, 414–417.

——, ——, ——, *et al* (1990b) Development of case vignettes to assess mental health training of primary care medical officers. *Acta Psychiatrica Scandinavica*, **82**, 174–177.

TAYLOR, H. R., KATALIA, S., MUNOZ, D., *et al* (1991) Increase in mortality associated with blindness in rural Africa. *WHO Bulletin*, **69**, 335–338.

VERGHESE, A., BAG, A., SENSEMAN, L. A., *et al* (1973) A social and psychiatric study of a representative group of families in Vellore Town. *Indian Journal of Medical Research*, **61**, 608–620.

VERMA, S. K. (1975) *Construction and Standardisation of PGI Health Questionnaire N-2*. Chandigarh: PGI.

WILLIAMS, P., TARNOPOLSKY, A., HAND, D., *et al* (1986) Minor psychiatric morbidity and general practice consultations: the West London Survey. *Psychological Medicine, Monograph supplement No. 9*.

WORLD HEALTH ORGANIZATION (1992) *The Tenth Revision of the International Classification of Diseases and Related Health Problems* (ICD–10). Geneva: WHO.

Index

Compiled by ELISABETH PICKARD

Page numbers in **bold** type refer to figures, and those in *italics*, to tables.